ATLAS OF EXPERIMENTAL

IMMUNOBIOLOGY AND IMMUNOPATHOLOGY

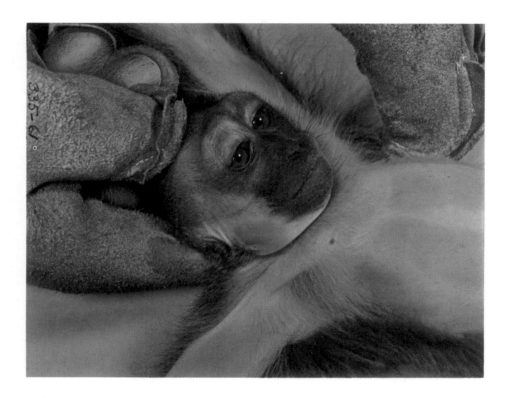

Frontispiece. Passive cutaneous anaphylaxis in cynomolgus monkey sensitized with 0.1-ml serum samples from employees of a castor bean processing factory who suffered from asthma and rhinitis. Challenge 27 hours after sensitization by iv injections of Evans blue (0.5 percent, 3.8 ml) followed by 1.5 mg ricin-free castor bean seed protein. Color developed at original injection sites in cheek, forehead, and chest within 2 minutes after antigen injection.

Courtesy of Dr. L. L. Layton.

ATLAS OF EXPERIMENTAL

IMMUNOBIOLOGY AND IMMUNOPATHOLOGY

BYRON H. WAKSMAN, M.D.

NEW HAVEN AND LONDON, YALE UNIVERSITY PRESS

1970

Library of Congress catalog card number: 73–81434

Standard book number: 300–01154–7

Designed by John O. C. McCrillis,
set in Times New Roman type
and printed in the United States of America by the Meriden Gravure Co.,
Meriden, Connecticut.
Distributed in Great Britain, Europe, Asia, and Africa by Yale
University Press Ltd., London; in Canada by McGill University Press,
Montreal; and in Latin America by Centro Interamericano de Libros
Académicos, Mexico City.

This atlas is dedicated to my mother Deborah, who gave me life and love, to my father Selman, who taught me that a systematic approach to the unknown is a fruitful and exciting way of life, and to Michael Heidelberger, who introduced me to immunology and taught me rigorous habits of thought and experimentation.

Preface

The author who today publishes a book on immunology must be an incurable optimist, since there has been a flood of excellent volumes in this field within a decade, some of them texts, some highly organized symposia, others collections of unrelated papers. All have demanded attention, and it is not certain that much time remains for the perusal of still another. Yet there is at present no unified source of pictorial material to which the student, professor, or investigator may turn which illustrates morphologic aspects of the many immunologic phenomena that are or may be significant. I venture to hope therefore that this book will fill a need.[1]

That immunology is important hardly needs stating. The mechanism whereby an organism produces on demand as many as 10^5 distinct antibody molecules, differing in primary structure, ranks as one of the most challenging problems in contemporary molecular biology. At the same time, immunologic mechanisms play a major role in pathogenesis of many important classes of disease: infectious, allergic, hematologic, dermatologic, endocrinologic, and the still poorly understood "autoimmune" and connective tissue disorders. Organ transplantation, a subject much in today's headlines, and tumor immunity are subheadings within cellular immunology (a point of view which will not, I hope, offend my surgical colleagues); and immunologic deficiency disorders and neoplasms of the immunologic (lymphatic) organs provide still other important problems in medicine and surgery.

This book, then, is intended to provide a convenient source of information for nonimmunologists (physicians, surgeons, molecular biologists) who work with immunologic entities, as well as for those immunologists who may lack familiarity with the morphologic or more purely biologic side of immunology. I hope it will be used by graduate students and fellows entering this field to familiarize themselves with the scope of immunology and with the anatomic and physiologic basis of immunologic events. Finally, it should prove useful to all teachers of immunology as a source of illustrative material for lectures and seminars.

The book contains illustrations of most of the major immunologic phenomena which are generally recognized today. It does not pretend, however, to completeness. The material is taken largely from animal experiments, but a few photographs of human subjects are included, to illustrate problems in autoimmunity and transplantation. In many instances the photographs are taken from the first published work in a given field or from work which first established a particular experimental point. I am infinitely grateful to the many friends and colleagues who have contributed to this collection. Many of the photographs are from my own experiments and were used here for convenience. Since the exciting work in immunobiology has, with a few notable exceptions, taken place since World War II, I include almost no photographs that antedate this period.

Each legend offers a description of the experimental setting and the technique used, together with some interpretation of the facts presented in the corresponding plate. An attempt is made to construe each problem in dynamic terms and to show how the morphologic techniques lend themselves to an analysis of mechanism. Lettering and arrows have been used sparingly, primarily as an aid to nonmorphologists. In each case a reference to the published source (if any) is given.

To complement the plates and legends and in part to explain their relation to larger problems, each group of plates is introduced by a brief discussion of the corresponding field. The synthesis is entirely personal and, of necessity, speculative in some degree. Since many of the areas discussed are the subject of active research, relationships are described here without qualification which may have to be reconsidered tomorrow; I hope that

[1] The author's recent personal research, reflected in many of the illustrations, was supported by United States Public Health Service grants AI–06112 and AI–06455. Preparation of the atlas was aided by grant LM–00519 from the National Library of Medicine and a grant from the Foundation for Microbiology.

I may be forgiven for offering hypotheses as unvarnished facts. In the sections that deal with the anatomy and physiology of the lymphoid organs and in the discussions of tolerance and cellular sensitivity, some of the ideas presented are quite new. This text nevertheless is offered principally as an aid to the study of the plates, and it is from the latter that the reader will gain the greatest reward. For certain classes of phenomena, e.g. neutralization and anaphylaxis, illustrations are clearly inadequate since the main changes are physiologic rather than anatomic. In these instances there are few plates, and the reader must fall back on the text for guidance. In other cases—cellular hypersensitivity is a good example—the principal findings to date are morphologic, and the student can grasp a large part of the subject by looking at the pictures.

In addition to the references that appear in the legends, a general bibliography is appended which is divided into sections corresponding to the grouping of the plates and explanatory text. However, no specific documentation is offered in the text; reference is rather made to the plates that illustrate a point than to the work that proved it. In the bibliography, a few individual articles of importance in each field are listed. Most of the references, however, are to recent books and general reviews which may be used as sources for a detailed survey of the literature in a given area.

My expression of gratitude to those who have kindly provided me with photographs must be accompanied by an apology to those—and there are many—whose pictures might or should have been included here. This atlas, as the work of a single author, inevitably shows omissions and errors of emphasis. I am grateful to my wife and children, who were no more than occasionally impatient during the prolonged period in which I sorted, cut, and pasted pictures. This activity, aside from its didactic purpose, could be justified as gratifying both a scientific and aesthetic impulse. Finally, I am deeply indebted to the Marine Biological Laboratory and its magnificent library for the opportunity to compose this volume in an atmosphere conducive to scholarship.

Woods Hole, Massachusetts   B. H. W.
July 1968

Contents

List of Plates

List of Abbreviations

Ab:	Antibody
Ag:	Antigen
AR:	Autoradiograph
BCG:	Bacille Calmette-Guérin
BGG:	Bovine γ-globulin
BSA:	Bovine serum albumin
CAM:	Chorioallantoic membrane
DNP:	Dinitrophenyl
EM:	Electron micrograph
Fluor.:	Immunofluorescence technique
GBM:	Glomerular basement membrane
GVH:	Graft-vs.-host
γG, γM, γA:	Various classes of antibody
HE:	Hematoxylin-eosin
HGG:	Human γ-globulin
HSA:	Human serum albumin
IE:	Immunoelectrophoresis
ip:	Intraperitoneal
iv:	Intravenous
LE:	Lupus erythematosus
MeG-P:	Methyl green–pyronine
OT:	Old tuberculin
PAS:	Periodic acid (Schiff reagent)
PCA:	Passive cutaneous anaphylaxis
PK:	Prausnitz-Küstner
PNS:	Peripheral nervous system
PPD:	Purified protein derivative of tuberculin
PTAH:	Phosphotungstic acid–hematoxylin
RA:	Rheumatoid arthritis
RBC:	Red blood cell
RE:	Reticuloendothelial

Introduction: The Immune Response

ANTIBODY

The first *antibodies* studied in modern immunology were antibodies to tetanus and diphtheria toxins. These were *formed in response to immunization*. Each neutralized toxin *in vitro* and protected living animals against its harmful effects, and each was *specific* for the toxin used to immunize. These antibodies play an obvious *role in immunity*.

Nontoxic materials also induce antibody formation, and it is clear that there is an enormous variety of specific antibodies. Antigen–antibody combination gives rise to many *effects in vitro*, among them precipitation, agglutination, complement fixation and cell lysis, opsonization, cytophilia, and neutralization of toxins or viruses. In each case there is a primary combination of specific determinants on the antigen molecule with antibody-combining sites which possess steric complementarity for those determinants. The secondary phenomena depend on the molecular character and amount of each reactant and on the nature of the system observed. A single antibody, against pneumococcal capsular polysaccharide, for example, can precipitate the specific antigen from solution, agglutinate encapsulated pneumococci, opsonize them (prepare them for phagocytosis), etc. Some of these effects have a defensive role, notably neutralization, opsonization, and cytophilia, and to a lesser extent agglutination and lysis (see Postscript). At the same time antigen-antibody aggregates formed *in vivo* have the property of damaging tissue and producing lesions (*hypersensitivity, allergy*).

It is now clear that each individual makes antibodies of different *molecular classes* (different immunoglobulins) in response to a single antigen. Well known classes are γG (or IgG), γM, γA, γD, and γE. These differ in molecular size, charge, and carbohydrate content, in antigenic determinants that distinguish them from each other, and in their biologic behavior. γE-immunoglobulin, for example, is the antibody responsible for the large class of human atopic allergies (see Section 11). γA-immunoglobulin is formed in large amounts in various mucosae and apparently is the principal protective antibody in mucosal secretions. Each immunoglobulin class has several subclasses, and there appear to be additional classes which have not been characterized or do not fit this simple list. Guinea pigs, for example, form two distinct γG molecules, one of which (γ_2) is complement-fixing and lyses cells coated with antibody (Section 10); the other (γ_1) does not fix complement but sensitizes guinea pig tissues for anaphylaxis (Section 11).

Each antibody molecule is constructed of pairs of *polypeptide chains*, one light (L) and one heavy (H). The γG and γA molecules are made up of two such pairs; γM is made up of 10. Two types of L chains (κ and λ) are found in all the immunoglobulin molecules examined so far. However each immunoglobulin class has its own characteristic H chain: γ in γG molecules, μ in γM, α in χA, δ in γD, and ϵ in γE, and these differ somewhat in the different subclasses. *Antibody combining sites* are formed by the interaction of the L and H chains making up a pair. Thus there are two combining sites in each γG molecule, 5 (or 10) in γM, and so on. The specificity of the combining site is determined by the primary amino-acid sequence in a variable part of the L chain and a corresponding variable portion of the adjacent H chain.

The extraordinary diversity of sequences actually found in different antibody molecules has been accounted for by hypothetical events, such as a rapid flux of somatic mutations in DNA which codes for the variable region of each chain, occurring at a particular moment in the development of precursor lymphocytes (Section 4), a partial breakdown of the DNA in this region with faulty repair, a recombinational event involving a "scrambler" gene, the formation of an extra set of t-RNA's which gives alternative readings to ambiguous triplets in m-RNA coding for the variable region, etc. Available evidence suggests that precursor cells undergo a *generation of diversity* at an early stage in their development and begin to form a specific immunoglobulin, and that antigen

1

used to immunize or to induce tolerance interacts only with cells making antibody of sufficiently high affinity for that particular antigen (the clonal or selective hypothesis).

The invariant regions of both L and H chains may show minor (allotypic) variations, which are genetically controlled. The *biologic properties* of each immunoglobulin molecule, e.g. its ability to fix complement, to fix to tissue, to opsonize, or to initiate anaphylaxis, are determined by unknown properties of the invariant portion of the H chain and its associated carbohydrate. The transport of γA-antibody through mucosal surfaces involves an additional polypeptide, the "transport piece" which is synthesized locally and binds two or more γA molecules to form a single larger unit.

In the response to a single antigen, there are *degrees of heterogeneity* beyond those inherent in the formation of different molecular classes of antibody. Within each class, antibody molecules of widely different electrophoretic mobility are formed, presumably by many different clones of cells. Antibodies with combining sites of different specificities are formed against many different determinants in or on the antigen used to immunize and against different portions of the same determinant group. Needless to say, antibodies are also formed against contaminating antigens. The immune response is characterized on the one hand by a progressive broadening of the spectrum of specificities being formed and, on the other, by a progressive increase in formation of antibody with high affinity for the antigen, as though cells making high affinity antibody are progressively selected for or stimulated.

So-called *natural antibodies*, present in the circulation of all individuals, appear to be formed in response to organisms present in the normal gastrointestinal and other flora as well as to foods and other antigenic stimuli. These increase from birth and are diminished or lacking in germ-free animals or animals thymectomized or bursectomized at birth (Section 8). They show an anamnestic rise in response to suitable secondary stimulation. Human "natural antibody" to *Escherichia coli* and *Neisseria gonorrhoeae* is found in γG, γM, and γA classes. In many sera, however, most natural antibody is γM. In the presence of chronic infection, there is a general rise in blood γG levels, presumably attributable to formation of multiple specific antibodies. In certain conditions, notably trypanosomiasis, there is a huge increase in γM, but it is not clear whether this is all specific antibody. A similar rise in γA is present in hepatic cirrhosis. Immunoglobulin levels and specific antibody formation are decreased in chronic lymphatic leukemia and the paraproteinemias (multiple myeloma, Waldenström's macroglobulinemia) (Section 8), and of course in hypogammaglobulinemia. There is a lowering of immunoglobulin levels in subjects with the nephrotic syndrome or protein loss enteropathy.

Finally attention is drawn to so-called *specifically sensitized cells* of the delayed or cellular type of sensitization (Sections 16–21). These are lymphocytes that appear to make a specific immunoglobulin, which either is not released from the cell or is made only in very small amount. It has not been identified convincingly with any of the known immunoglobulins. The exact relationship of sensitized cells to memory cells for one or more of the humoral antibody classes is still being explored (Sections 4, 6).

Antibody Formation

The *primary antibody response* is characterized by an inductive phase during which little or no antibody is formed, a productive phase during which antibody increases to a peak titer, and a declining phase. The *secondary or anamnestic antibody response* can be elicited with a smaller dose of the same antigen and has a shorter latent period, and the antibody titer rises more rapidly to a higher peak.

During the *inductive phase* there actually are few or no antibody-forming cells, and this phase represents a period during which *memory cells* are recruited. The primary response is attributed to the action of residual antigen on newly formed memory cells and induction of a secondary response. This phase is sensitive to agents that affect the processing of antigen (Section 2) or destroy precursor lymphocytes (Section 4) and to inhibitors of nucleic acid synthesis (Section 6). It is no more than a few hours in the case of γM-globulin synthesis but may be several days to weeks in the case of γG-antibody.

In the *productive phase* there is a logarithmic rise in antibody titer corresponding to rapid replication of *antibody-forming cells*. and an increase in protein synthetic machinery (Section 6). The antibody released is all formed by *de novo* synthesis, as can be shown by incorporation studies with labeled amino acids. This phase is sensitive to inhibitors of cell multiplication and of nucleic acid and protein synthesis. It is usually brief in the case of γM synthesis and prolonged in the case of γG. However, where γG is not formed and there is therefore no homeostatic inhibition of γM formation, the latter may continue for long periods of time.

The *declining phase* represents the sum of two independent events: continuing antibody synthesis (if any) and the catabolism of antibody already formed. It can be analyzed by comparing the rate at which antibody titer decreases with that of passively administered labeled antibody and by measuring incorporation of amino acids into new antibody molecules. The prolonged continuation of antibody synthesis, in some instances, depends on persistence of the antigenic stimulus, as with living organisms (viruses, rickettsiae) or molecules which are poorly catabolized (pneumococcal polysaccharides) or indeed on repeated stimuli (diphtheria). It depends, in other cases, on persistence of small numbers of antibody-forming cells for prolonged periods.

Memory also increases with time to a peak, persists at the peak level for a variable period, then declines. With protein antigens like diphtheria toxoid, BSA, and hemocyanin, the time scale of this process is measured in months or years, and its duration is clearly related to the dose of immunizing antigen. It is tempting therefore to relate it to the actual persistence of antigen. However, it depends as well on the fact that memory cells are long-lived, nondividing cells (Sections 4, 6). Memory may be boosted by repeated antigenic stimulation, but it is not clear whether this represents recruitment of new memory cells from precursors or from memory cells already present (these may in fact be the same; Sections 4, 6).

The primary and secondary responses and formation of immunologic memory are all related to the *dose of immunizing antigen* and its *immunogenicity or antigenicity* (Section 1). They are increased by the use of particulate antigens, multiple inoculation sites, and continued or repeated antigenic stimulation. With the latter, a maximal level of antibody is reached, which has been attributed to the saturation of available target (precursor) cells of a given specificity or, alternatively, to homeostatic limitation of antibody formation by antibody already present. With many antigens, continuing antigenic stimulation leads to a refractory phase or tolerance (see below). With noncatabolizable antigens like pneumococcal polysaccharide, one sees persistent maximal antibody formation, lack of a secondary response, and, with increasing antigen dose, a rapid production of tolerance. The commonly used *adjuvants* (e.g. alum precipitation, water-in-oil emulsification) have the effect of prolonging and intensifying the antigenic stimulus but may also act by production of an antibody-forming *granuloma* at the injection site.

The responses considered so far are all highly *specific* in that a secondary stimulus must be the same as a primary to be effective and that only antibody is formed that can react with the antigen used to stimulate. When a secondary response is induced with antigen different from but cross-reactive with that used for the primary, only antibody reactive with both antigens is formed secondarily ("original antigenic sin"), though there may be a primary response as well to non-cross-reactive determinants of the second antigen. There has not as yet been a convincing demonstration that secondary antibody formation is elicited by nonspecific agencies.

Certain circumstances favor the induction of one type of antibody response as compared with another. The chemical nature of the antigen is an important factor (Section 1). With proteins, a transient γM response occurs early and is followed by γG, and the anamnestic response is largely or entirely γG. Delayed sensitivity is induced if a small antigen dose is given intradermally or if mycobacterial adjuvant is used. With carbohydrate antigens, the response may be largely or entirely γM, γG formation occurring late and there being no delayed sensitivity. The physical form of the antigen is important. Very large molecules, such as keyhole limpet hemocyanin, or particles, such as intact flagella or soluble protein coated on acrylic resin particles, give a greatly enhanced γM response. Use of certain helminth antigens or of pertussis as an adjuvant favors formation of γE and other anaphylactic antibodies. Immunization by way of mucosal surface(s) favors γA-antibody production locally. The different responses are seen with qualitatively different stimuli, each has a different and characteristic time course, and each appears at a different time in phylogeny and ontogeny (Section 7). Each may be separately affected by such agencies as X ray, antimetabolites, thymectomy, bursectomy, and appendectomy (Sections 4, 8), and split tolerance may be produced, affecting one but not another. Finally, genetic defects and paraprotein-emias are found which affect one type of response but not another (Section 8). It is therefore a justifiable presumption that the different responses are functions of different families of cells.

Control Mechanisms

In addition to nonspecific agents, which affect immune responses by increasing or decreasing the antigen-processing function of phagocytic cells, the supply of precursor lymphocytes or nucleic acid synthesis, three specific mechanisms for controlling the immune response are significant. *Competition of antigens* appears to act at the level of the processing cell, either by competition for receptor sites at the cell surface or by competition for "space" at the site of interaction of the processing cell with precursor lymphocytes. The effect is determined by the relative dose and timing of the two antigenic stimuli and the relative intensity of the response to each. With an antigen that induces a secondary response, the suppressive effect on the response to a second antigen is enhanced; and with an antigen to which the subject is tolerant, competition with a second antigen is decreased or absent.

The second mechanism, the *homeostatic control* of antibody synthesis *by antibody* already present, may play an important role in determining the character of the normal immune response. This mechanism too appears to affect either the afferent or efferent steps of antigen processing or both. Antibody, by combining with antigen, may enhance its local uptake and destruction and prevent its reaching processing cells in the regional lymph nodes or the spleen. In general, however, antibody appears to act at the surface of the processing cell (Sections 2, 6), perhaps by reacting specifically with the antigen–RNA complex formed there and inhibiting its interaction with precursor lymphocytes. Antibody given passively, even a considerable time after antigenic stimulation, has been shown to turn off existing antibody synthesis, and added antibody prevents specific cell clustering essential to primary immunization *in vitro* (Fig. 6.5). In general only formation of antibody of lower affinity than that given is inhibited. The mechanism has been shown to affect both γM and γG formation as well as the development of memory. It is suggested that this process accounts for the prompt arrest of γM-antibody formation when γG begins to be formed in many systems, drives the individual to the formation of antibody of ever-increasing affinity over a period of weeks or months, and limits the level of circulating antibody that may be attained to any given antigen. Low-affinity γM antibody, by forming immunogenic antigen–antibody aggregates, may sometimes act to enhance rather than interfere with immunization.

The third control mechanism is specific *immunologic tolerance or paralysis* (Figs. 19.1,2). Antigen, introduced in fetal or early postnatal life, induces a state of specific nonreactivity to that antigen, which appears to be determined by the ablation (functional or actual) of clones of precursor lymphocytes capable of producing antibody reactive with the specific antigen. The state of tolerance is related to persistence of antigen, and its duration is therefore determined by the initial dose given. When it wanes, it may be followed temporarily by a state of immunologic memory. Tolerance to protein antigens is readily maintained by giving repeated small doses of antigen. With slowly catabolized polysaccharides, e.g. pneumococcal SIII, it may be nearly permanent. With cellular antigens, lymphoid cells of the donor populate lymphoid organs of the tolerant host, which is therefore a chimera; tolerance lasts as long as these cells continue to replicate and the chimeric state is maintained. The persistence of antigen does not serve as a "treadmill" on which newly formed antibody is continually destroyed but rather as a mechanism for the ablation of newly formed "uncommitted" lymphocytes of the appropriate specificity.

Tolerance may be broken by doses of X-irradiation sufficient to destroy a large proportion of the functional lymphocyte population, by unusually intensive immunization, and by the use of cross-reacting antigen for stimulation. In the last case, the antibody formed is directed at minor determinants of the tolerated antigen. "Split tolerance," also known as "immune deviation," designates tolerance for some immune responses but not for others. "Partial tolerance" is a state of lessened reactivity for the specific antigen. With histocompatibility antigens, tolerance is observed following natural embryonic parabiosis (as in cattle), artificial embryonic para-biosis (e.g. with eggs of different strains or species of birds), the maternal–fetal relationship (which is a form of parabiosis), pre- or postnatal transfusion of living lymphoid cells of donor type, or sometimes grafting of other tissues such as skin to fetus or newborn. In all these instances the tolerant animal becomes a lymphoid chimera. Tolerance produced by transfusion of adult lymphoid cells, if these are immunologically competent, may be complicated by graft-vs.-host reactions (Section 20). This problem is avoided by using embryonic donor cells, donor cells genetically unable to react against the recipient's antigens, or donor cells tolerant of the recipient.

Tolerance is readily produced in adult animals when the elicitation of an immune response is prevented by X-irradiation, treatment with antimetabolites, blockade, or other means. In untreated animals, with protein antigens, use of nonaggregated material which is lacking in adjuvanticity, or of single or repeated doses of antigen below the threshold required for immunization, leads to tolerance. Conventional doses of protein give partial tolerance, but this is usually masked except at very high dose levels by a simultaneous immune response elicited by the aggregated antigen included in the immunizing dose. With many polysaccharides, with increasing dose, the immune response is rapidly overshadowed by the production of tolerance. In general, agents leading to enhanced macrophage function favor the immune response and interfere with the development of tolerance (Section 2). With histocompatibility antigens, production of tolerance in adults requires prolonged parabiosis, repeated pregnancy (the fetuses acting as source of tolerance-inducing antigen), or persistent grafts (e.g. in the hamster cheek pouch).

Tolerance is the mechanism whereby the organism avoids *autoimmunization*. With most or all widely dis-seminated body constituents, tolerance is induced and maintained by continuous exposure of lymphocytes to antigen. This mechanism may be bypassed in special situations which lead to autoimmunization (Sections 21, 22).

HYPERSENSITIVITY

The production of humoral or cell-bound antibody is unavoidably associated with the development of hypersensitivity (allergy), manifested by characteristic response(s), usually harmful to the hosts, upon re-exposure to antigen. The allergic manifestations may result from any of several *mechanisms*, considered in greater detail in subsequent sections: neutralization, single cell damage, anaphylaxis, Arthus (immune complex), or delayed (cellular). At the same time and quite independently, they may conform to any of a number of dis-tinct *patterns*. With exogenous antigens, lesions may depend upon the host's own antibody or "sensitized cells," formed as a result of active immunization, or upon antibody or "sensitized cells" passively transferred from an immunized individual. With autogenous antigens, lesion formation may involve antibody or cells formed by the host (autoimmunization) or transferred antibody or cells. The latter categories include such conditions as erythroblastosis, in which maternal antibody attacks fetal cells, and graft-vs.-host lesions pro-duced by transferred immunocompetent lymphocytes. Finally, complex antigens, formed by combination of exogenous hapten with host carrier macromolecules, elicit reactions of partial autoimmunity in that antibody (or cells) formed by the host may be directed in part to the host component of the antigen. Again, another pattern is provided by experiments with complex antigens and transferred antibody or cells.

The mechanism of any given lesion determines not only its morphologic character but also whether it can be transferred passively with serum or only with suitable cells, whether it can occur in subjects with agammaglo-bulinemia, sarcoid, etc., and how it is affected by such agents as X ray, steroids, nitrogen mustards, anti-metabolites, antihistamines, and anticlotting agents or by such manipulations as thymectomy. The pattern, on the other hand, affects the time course of lesion formation, the distribution of lesions, and the need for ad-ministration of exogenous material (antigen, hapten) during immunization, to induce tolerance, or to elicit lesions in actively or passively sensitized hosts.

1. Antigens

Antigens involved in immunobiologic and immunopathologic phenomena may be studied by classic quantitative immunochemical methods such as precipitation or agglutination. However, much of the recent development in our knowledge, of tissue antigens in particular, has been based on the application of three distinct groups of new techniques. First, the use of *sensitive serologic methods* (among them passive hemagglutination or agglutination of antigen-coated particles such as collodion, latex, or bentonite; the Coombs technique and the closely related antiglobulin consumption test; and complement fixation) has permitted identification of many previously unrecognized antigen–antibody systems. Second, *gel diffusion analysis* has provided a means of enumerating the antigens participating in a given biologic situation. Immunoelectrophoresis (illustrated in Figs. 1.1,2) offers the most subtle and widely applicable of the gel diffusion methods. Third, *immunologically specific morphologic techniques* have made it possible to localize specific antigens in tissues, in cells, or indeed in cell organelles or other ultrastructural components. The simplest and the most versatile morphologic method is specific immunofluorescence (illustrated in Figs. 1.3–16), which is used at the level of the light microscope. Ferritin-labeled antibody provides a similar specific means of localizing antigens at the electron microscopic level. Other morphologic approaches, less widely utilized, are autoradiography of material containing isotopically labeled antigen (Figs. 1.17,18) and the specific hemadsorption technique. The same methods are used to supplement conventional morphologic studies of stained material and histochemical and electron microscopic preparations in the analysis of antigen uptake, antibody production, and the mechanism of lesion formation in various immunopathologic states, as will be seen in later sections.

The *specificity* of antigens is determined by the stereochemical configuration of limited areas of the molecular surface, so-called *antigenic determinants*. These may be sequences of sugars or amino acids, three-dimensional arrays of such subunits determined by the secondary and tertiary structure of the antigenic molecule, or attached small molecules, *haptens*. The ability of the molecule to induce an immune response, its *immunogenicity*, depends on a number of factors. These include molecular size, possibly digestibility by enzymes present in host cells, and a poorly defined but essential *carrier function*, which appears to reflect the presence of molecular configurations for which the processing cells of the host (Section 6) possess suitable receptors. The specificity defined by the carrier and the complementary configuration of the processing cell surface is much broader than that inherent in the antigenic determinant and its complementary configuration in the lymphon (Section 4). An antigen, to be immunogenic, must also possess *foreignness*, i.e. antigenic determinants to which the host is not tolerant and for which reactive lymphons are available. The intensity with which an antigen immunizes, reflects additional properties of the molecule subsumed under the term *adjuvanticity*. This may express the "stickiness" of the molecule for processing cells or some other quality that affects the number or activity of processing cells. The adjuvanticity of an antigen is greatly enhanced by the particulate form or by the additional use of adjuvants which affect the RE system. Immunogenicity and the carrier function are requisite for primary immunization, for secondary stimulation, and for the elicitation of a delayed (cellular) hypersensitivity reaction (Sections 16–18). These requirements may be bypassed in the case of systems which involve an antigenic determinant able to combine at very high affinity with certain lymphons. For the induction of tolerance, the molecular requirements appear to be similar to those for immunization, but without adjuvanticity.

All antigens fall within one of three broad categories. Many are exogenous materials; others are constituents of the tissues or body fluids, i.e. iso- or autoantigens; and still others are complex antigens resulting from the interaction of exogenous materials with body constituents. Of the *exogenous antigens*, the most important is the group of infectious agents, including bacteria, viruses, fungi, protozoa, and metazoan parasites. These must enter the body through one of its many portals, i.e. skin, mucous membranes, gastrointestinal tract, etc. All contain a multiplicity of potential antigens (Fig. 1.1 shows the presence of approximately twenty distinct antigens in the group A streptococcus which induce antibody formation in man). Each antigen molecule, furthermore, may possess an equal multiplicity of specific determinants. Another major group of exogenous antigens is found in foods, plant pollens, animal danders, insect "emanations," dusts etc., which enter the body generally by way of the respiratory or gastrointestinal mucosa or the conjunctiva. Again each is made up of many distinct components. Insect bites and stings, which may introduce intensely active pharmacologic agents into the skin (among them phospholipases, 5-hydroxytryptamine, and histamine-releasing substances), also commonly introduce antigenic molecules which may lead to anaphylactic or delayed sensitization. Finally, serum and many drugs injected by physicians are antigenic and frequently lead to sensitization which may be of any type.

Endogenous antigens may be present in any cellular element, in extracellular tissue components, or in the body fluids. The cell nucleus, for example, possesses distinct antigens in the nuclear membrane and the nuclear sap; and both the DNA and protein constituents of the chromosomes may give rise to formation of specific antibodies (Figs. 1.3,4). Other membrane systems of the cell contain polysaccharide antigens such as the blood group substances (Figs. 1.7,8), cytosides such as cardiolipin (these are lipid molecules whose specificity may be determined by simple sugars), protein or lipoprotein antigens such as the H-2 histocompatibility antigen of the mouse cell (Fig. 3.13), or more complex antigenic material containing lipid, carbohydrate, and protein such as myelin (Fig. 1.9). The cytoplasm contains many soluble enzymes, which are potential antigens, and may contain additional special antigenic substances such as hemoglobin. Cytoplasmic organelles, such as ribosomes, have RNA which can act as a hapten. Extracellular antigens are found in the fibrillar elements of connective tissue (collagen for example), in the ground substance, and in basement membranes (Fig. 1.11). These in general are proteins or mucopolysaccharides. Finally the body fluids, serum for example, may contain as many as thirty distinct protein and polypeptide antigens (Fig. 1.2).

While distinct antigens are present in different parts of an organ such as the thyroid (Fig. 1.5) or the cell (Fig. 1.6), or indeed within an organelle like the nucleus (Fig. 1.3), cross-reacting or identical antigens, many of the membrane antigens in particular (Figs. 1.7,8; 3.13), are found in cells throughout the body. Other antigens may be found in a limited number of special locations, e.g. the similar basement membrane antigens of the placenta and the renal glomerulus (Fig. 1.11) or the common antigen in muscle and in the "myoid" reticulum cell of the thymus (Figs. 1.12–14). Such limited cross-reactivity may be significant in determining patterns of disease in toxemia of pregnancy, for example, which affects both the placenta and kidney, or in myasthenia gravis, affecting thymus and muscle, though these relationships are by no means well worked out. A similar cross-relationship between a tissue component and an exogenous material, as in the case of heart antigen and group A streptococcal cell wall components (Fig. 1.10), may also be a highly significant pathogenetic mechanism in such a disease as rheumatic fever.

A convenient distinction has been made in the past between "species specificity," a term that designates evolutionary changes in specificity of a single molecule such as serum albumin in different species; "group or type specificity" and "allotypic specificity," which designate differences in specificity of a single molecule between different members of the same species; "organ specificity," which refers to essential identity or a close relationship of certain specialized materials such as lens protein or myelin in members of different species; and "heterophile specificity," which indicates coincidental antigenic relationships between biologically unrelated substances (as in the heart-streptococcus case). In any situation, the number of antigens playing a role is determined by whether a response is elicited in a member of another species, a member of the same species, or indeed in the same individual.

The category of *complex antigens* includes mainly cases in which an exogenous material, usually a natural substance or a drug acting as hapten, forms a conjugate with a normal body constituent and renders it antigenic in the host. The classical example is contact allergy in which a reactive small molecule, placed on the surface of the skin, reacts with an unknown protein of the epidermis to form the sensitizing antigen (Figs. 1.17,18).

Other well-recognized cases include such drugs as quinidine, Sedormid, or amidopyrine reacting with erythrocytes, platelets, or leukocytes and penicillin or aspirin reacting with serum proteins. Any class of immune response may be produced.

An additional important category of antigenic substances is represented by *neoantigens*, appearing in virus-infected cells and apparently coded for by part of the virus genome. These are major determinants of the immune response (and tolerance) in relation to virus-induced tumors (Fig. 1.15), and may possibly play a role in certain autoimmune states.

The *location of antigen* determines the *distribution of lesions* which it may elicit (see next section). Thus an antigen fixed at a site of injection (Fig. 1.16) or produced by a local interaction of exogenous allergen with body protein (Figs. 1.17,18) will elicit only a local lesion. An antigen present throughout an organ system, as in myelin, can elicit lesions throughout that system, as in autoallergic encephalomyelitis (Section 21). The mechanism of lesion formation (neutralization, single cell, anaphylactic, Arthus, delayed) does not depend on whether the antigen is restricted to a single cell, as with lens protein, or is present in cells throughout the body, as in the case of transplantation antigens.

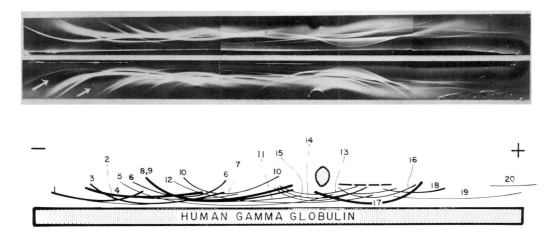

Fig. 1.1. Immunoelectrophoretic assay of streptococcal antigens detectable with naturally occurring antibodies present in pooled normal human γ-globulin (in trench). (Above) Top well contained the standard reference crude group A streptococcal culture supernate concentrate; lower well contained a different lot of crude concentrate. (Below) Diagrammatic representation of the results noted with the reference group A system.

Identification of the antigens associated with the following arcs. 1, Proteinase precursor. 4, C carbohydrate (complexed with protein?). 5, An antigen related to erythrogenic toxin (?). 10, Streptolysin 0. 11, Streptokinase. 17, Deoxyribonuclease B. 19, Rapidly migrating, purified, but unidentified antigen.

From Halbert and Keatinge, *J. Exp. Med. 113*:1013–28 (1961).

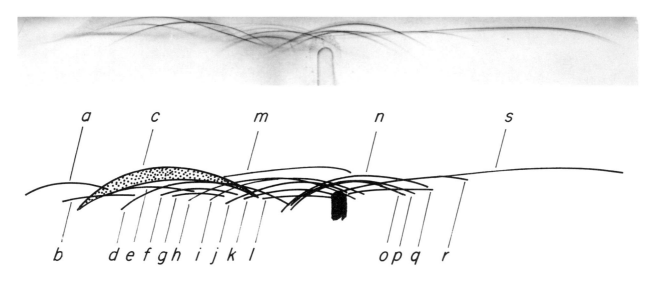

Fig. 1.2. Immunoelectrophoretic pattern of normal human serum showing some, but by no means all, of the recognized constituents active as heteroantigens. (Below) Individual lines have been designated: (a) 1; (b) 2; (c) albumin; (d) principal α_1; (e) orosomucoid; (f, g) α_1; (h) haptoglobin; (i) α_2; (j) ceruloplasmin; (k) α_2 macroglobulin; (l) α_2 lipoprotein; (m) Gc; (n) transferrin; (o, p) β_1; (q) β_{2M} (γM); (r) β_{2A} (γA); (s) γ (γG).

Courtesy of Drs. P. Grabar and J. Courcon.

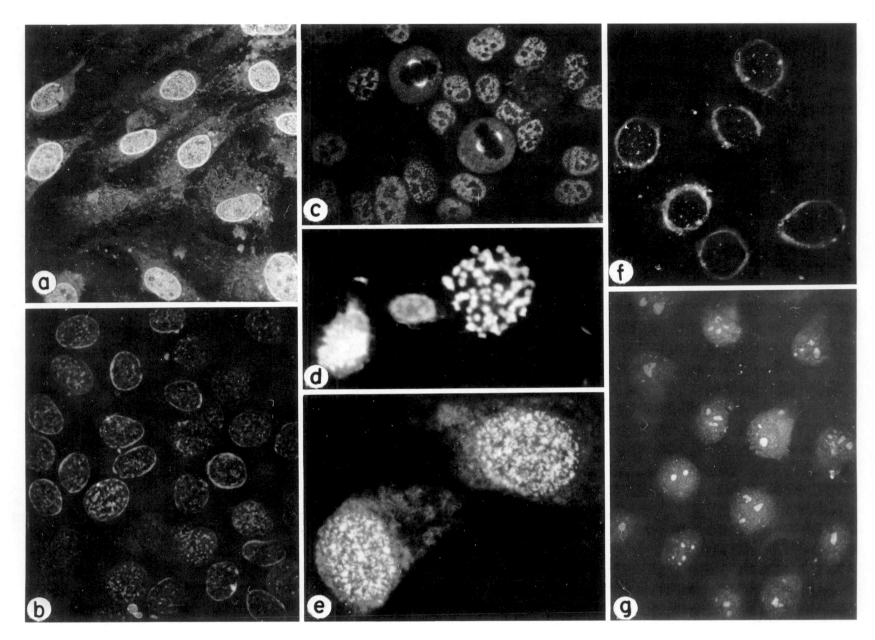

Fig. 1.3. Distinct patterns of nuclear staining produced by antibody to different constituents of the nucleus. HeLa cells in tissue culture, stained with various human sera (from patients with such "collagen" diseases as systemic lupus erythematosus, scleroderma, dermatomyositis, and rheumatoid arthritis) containing antinuclear antibody. Cells were washed and then treated with horse antihuman-globulin antibody conjugated with fluorescein isothiocyanate. (a) Strong reaction with nuclear membrane and chromatin; ×480. (b) Weak reaction of same type; ×560. (c) Reaction with chromatin only. Dark negative areas appear to correspond to nucleoli. Two center cells are in mitosis; ×550. (d) Similar reaction in preparation pretreated with colchicine to arrest mitosis and swollen in hypotonic solution; ×350. (e) Predominant reaction with chromatin or associated structures; ×1,150. (f) Reaction primarily with nuclear membrane; ×700. (g) Reaction with nucleoli; ×480.

From Rapp, *J. Immunol.* *88*: 732–40 (1962).

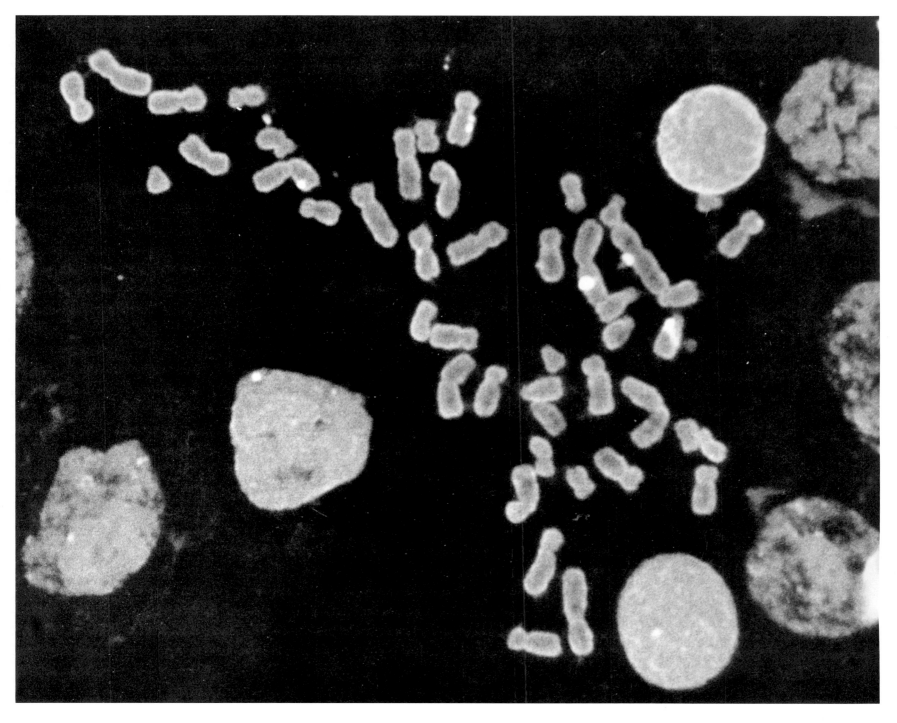

Fig. 1.4. Chromosome preparation from tissue culture of human blood, arrested in mitosis with colchicine and subsequently stained by the indirect technique with serum from a patient with systemic lupus erythematosus, followed by a fluorescent conjugate of horse antihuman globulin. Fluorescent staining shows uptake of antinuclear factor by several nuclei in the field as well as by individual chromosomes of the mitotic figure.

Courtesy of Dr. John E. Tobie (see Krooth, Tobie, Tjio, and Goodman: *Science 134*:284–86, 1961).

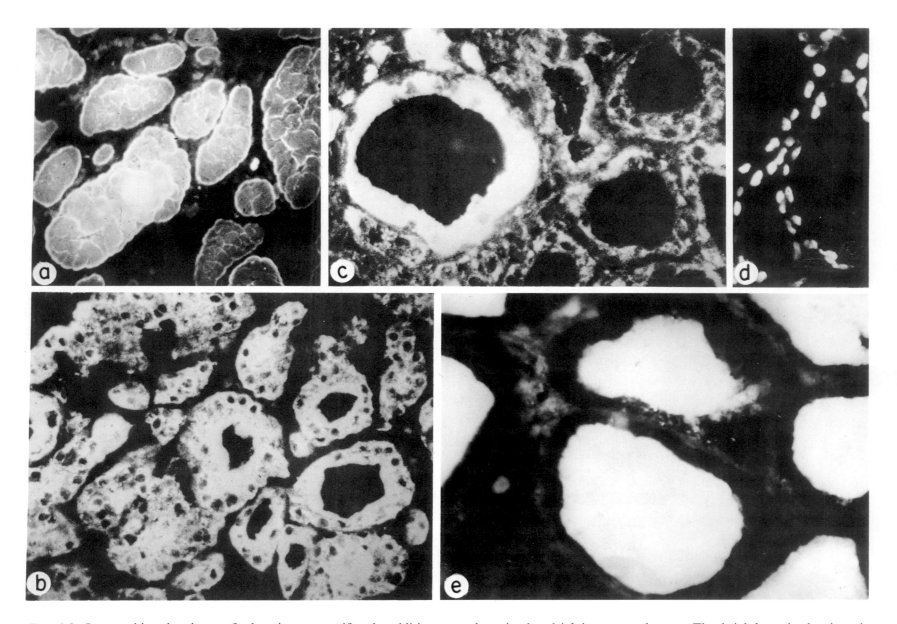

Fig. 1.5. Immunohistochemistry of chronic nonspecific thyroiditis in man. All sections were treated with the patient's serum followed by a fluorescein-conjugated antihuman immunoglobulin. (a) Floccular pattern of colloid fluorescence obtained on treatment of methanol-fixed human thyroid sections with serum containing thyroglobulin autoantibodies. The cytoplasm is unstained even when microsomal antibodies are also present, since the microsomal antigen is destroyed by fixation. (b) Unfixed frozen section of human thyrotoxic thyroid gland treated with Hashimoto serum containing complement-fixing microsomal antibodies. The cytoplasm of the acinar epithelial cells is stained, fluorescence being maximal at the apical margin; nuclei are unstained. Colloid is normally leached out from unfixed sections during the treatment, but when thyroglubulin antibodies are present, the colloid is sometimes retained in the small acini. (c) Unfixed human thyrotoxic thyroid treated with serum from a patient with primary biliary cirrhosis containing nonorgan-specific antibodies directed against the mitochondrial inner membranes. The brightly stained acinus is composed of "Askenazy cells" which are rich in mitochondria with extensive cristae. The other acini in which the cells have not undergone eosinophilic metaplasia also give a positive reaction, but the sparser population of mitochondria gives a less intense granular fluorescence. (d) Fluorescent staining of unfixed thyroid section with nuclear antibodies in serum from a patient with systemic lupus erythematosus. Staining of nuclei in the glandular epithelium as well as the connective tissue elements is in evidence. (e) Uniform pattern of colloid staining in fixed thyroid section treated with a Hashimoto serum containing antibodies to the second colloid antigen but lacking thyroglobulin antibodies.

Indirect immunofluorescence technique; (a, b, d) ×260; (c, e) ×400. (a–c, e) Courtesy of Drs. I. Roitt and D. Doniach. (d) From Beutner and Witebsky, *J. Immunol.* *88*: 462–75 (1962).

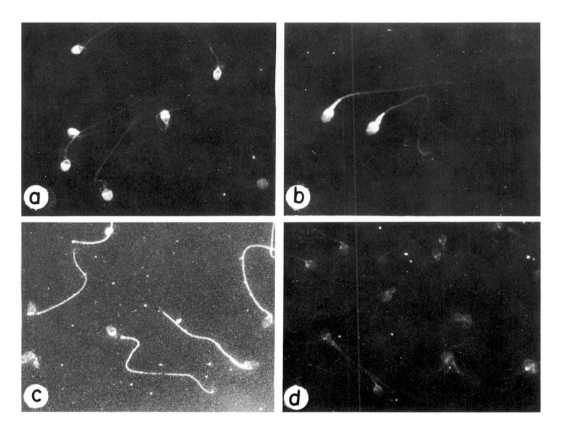

Fig. 1.6. Antigens of human sperm, demonstrated by the indirect fluorescence technique with various human sera containing sperm autoantibody and normal sperm. (a) Fluorescent staining of head. (b) Staining of posterior part of head and midpiece. (c) Staining of tail. (d) Absence of staining with normal serum.

P. Rümke: "Autoantilichamen tegen Spermatozoën als Oorzaak van Onvruchtbaarheid bei de Man," Thesis, 1959.

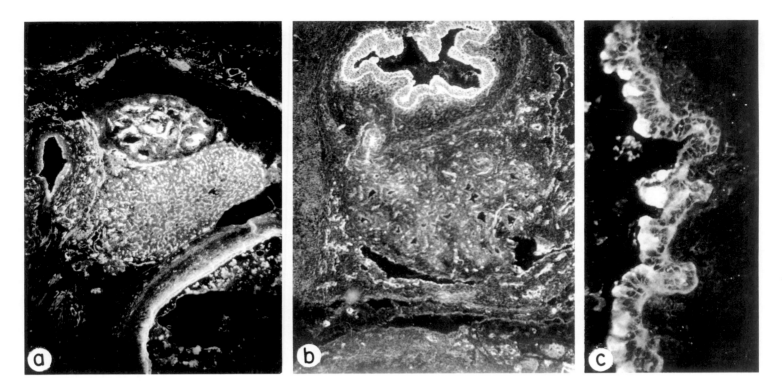

Fig. 1.7. Distribution of blood-group mucopolysaccharides in epithelia and mucous secretions during development. (a) Early human fetus (27 mm): section showing stomach, adrenal, kidney, and aorta, stained with rabbit anti-A and overlaid with fluorescent goat antirabbit globulin conjugate; ×35. (b) Same fetus: section showing duodenum, pancreas, and pancreatic duct, stained similarly; ×70. (c) Stomach mucosa of older fetus (7/10 cm crown–rump/crown–heel) of blood group O, stained with conjugate of human Bombay (anti-H) serum and overlaid with horse anti-human globulin conjugate; ×300.

Fresh frozen specimens, sectioned in cryostat and stained by indirect fluorescence technique. From Szulman, *J. Exp. Med. 119*: 503–16 (1964).

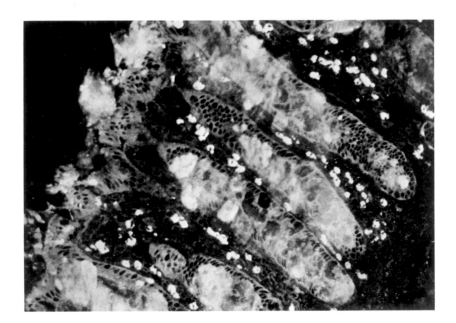

Fig. 1.8. Adult human colon from subject of type O, stained with human anti-H. Intense staining of mucus in goblet cells of crypt epithelium.

Cryostat section, indirect fluorescence technique; ×170. From Szulman, *J. Exp. Med. 115*: 977–96 (1962).

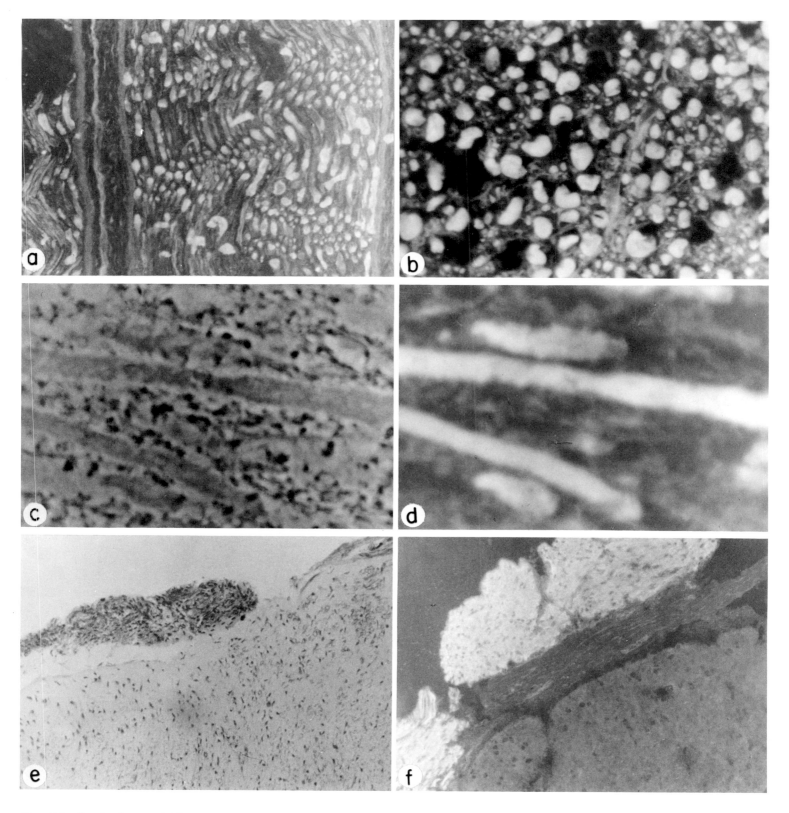

Fig. 1.9. Serologic specificity of antibodies against myelin. (a) Rabbit sciatic nerve stained by indirect fluorescence technique, with rabbit antibody against sciatic followed by fluorescent antibody to rabbit γ-globulin. Bright staining of myelin sheaths is clearly shown. (b) Cross section of rabbit spinal cord, similarly stained with rabbit antibody against cord. (c, d) Longitudinal section of rabbit cord, in phase contrast and stained with anticord as in (b). (e, f) Human neonatal (10 days old) spinal cord and dorsal spinal root, stained with Luxol fast blue and with same rabbit anticord serum as (b) and (d) respectively. (e) At this stage of development, myelin is present in root but not in cord, and antibody stains this myelin specifically. Interspecies cross-reactivity of responsible antigen is also demonstrated by the staining.

(a, b, d, f) Frozen sections, stained by indirect fluorescence technique; ×100, ×200, ×400, ×100. (c) Same as (d) in phase contrast. (e) Paraffin section of block adjacent to (f), stained with Luxol blue; ×100. From Sherwin, Richter, Cosgrove, and Rose, *Science 134*:1370–72 (1961). Copyright 1961 by the American Association for the Advancement of Science.

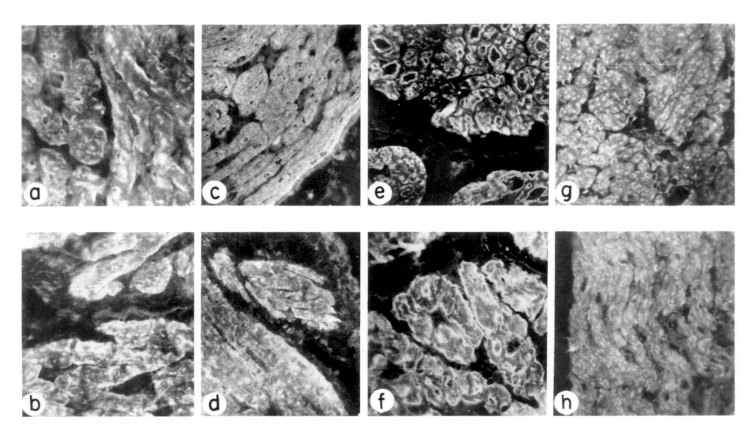

Fig. 1.10. Cross-reactions of heart antigens. (a–d) Normal rabbit heart, stained by fluorescence technique with rabbit antiserum prepared against beef heart. (a, b) Sections of left auricle and left ventricle respectively; (c) and (d) include endocardium. Myocardial cells are more or less diffusely stained. Endocardial connective tissue shows autofluorescence (blue). (e, f) Normal rabbit heart, similarly treated with rabbit antiserum against rat heart, also shows sarcoplasmic staining, especially around nucleus, between myofibrils, and at periphery of myofiber. (g, h) Normal rat heart, stained with rabbit antibody against group A streptococci, shows staining largely limited to sarcoplasmic sites between myofibrils.

(a, b, e–h) ×260, (c, d) ×130. From Kaplan, *J. Immunol.* *80*: 254–67 (1958).

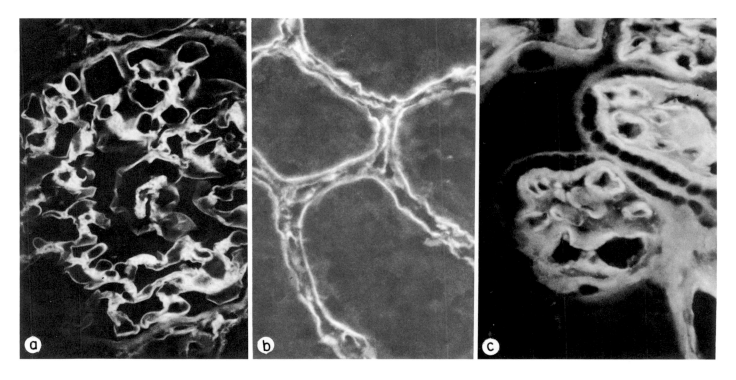

Fig. 1.11. Localization of nephrotoxigenic antigen. Human tissues stained by fluorescent sheep antihuman placenta serum (absorbed with whole human blood and mouse liver powder). (a, b) Kidney showing staining of glomerular basement membrane (a), tubular basement membranes, basement membranes of intertubular capillaries, and possibly intertubular reticular fibers (b). (c) Placental villi showing staining of subsyncytial connective tissue and basement membranes of small vessels. Paler fluorescence at surface of trophoblast is blue-grey (nonspecific) autofluorescence. Sheep antibody against human glomerular basement membrane stains apparently identical antigen in the same distribution. All ×570. From Steblay, *J. Immunol. 88*: 434–42 (1962).

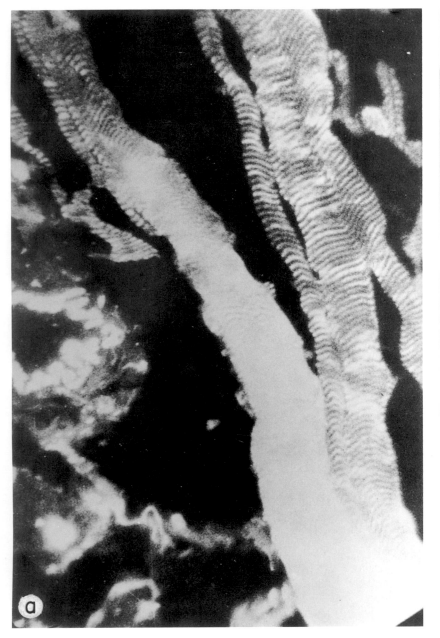 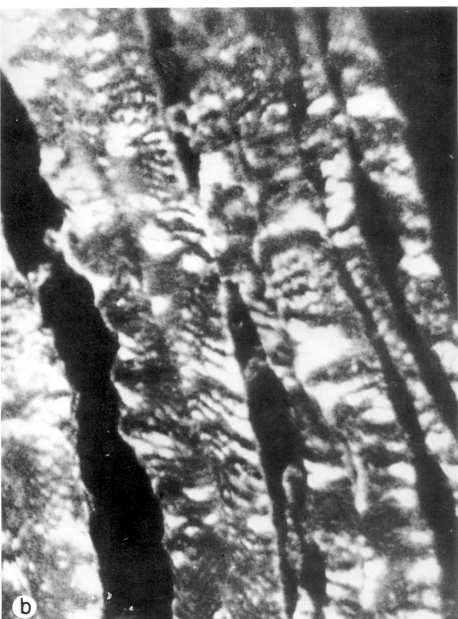

Fig. 1.12. Immunohistochemistry of myasthenia gravis. (a) Section of human skeletal muscle stained with globulin pool from ten myasthenic sera conjugated with fluorescein isothiocyanate (direct immunofluorescence). There is delicate staining of striations in myofibers. Tunica elastica of small vessel at left shows autofluorescence. (b) Section of same muscle biopsy, treated sequentially with untagged myasthenic serum globulin, guinea pig complement, and fluorescent conjugate of rabbit antiguinea pig complement (complement fixation immunofluorescence). Note irregular character of complement staining in alternate striations. ×850. From Strauss, Seegal, Hsu, Burkholder, Nastuk, and Osserman, *Proc. Soc. Exp. Biol. Med. 105:* 184–91 (1960).

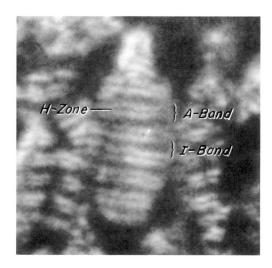

Fig. 1.13. Immunohistochemistry of myasthenia gravis. Bovine skeletal muscle treated successively with reactive myasthenic serum, diluted 1:16, and rabbit antihuman γ-globulin conjugate (indirect immunofluorescence). Staining is seen in the lateral portions of A bands but not in central H zones. The lateralization of fluorescence appears related to the state of contraction of a given segment of muscle. ×900. From Strauss, van der Geld, Kemp, Exum, and Goodman, *Ann. N.Y. Acad. Sci. 124*:744–66 (1965).

Fig. 1.14. Immunohistochemistry of myasthenia gravis. Patterns of immunofluorescence in human skeletal muscle (mu.) and thymus (thy.) encountered in a coded, randomized study of sera from 1,139 individuals. Sections were fixed with 95 percent ethanol, washed in repeated changes of phosphate-buffered saline, incubated with test serum 1:60, washed again with buffered saline, treated with a 1:200 dilution of specific fluorescent antibody to human γ-globulin, and finally washed and mounted in buffered glycerol. (a) Negative pattern observed with sera of some subjects with myasthenia gravis, normal controls, and "disease controls," as well as subjects with thymomas unassociated with myasthenia gravis. No fluorescence of muscle striations or of thymic epithelial cells was seen. (b) Pattern of concurrent immunofluorescence in alternate skeletal muscle striations and thymic epithelial cells, seen with sera of certain patients with myasthenia gravis, with thymomas unassociated with myasthenia gravis, in one normal individual, and in one patient with a thymoma associated with an aregenerative anemia (no myasthenia gravis). Sera from twelve of thirteen patients with thymomas with myasthenia gravis produced this pattern. The cell margins and granular cytoplasmic material of thymic epithelial cells are most intensely stained. (c) Pattern of nuclear immunofluorescence produced by sera from individuals with systemic lupus erythematosus, rheumatoid arthritis, and scleroderma, and from a small number of patients with myasthenia gravis. (d) Staining reactions revealing *both* antinuclear and concomitant antistriational, antithymic epithelial cell antibodies, with sera from six patients with myasthenia gravis and five patients with thymomas unassociated with myasthenia gravis. In this group, reactivity with thymic epithelial cells was obscured by the diffuse reaction with thymocyte nuclei at the 1:60 screening dilution of test serum. At dilutions of 1:120, 1:240, etc., anti-nuclear reactions diminished, while fluorescence in epithelial cell cytoplasm persisted. Arrows in photomicrograph of thymus denote thymic epithelial cells against faint backgrounds of fluorescent thymocyte nuclei, at serum dilution 1:240.

All ×900. From Strauss, Smith, Cage, van der Geld, McFarlin, and Barlow, *Ann. N.Y. Acad. Sci. 135*: 557–79 (1966).

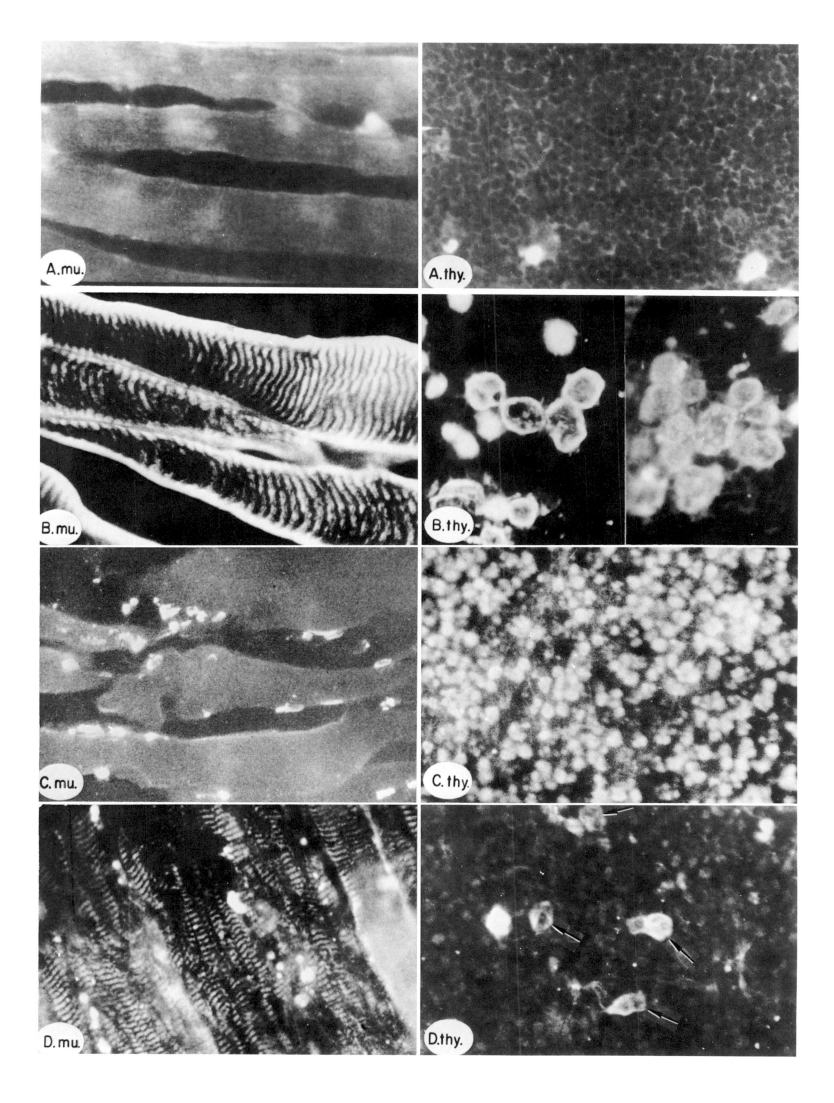

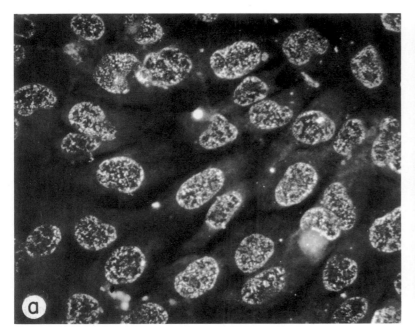 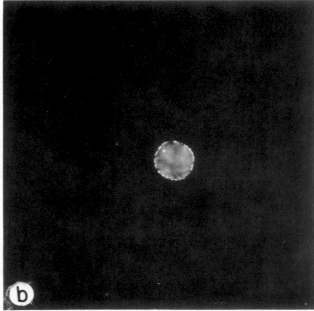

Fig. 1.15. Neoantigens coded for by virus genome. Two different antigens in hamster cells transformed *in vivo* by SV40 virus. (a) Demonstration of the SV40 tumor (T) antigen by serum from hamsters bearing tumors induced by the virus. T antigen is localized in the nuclei of the transformed cells. × 500. (b) Demonstration of a new cell surface antigen by serum from hamsters challenged with trans-formed cells. Antigen–antibody reaction gives a "necklace" effect in the fluorescence photomicrograph. No antigen is seen within the cell. × 400.

Indirect fluorescence technique. (a) From Rapp, Butel, and Melnick, *Proc. Soc. Exp. Biol. Med. 116*: 1131–35 (1964). (b) From Tevethia, Katz, and Rapp, ibid. *119*: 896–901 (1965).

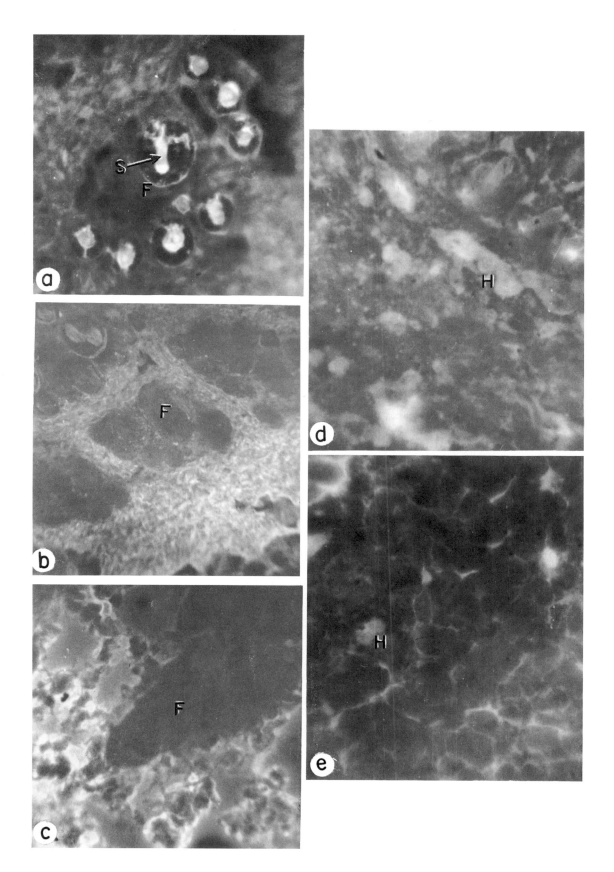

Fig. 1.16. Distribution of protein antigen injected intradermally. Ovalbumin (2 or 10 mg) injected into normal rabbit (a), rabbit sensitized passively with specific antibody (4 mg N) (b), or rabbit sensitized 2 weeks earlier with ovalbumin in Freund adjuvant (c–e). Sacrifice at 1 hour (a–c) or 24 hours (d, e). (a) Antigen is seen around and between hair follicles (F) in upper dermis. Follicles themselves show reddish autofluorescence (S, hair shaft). (b) Antigen is widely distributed in connective tissue of deeper dermis between and below follicles. None is present within the follicles. (c) Lakes of extracellular antigen are present in edematous connective tissue near follicles. (d) In upper dermis at 24 hours, antigen is almost entirely within cytoplasm of numerous histiocytes (macrophages) (H). (e) In deeper dermis at this time, there is persistent extracellular antigen between bundles of collagen and some within histiocytes.

Direct fluorescence technique; (a–c) ×200, (d, e) ×400. From Waksman and Bocking, *Proc. Soc. Exp. Biol. Med. 82*: 738–42 (1953).

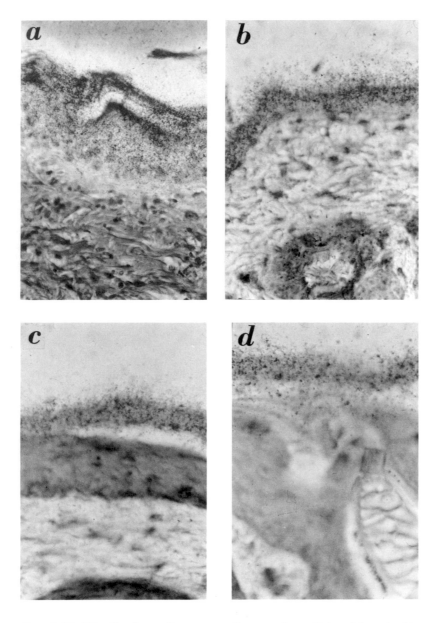

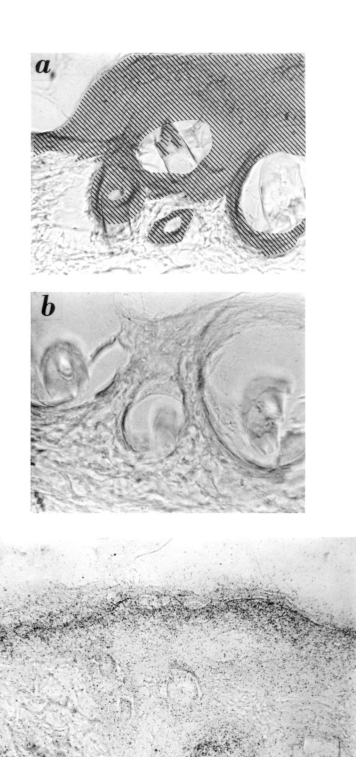

Fig. 1.17. Distribution of contact allergen that elicits delayed skin reaction. Two drops of 1-C¹⁴-labeled 2,4-dinitrochlorobenzene, 0.012 M in Methyl Cellosolve, applied to surface of guinea pig skin. Sites sectioned 1, 2, 3, and 4 days after application (a–d) show original appearance of label throughout epidermis and its progressive movement toward superficial epidermal layers as basal cells multiply and push older cells toward surface.

Ten-μ paraffin sections on NTB nuclear track plate, exposed 3.5–5 months, developed, and stained with metanil yellow and iron hematoxylin; all ×430. From Eisen and Tabachnik, *J. Exp. Med. 108*: 773–96 (1958).

Fig. 1.18. Distribution of contact allergen that elicits delayed skin reaction. (a, b) Labeled dinitrofluorobenzene (0.5 M, in 1:1 acetone-corn oil) applied to surface of guinea pig skin. Sections taken at 24 hours are stained for nitrobenzenes (by reduction, diazotization, and coupling with N-1-naphthylethylene diamine dihydrochloride). Cross-hatching in (a) shows distribution of hapten (brilliant purple color). (b) Adjacent section, similarly treated but with reduction step omitted, shows no staining. (c) Autoradiograph prepared 24 hours after intradermal injection of labeled dinitrochlorobenzene (11.3 μg). There is a relative concentration of hapten (silver grains) in epidermis and hair follicles (arrows).

All ×430. From Eisen and Tabachnik, *J. Exp. Med. 108*: 773–96 (1958).

2. Phagocytic Cells and Antigen Uptake

The disposition of foreign materials that enter the body, as well as the endogenous components of tissues or body fluids, has importance from four points of view. The primary problem is one of scavenging or, as it is frequently referred to, *clearance*. This function has no necessary relation to specific immunologic mechanisms. The remaining problems are immunologically significant. One concerns that aspect of antigen distribution and uptake which leads to *immunization* or *sensitization*. Another concerns the *induction of* specific immunologic *tolerance*. The last has to do with the localization of antigen in *eliciting* different classes of immunologically induced *lesions*. There is no evidence that the role of foreign and endogenous antigens, or of antigenic complexes of foreign hapten with host carrier, differs in respect to these various functions.

Exogenous haptens or antigens may enter the body by way of the classic *portals*—skin, conjunctiva, respiratory mucosa, gastrointestinal tract, or genitourinary tract—each of which is provided with special clearing mechanisms, e.g. cilia and mucus, which interfere with penetration. The exogenous materials then find themselves in a local tissue, in one of the body cavities (pleura, peritoneum, pericardium, joint, meninges, etc.), in lymphatics draining the local site or cavity, or in the blood stream. Endogenous and complex antigens may, of course, have a similar distribution. *Antibacterial* and *antiviral substances*, such as lysozyme, are present on the skin and mucosal surfaces as well as in the blood, lymph, and tissue fluids. These are not discussed further here.

The principal means of disposing of foreign substances is *pinocytic* or *phagocytic uptake* in the two general types of cell specialized for this purpose, *neutrophilic and eosinophilic granulocytes* (polymorphonuclears) (Figs. 2.17,18), and *reticuloendothelial (RE) cells* (Figs. 2.3,12,13). The former are essentially limited to the blood stream except in inflammation. The latter appear to be derived largely, if not entirely, from rapidly dividing precursors in the bone marrow. They include small, immature forms in the blood stream and lymph, known as monocytes; some of these, in such species as the rat, may be indistinguishable by light microscopy from small to medium lymphocytes, but in all cases they share the histochemical and ultrastructural features of the RE group of cells. In vessel walls they take the form of adventitial cells, and in the tissues of resting or wandering histiocytes. They may have special names: microglia in the central nervous system, alveolar cells in the lungs. In reticular and lymphoid organs, they are seen as a phagocytic "endothelium" which lines sinuses and sinusoids. Again specialized names are applied to the same cells in different places, e.g. the Kupffer cells of the liver. Finally, they make up at least part of the population of reticulum cells in these organs. It is not certain, however, that the dendritic reticulum cell of the lymphoid follicle, in spleen and lymph nodes, is a reticuloendothelial cell, since it is not phagocytic; and the thymic reticulum cells that are derived from branchial cleft epithelium are also clearly not of this type.

Reticuloendothelial cells share a number of properties. They stick to wettable surfaces like glass, unlike lymphocytes. They show vigorous pinocytosis (Figs. 2.14,16) and by this means take up proteins in solution in the ambient medium (Fig. 2.15; see also 18.7,15). Activated cells are phagocytic (Figs. 2.2,3,9). They contain a battery of hydrolytic enzymes such as acid phosphatase within their lysosomes, and the discharge of lysosomal contents into phagocytic vacuoles (Figs. 2.17–19), with activation of the released hydrolases at the acid pH of the vacuole, leads to rapid digestion of phagocytized materials. They are metallophilic, i.e. easily stained by silver and other impregnation techniques (Fig. 2.12). They respond to a heavy phagocytic load by replication (Fig. 2.11). Certain well-defined types of molecules, acting at the surface of RE cells, trigger striking changes in their size and functional state, from the small lymphocyte-like monocytes to mature, highly activated macrophages filled with phagocytized material. Epithelioid and giant cells, resulting from fusion of many epithelioid cells, are formed in certain types of lesions from precursors in the same cell series. Artificially induced cell exudates, in the peritoneal cavity for example, consist after the first few hours largely of cells of RE type, with an admixture of true lymphocytes.

An additional mechanism that plays an important role in the disposition of antigenic materials is *inflammation*. Substances with toxic or irritant properties may induce changes in vascular permeability and edema, accompanied by a local accumulation of nonspecific antibacterial and antiviral agents coming from the blood stream and specific agents, notably humoral antibody and complement. A greater degree of vascular damage leads to successive diapedesis of polymorphonuclears and of monocytes from vessels in the inflamed area and activation of resting histiocytes in the tissue itself. In immunized hosts, similar inflammatory changes may be elicited by small quantities of substances which lack toxic or irritant properties entirely but are antigenically active. The anaphylactic mechanism, in this instance, leads to increased vascular permeability, the Arthus mechanism to more severe vascular damage and to polymorph diapedesis, and the cellular sensitivity mechanisms to rapid accumulation of highly activated mononuclear phagocytes (monocytes).

Antigens situated in a local tissue or in one of the body cavities play no role in the induction of tolerance and a minimal role in immunization (see below). Clearance depends entirely on phagocytosis by local histiocytes (Fig. 1.16) or the production of inflammation and phagocytosis by hematogenous cells. Their ability to elicit one or another type of specific immunologic lesion at the local site depends not only on the host's state of sensitization and the location of the antigen (Figs. 1.16–18) but also on additional factors such as the degree of vascularization of the tissue, the diffusibility of the antigen, its concentration, and so on. The precise localization of Arthus reactions at a local site, for example, is strongly influenced by the size and consequent diffusibility of the antigenic molecule injected into the dermal connective tissue. With highly diffusible antigen, antigen–antibody complexes may be formed almost entirely in the vessel lumen; with poorly diffusible antigen, they may be largely extravascular.

Antigens that enter the systemic circulation may, depending on their colloidal properties, be deposited in or beneath vascular basement membranes in a number of sites, particularly those in which filtration occurs, such as the glomerular basement membrane or the synovia (Figs. 2.8–10). Here they may elicit striking lesions in immunized hosts. Perhaps the best known example is the glomerulonephritis of immune complex disease (Section 13). Alternatively, they may be taken up by granulocytes within the circulation (Fig. 2.8) or cleared by RE cells lining sinusoids in the liver, spleen, lungs, and bone marrow (Figs. 2.2,3,9). The rate of clearance of particulate materials is determined by concentration and by particle size and surface charge, on the one hand, and by the number and activity of RE cells on the other. It may be markedly enhanced by antibody, which coats and opsonizes the particles, by agents such as zymosan or endotoxin, which lead to RE cell proliferation, or by tuberculous infection which leads to proliferation but also increases the phagocytic activity of individual RE cells. It is depressed by blockade of RE cells. Blockade shows a certain degree of specificity; a given agent such as carbon may block RE uptake of some particulates but not others. Agents like cortisone do not affect RE cell activity as such but depress the ability of these cells to replicate in response to an increased phagocytic load or to endotoxin. Others, such as silica or methyl palmitate and similar esters, may actually destroy RE cells. The distribution of cleared particles depends on the character of the particle surface as well as on particle concentration. Red cells coated with antibody may be taken up and destroyed in either the liver or the spleen, depending on the type of antibody employed. The RE clearance function is readily measured and has been subjected to thorough mathematical analysis.

Soluble materials, which are taken up by pinocytosis, are cleared and catabolized at a slow exponential rate, which varies with molecular size and possibly other factors and with the metabolic rate of the host. Clearance proceeds until antibody is produced in the host, at which point antigen–antibody complexes are formed and rapidly cleared (immune clearance) by the RE system in a manner similar to that of other particles. In irradiated or specifically tolerant hosts, or in hosts injected with autologous or homologous protein, no phase of immune clearance is seen. Antigen–antibody complexes formed in the circulation are themselves important pathogenic agents (Section 13).

Immunization is largely a function of antigen uptake by certain phagocytic cells in peripheral lymphoid organs

(Fig. 2.1). Antigens entering the body across a mucosal surface are taken up in such *surface organs* as the tonsils and Peyer's patches; here the afferent limb of immunization occurs by way of crypts in the mucosa. Antigens entering the skin, extremities, or the respiratory or gastrointestinal mucosae rapidly find their way into lymphatics and a series of *draining lymph nodes*; here the afferent lymph serves as the pathway of immunization. Finally, antigens entering the blood stream induce immunization primarily in the *spleen*, the blood itself providing the afferent pathway. These organs have a triple function. First they provide for the clearance and *processing of antigen* by their anatomic location and the provision of widely dilated sinuses or sinusoids lined with phagocytic cells through which the blood or lymph must pass. Second, they contain *immunocompetent lymphocytes* and provide a physiologic pathway for the continuous recirculation of these cells between the peripheral pool in the blood and the lymphoid parenchyma (Section 4). Third, by bringing the cell containing processed antigen into close *juxtaposition* with the immunocompetent lymphocyte, they effect immunization. The lymphocytes are transformed into replicating differentiating forms and ultimately into plasma cells and other cells making antibody, memory cells, or the "sensitized" lymphocytes of cellular hypersensitivity.

During primary immunization, i.e. in hosts not possessing antibody, soluble or particulate antigen is taken up by RE cells lining the cortical and medullary sinuses of lymph nodes and present in large numbers in the marginal zone, about the white pulp, of the spleen (Figs. 2.2,5–7). In these cells it is found within secondary lysosomes and is rapidly catabolized. Particulate antigen, especially in the presence of small amounts of antibody or in animals primed by earlier immunization, is taken up in lymphoid follicles where it is found closely adherent to the surface membranes of large, nonphagocytic reticulum cells (Figs. 2.5–7) which form a "dendritic" reticulum network in each follicle. Here it may remain unaltered for days or weeks. Antigen is never found inside these cells, nor is it ever found inside lymphocytes or end cells such as plasma cells (Figs. 2.5,6). It is not known with certainty in which cell the processing of antigen occurs, nor if it is essential to each type of immune response. Present evidence suggests that a fragment of antigen at the cell surface, possibly attached to a special small RNA molecule, is the effective immunizing agent which triggers the immunocompetent lymphocyte to initiate its differentiation. As in clearance, the uptake and processing of antigen is diminished by blockade, presumably affecting receptor sites on the surface of the phagocytic cell; by competition of antigens, which also may involve competition for receptor sites or may have an entirely different mechanism; by the effect of specific antibody, which (depending on its concentration) may interfere with or promote uptake; and finally by agents such as X ray to which the processing cell is sensitive. It is enhanced by agents which either stimulate formation of increased numbers of RE cells or lead to increased activity of individual cells. Tuberculous infection and endotoxin are the best-known agents of this type. The processing function of the RE cell, however, is distinct from its role in clearance.

Finally, *tolerance* is induced in situations in which *antigen processing does not take place* and antigen can react directly with lymphocytes. This can occur at any age in central lymphoid organs like the thymus, which lack a suitable antigen-trapping apparatus. In the spleen and lymph nodes it occurs readily in the perinatal period, when antigen trapping is imperfectly developed. However, it can occur at any age, if antigen is introduced by an unphysiologic route (i.e. to the nodes by way of the blood stream) or in a form that is not easily phagocytized (monomeric bovine γ-globulin). It requires that *antigen encounter all available peripheral lymphocytes and their precursors*. Therefore, in intact animals it must be widely disseminated and must be able to enter all lymphoid organs across blood–tissue barriers. In adults, this can occur with antigens of the size of common proteins and polysaccharides (Fig. 2.4). In the perinatal period, even particulates and cells can penetrate readily from the blood stream into the thymus and other lymphoid organs. In adults rendered lymphopenic by X ray or other agents, tolerance results from entry limited to central organs such as the thymus, as by direct local antigen injection. The persistence of tolerance in all situations appears related to the persistence of antigen, probably extracellular, in e.g., the thymus. This may be long lasting with noncatabolizable materials such as pneumococcal polysaccharide or living lymphoid cells (in chimeric states) or temporary and dose-related with proteins. The simultaneous induction of tolerance in some lymphoid cells and immunization in others, with the production of partial tolerance, appears to be a common state of affairs, especially with antigens introduced by a systemic route.

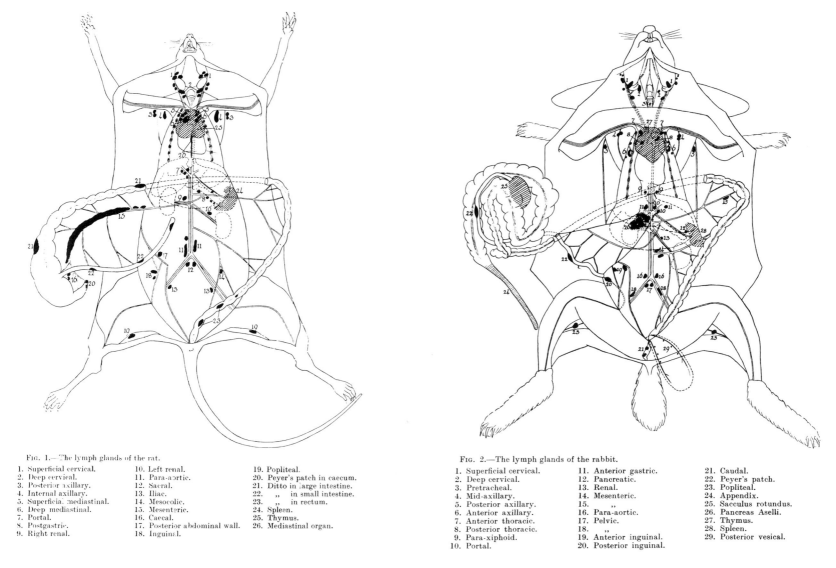

Fig. 1.—The lymph glands of the rat.

1. Superficial cervical.
2. Deep cervical.
3. Posterior axillary.
4. Internal axillary.
5. Superficial mediastinal.
6. Deep mediastinal.
7. Portal.
8. Postgastric.
9. Right renal.
10. Left renal.
11. Para-aortic.
12. Sacral.
13. Iliac.
14. Mesocolic.
15. Mesenteric.
16. Caecal.
17. Posterior abdominal wall.
18. Inguinal.
19. Popliteal.
20. Peyer's patch in caecum.
21. Ditto in large intestine.
22.   ,,   in small intestine.
23.   ,,   in rectum.
24. Spleen.
25. Thymus.
26. Mediastinal organ.

Fig. 2.—The lymph glands of the rabbit.

1. Superficial cervical.
2. Deep cervical.
3. Pretracheal.
4. Mid-axillary.
5. Posterior axillary.
6. Anterior axillary.
7. Anterior thoracic.
8. Posterior thoracic.
9. Para-xiphoid.
10. Portal.
11. Anterior gastric.
12. Pancreatic.
13. Renal.
14. Mesenteric.
15.   ,,
16. Para-aortic.
17. Pelvic.
18.   ,,
19. Anterior inguinal.
20. Posterior inguinal.
21. Caudal.
22. Peyer's patch.
23. Popliteal.
24. Appendix.
25. Sacculus rotundus.
26. Pancreas Aselli.
27. Thymus.
28. Spleen.
29. Posterior vesical.

Fig. 2.1. Distribution of lymphatic organs in the normal rat and rabbit. The distribution of lymph nodes in relation to extremities, the oropharyngeal cavity, and the gastrointestinal tract is noteworthy.
From Sanders and Florey, *Brit. J. Exp. Path. 21*: 275–87 (1940).

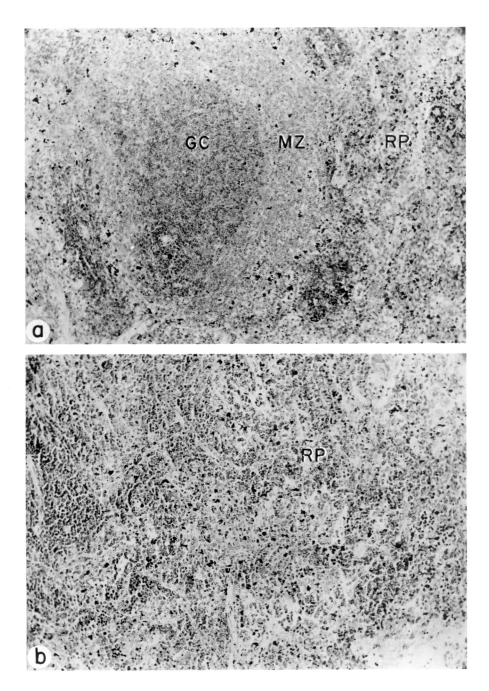

Fig. 2.2 Carbon uptake by reticuloendothelial cells in rat spleen. (a) Malpighian corpuscle and red pulp 33 hours after iv injection of mixed typhoid vaccine and carbon particles. Germinal center (GC) contains many faintly pyroninophilic cells. Carbon is seen largely in phagocytic cells of marginal zone (MZ) and red pulp (RP). Note its absence in germinal center. (b) Red pulp 56 hours after similar injection, showing heavy carbon concentration in close juxtaposition to pyroninophilic blast cells.

Methyl green–pyronine; ×230. From Gunderson et al., *J. Am. Med. Ass. 180*: 1038–47 (1962).

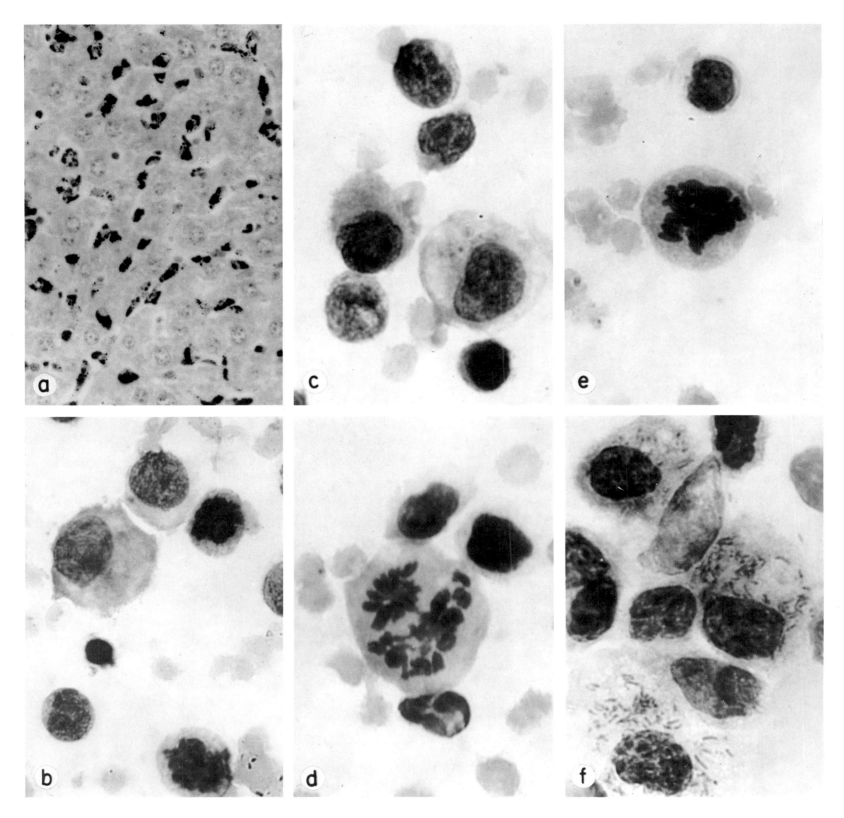

Fig. 2.3. Character of liver macrophages (Kupffer cells) in specific inflammation. (a) Liver of mouse undergoing graft-versus-host reaction, produced by injecting young adult (C57Bl x CBA-T6T6)F1 mice iv with 10⁸ C57Bl spleen cells. At 11 days, carbon-containing macrophages are strikingly increased. (b–e) Macrophages extracted from similarly affected livers of mice, with GVH produced by spleen cells or thoracic duct lymphocytes, by successive use of collagenase and trypsin. Mitosis arrested by dose of Colcemid 2 hours before sacrifice. A variety of morphologic forms is seen, and several dividing cells with nonbasophilic cytoplasm are shown. Lymphocytes are also present in (c) and (e). Karyotype analysis shows that almost all the dividing macrophages are of donor origin and must come from cells with morphology of small lympho-cytes (in thoracic duct lymph). (f) Phagocytic activity of similar cells extracted from liver of *Corynebacterium parvum*-treated radiation chimera. Use of both H³-thymidine labeling and T6 chromosomal marker has indicated that these cells, like those in conventional delayed reactions, come largely from the bone marrow by way of the blood stream.

(a) Hematoxylin-eosin; × 530. (b–f) Leishman's stain; (b, f) × 1,700, (c–e) × 2,100. (a–e) From Howard, Christie, Boak, and Evans-Anfom, in *La Greffe des Cellules Hématopoïétiques Allogéniques*, Centre Nationale de Recherche Scientifique, Paris, 1965, pp. 95–102. (f) From Howard, Boak, and Christie, *Ann. N.Y. Acad. Sci. 129*: 327–39 (1966).

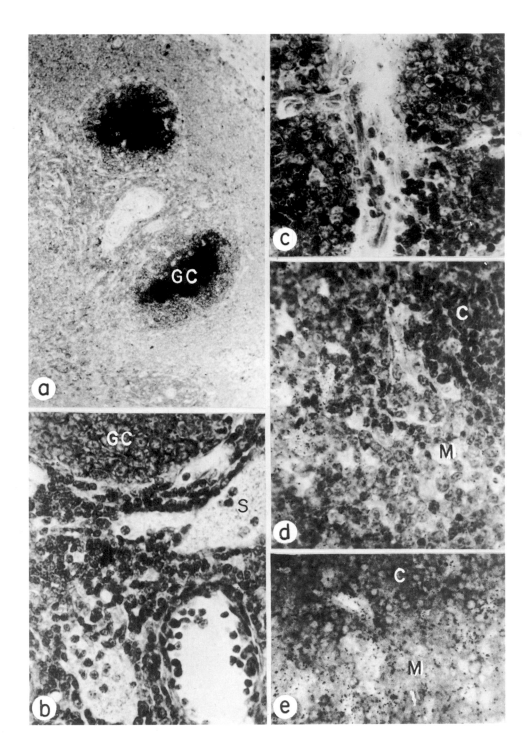

Fig. 2.4. Localization of soluble antigen in relation to production of tolerance in the rat. (a) Uptake of I^{125}-labeled heat-aggregated bovine γ-globulin (BγG), injected iv 24 hours earlier, in Malpighian follicles of adult spleen. This type of uptake characteristically is associated with an immune response (see Fig. 6.5). (b) Soluble, "monomeric" I^{125}-BγG in sinuses (S) and cortical parenchyma of adult lymph node 36 hours after ip injection. Germinal center (GC) is seen at top of figure. (c, d) Extravascular antigen in newborn thymus, 7 days after ip injection of labeled crude BγG. (c) Label near vessel in the cortex. In (d), more label is seen in medulla (below) (M) than in cortex (C). (e) Distribution of labeled BγG similar to that shown in (d), in adult thymus 24 hours after ip injection of crude material. Again much more label is seen in medulla. Extracellular location, in direct contact with lymphoid cells in thymus and lymph nodes, appears to favor induction of tolerance.

Stripping film autoradiographs, counterstained with May-Grünwald–Giemsa, (a) ×80, (b–e) ×300. From Horiuchi, Gery, and Waksman, *Yale J. Biol. Med.* *41*: 13–32 (1968).

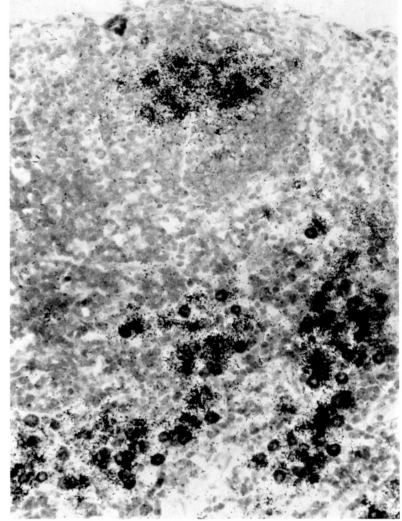

Fig. 2.5. Uptake of particulate antigen in the lymph node. Autoradiograph showing localization of I¹²⁵-labeled flagella (*Salmonella adelaide*) in the rat popliteal node, 7 days after footpad injection. Note the young germinal center (above) showing labeling in its outer aspect and the medullary macrophages heavily labeled in the lower portion of the figure.

×270. Courtesy of Dr. G. J. V. Nossal.

Fig. 2.6. Absence of antigen within antibody-forming cells in the lymph node. A medullary cord of plasma cells 7 days after antigenic stimulation with labeled flagella. Note that the plasma cells themselves (Pl) show only background labeling.

×400. From Nossal, Ada, and Austin, *Austral. J. Exp. Biol. Med. Sci. 42*: 311–30 (1964).

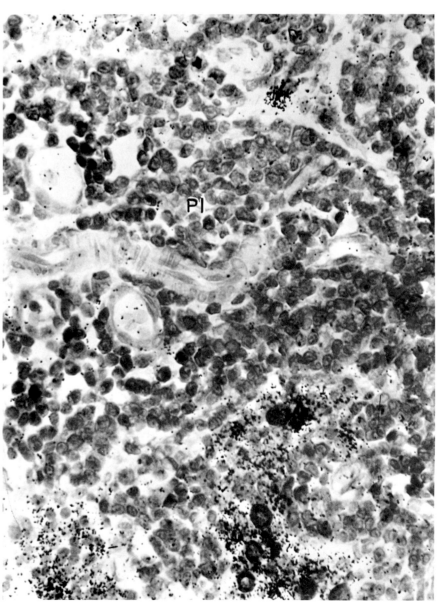

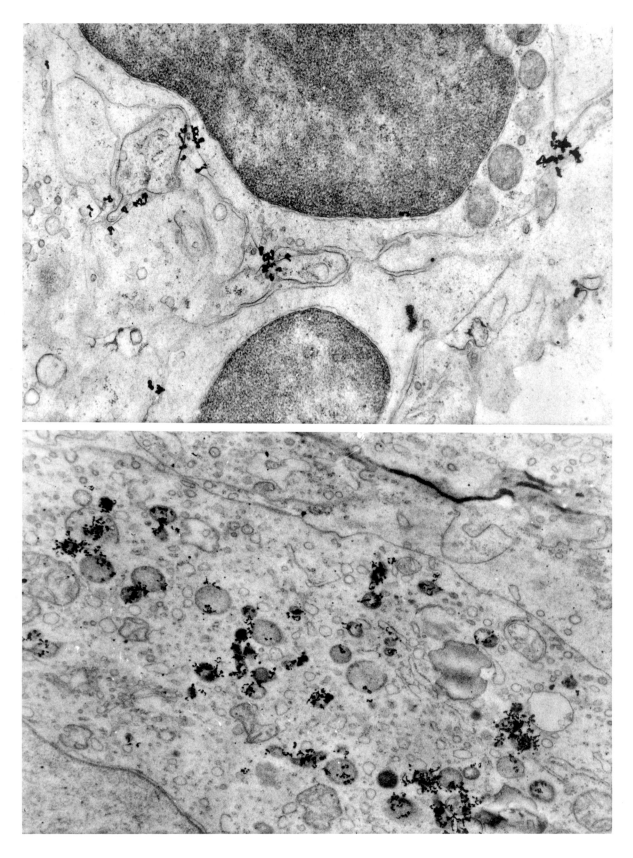

Fig. 2.7. Electron microscopic autoradiographs of cells showing uptake of antigen 24 hours after the injection of I^{125}-labeled flagella. (Above) Portion of a lymphoid follicle. The label is membrane-associated. Examination of serial sections shows that much of this material is on the surface of dendritic processes of reticular cells. (Below) Portion of a medullary macrophage from the same animal. Virtually all the antigen is in lysosomes and other phagocytic vacuoles.

$\times$ 20,000. From Mitchell and Abbot, *Nature 208*: 500–01 (1965).

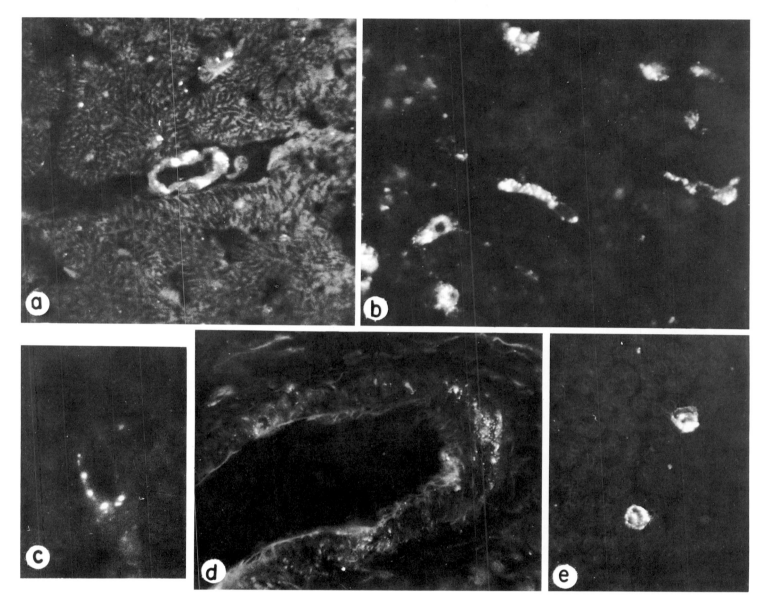

Fig. 2.8. Distribution of *E. coli* endotoxin in dogs after iv injection of a minimum lethal dose (4 mg/kg). Animals sacrificed at 10 minutes (b, e) and 13 hours (a, c, d). (a) Myocardium. Dense deposits of endotoxin are present in the wall of a small vessel, probably a venule; × 500. (b) Liver. Endotoxin particles are in the cytoplasm of the Kupffer cells; × 350. (c) Medulla oblongata. Endotoxin particles in a large capillary typically resemble a constellation; ×1,800. (d) Pulmonary artery. A large patch of endotoxin particles is in the media; ×350. (e) Peripheral blood smear. Two polymorphonuclear leukocytes with their cytoplasm engorged with endotoxin; ×350.

Frozen sections, stained by indirect fluorescence technique with rabbit antibody and fluorescent horse-antirabbit serum. From Rubenstein, *Proc. Soc. Exp. Biol. Med. 111*: 458–67 (1962).

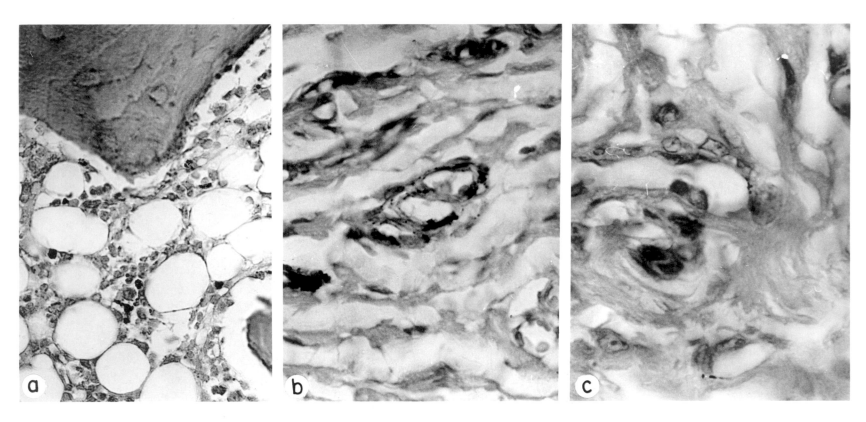

Fig. 2.9. Localization of particulate materials. Deposition of carbon, 24 hours after iv injection into adult rats, in bone marrow (a) and subendothelially in small veins of the ankle joint synovia (b, c). Conventional uptake in marrow is by phagocytic cells of the reticuloendothelial system. Deposition in synovia may depend on anatomic peculiarities of synovial vessels and provide an explanation for frequent occurrence at this site of allergic reactions produced by antigen–antibody complexes or by delayed reactions to foreign particulate antigens disseminated by way of the blood stream.

Hematoxylin-eosin; (a) ×180, (b) ×240, (c) ×480. Courtesy of Dr. M. Mueller.

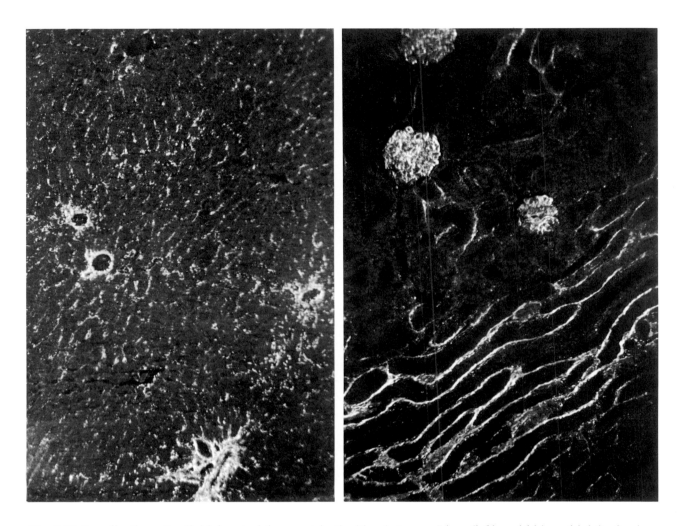

Fig. 2.10. Localization of colloidal material present in the blood stream. Liver (left) and kidney (right) of guinea pig which received 0.15 per cent silver nitrate in drinking water over a period of several months. Uptake of colloidal silver hydroxide in RE (Kupffer) cells of the liver sinusoids and deposition of the colloid in basement membranes of the renal glomeruli and tubules. Similar RE uptake is seen in other organs. Basement membrane deposition is found principally at sites of filtration: in kidney, choroid plexus of the central nervous system, and ciliary body of the eye.

Dark field; ×125. From Waksman, *J. Neuropath. Exp. Neurol. 20*: 35–77 (1961).

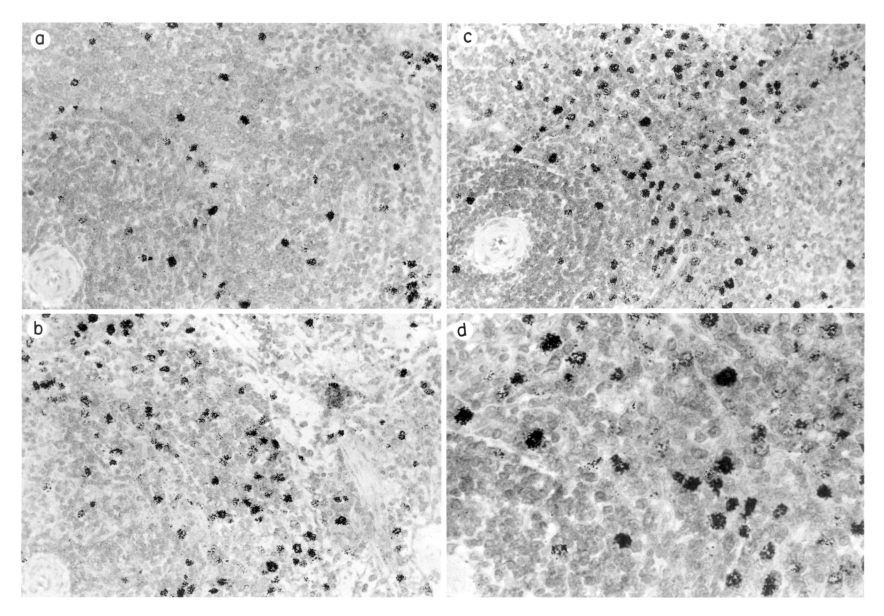

Fig. 2.11. Reticuloendothelial proliferation under the influence of increased work load. In rats given a single iv injection of homologous, heat-injured (49.5°C, 1 hour) erythrocytes, 42 per cent of the injected red cells are sequestered in the spleen by 2 hours, 18 per cent in the liver, and 9 per cent in the bone marrow. The marginal zone of phagocytic cells about the splenic white pulp, the major site of sequestration, shows several cycles of cell division in response to this stimulus, the effect being maximal at 1–2 days, as shown by increase of total DNA and increased rate of incorporation of H³-thymidine into DNA. Low-power views are shown here of the central arteriole (at lower left), white pulp, marginal zone, and adjacent red pulp (at right), before (a) and at 24 hours (b) and 96 hours (c) after the injection; (d) shows the same field as (c) under higher power. All are autoradiographs, prepared 2 hours after a systemic dose of labeled thymidine. Little change is seen in the white pulp, but there is a marked increase in the number of labeled cells in the marginal zone.

(a, b, c) ×160, (d) ×320. From Jandl, Files, Barnett, and MacDonald, *J. Exp. Med. 122*: 299–326 (1965).

Fig. 2.12. Metallophilia of RE cells, which may take up antigen in different situations. (a) Resting reticulum cells (histiocytes) in normal rabbit bone marrow. (b) Activated histiocytes in zone of inflammation, migrating from granulation tissue (right) into periphery of a tuberculous nodule (left). (c) Activated reticulum cells in sinuses of lymph node with chronic inflammation. (d) Metallophil cells (reticulum cells) in Malpighian corpuscle in rat spleen (see Fig. 6.4). Note central zone of ameboid forms within the germinal center.

Silver impregnation; ×450. From Marshall. Courtesy of Dr. R. G. White.

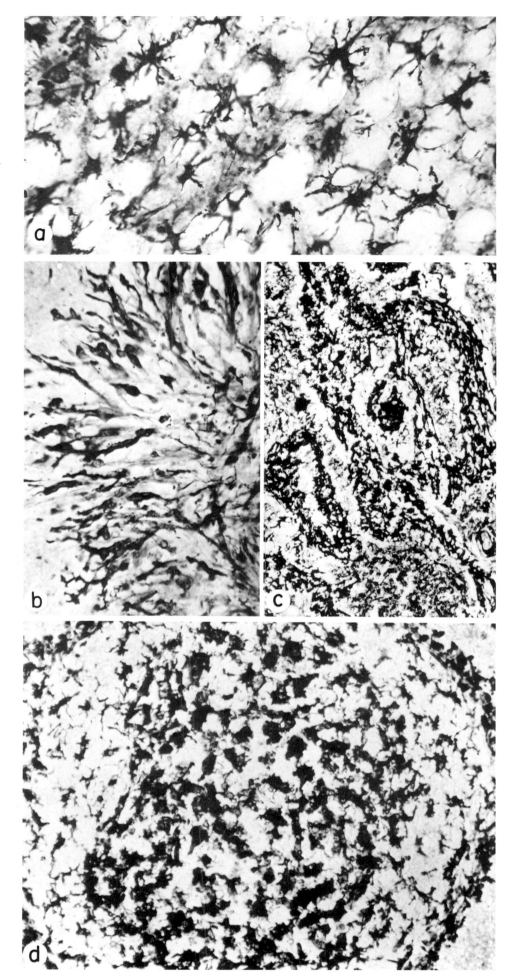

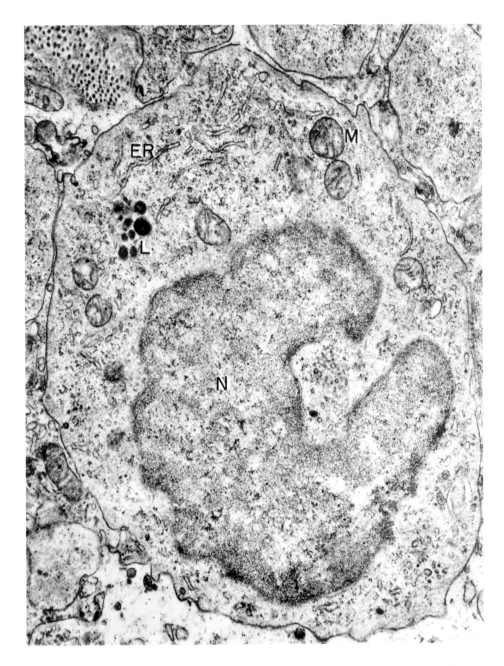

Fig. 2.13. Normal monocyte. Note pleomorphic nucleus (N) lacking a nucleolus but with chromatic condensations along nuclear membrane, mitochondria, (M), conspicuous lysosomes (L), and limited amount of ergastoplasm (ER) and phagocytized debris.

Electron micrograph; ×10,000. From Bessis, in *Electron Microscopic Anatomy,* S. M. Kurtz, ed., Academic Press, New York, 1964.

Fig. 2.14. Pinocytosis in two large reticular cells of chicken embryo spleen photographed in tissue culture. Successive frames of the film show movement of large pinocytotic vesicles (V) from a hyaloplasmic extension of the surface into cytoplasm toward the Golgi area and their rapid resorption.

Interference microscopy (Nomarski's system). Courtesy of Drs. R. Robineaux and J. Pinet, in *CIBA Symposium on Cellular Aspects of Immunity*, G. E. W. Wolstenholme and M. O'Connor, eds., Churchill, London, 1960, pp. 5–40.

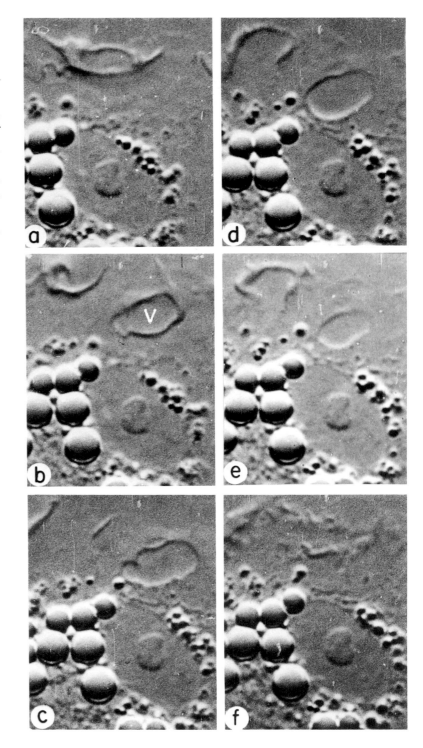

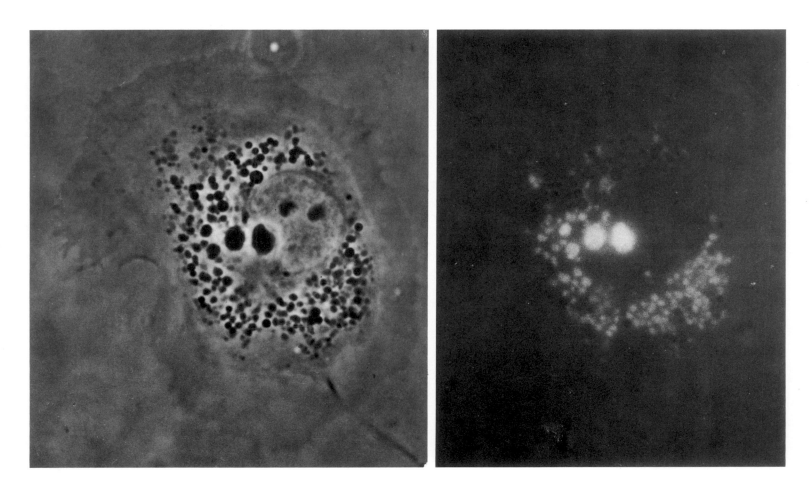

Fig. 2.15. Pinocytosis. Macrophage in culture of chick embryo spleen, to which fluorescein-labeled human α- and β-globulins have been added 48 hours earlier.

(Left) Phase contrast. (Right) Fluorescence microscopy; both ×6,000. Courtesy of Drs. R. Robineaux and J. Pinet, in *CIBA Symposium on Cellular Aspects of Immunity*, G. E. W. Wolstenholme and M. O'Connor, eds., Churchill, London, 1960, pp. 5–40.

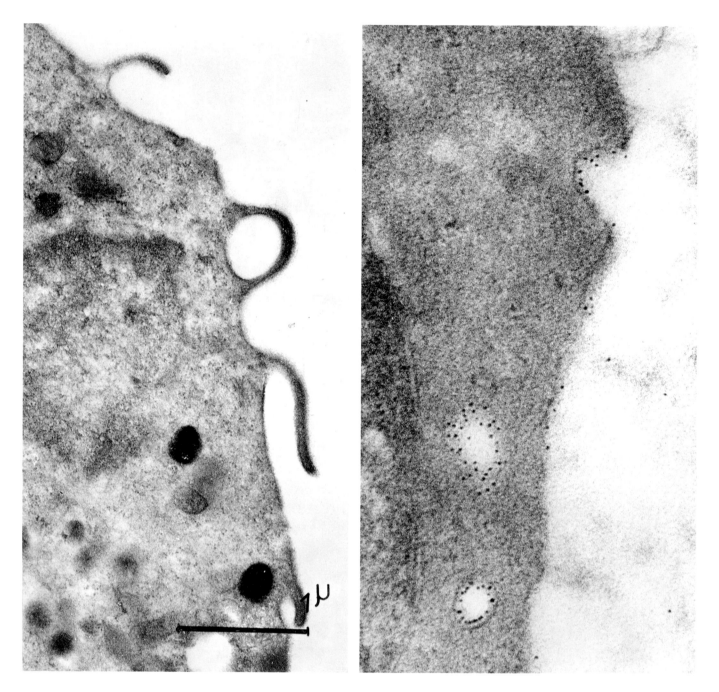

Fig. 2.16. Electron micrographs of spleen cells in culture, showing formation of micropinocytotic vesicles (left) and ingestion of ferritin molecules by "rhopheocytosis" (right).

   × 35,000. From Policard and Bessis *Nature 194*: 110–11 (1962).

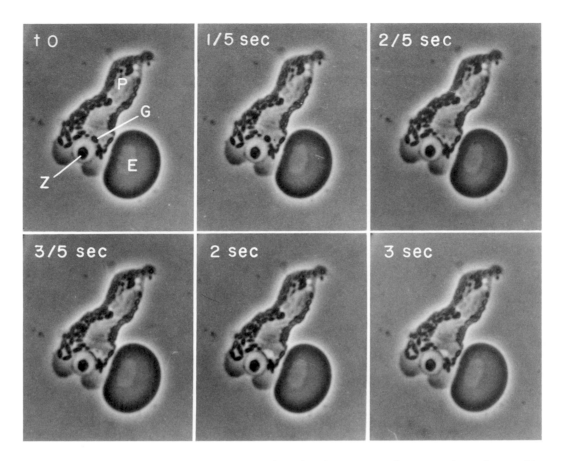

Fig. 2.17. Degranulation with phagocytosis. Timed sequence from motion picture film showing a chicken polymorph (P) ingesting a zymosan body (Z). The granule (G) and its lysis are clearly seen. An erythrocyte (E) lies alongside the poly.

Unpublished photograph, courtesy of Dr. J. Hirsch.

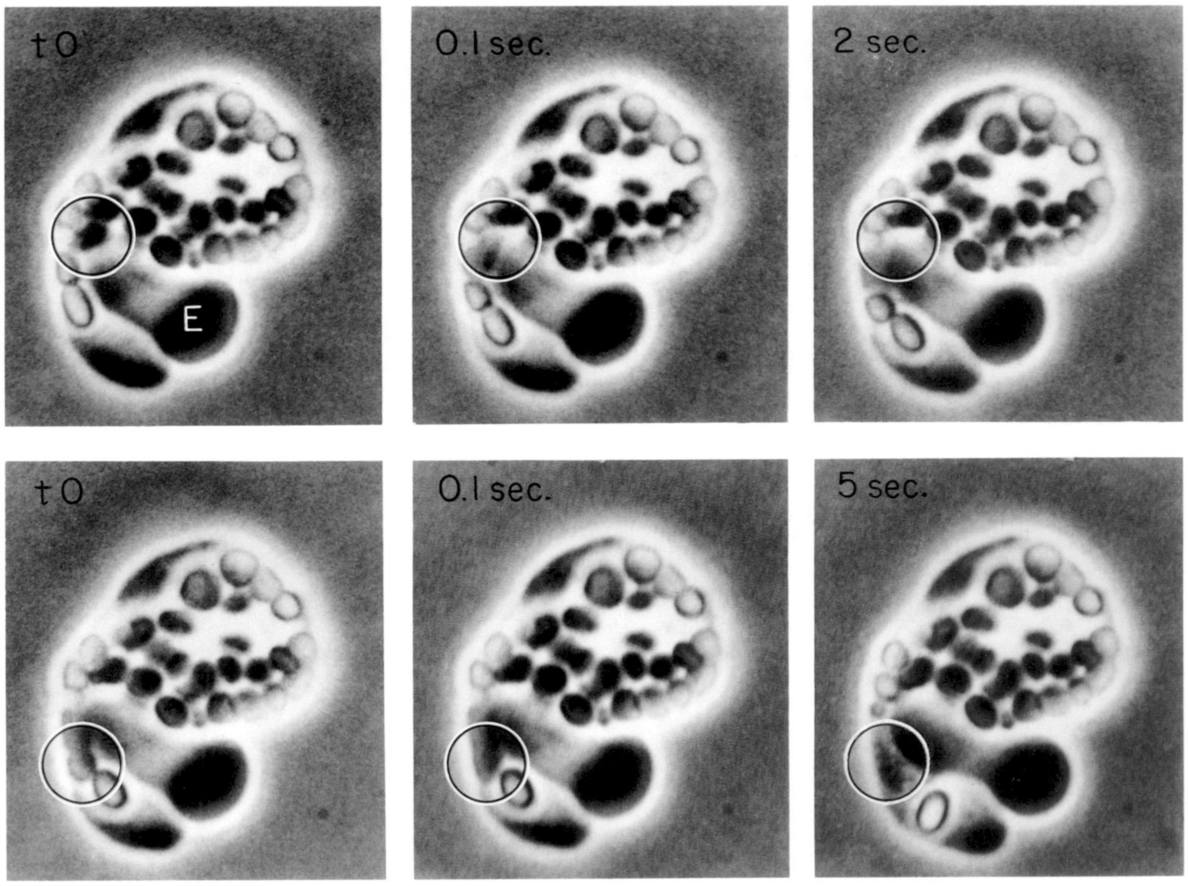

Fig. 2.18. Degranulation with phagocytosis. Two sequences showing a single horse eosinophil immediately after ingestion of a human erythrocyte. Successive lysis of two granules showing their fusion with the phagocytic vacuole and its contents.

From Archer and Hirsch, *J. Exp. Med. 118*: 287–94 (1963).

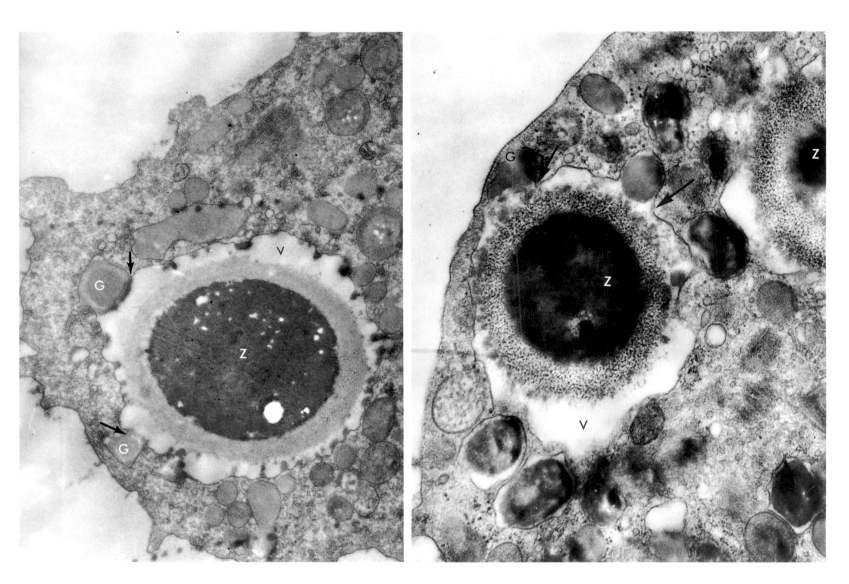

Fig. 2.19. Discharge of lysosomes following phagocytosis. Rabbit polymorphonuclear leukocytes incubated with zymosan in Hanks' solution for
1½ minutes. In both photographs several granules are shown discharging their
contents (hydrolytic enzymes) into phagocytic vacuoles containing zymosan
particles.

From Zucker-Franklin, and Hirsch., *J. Exp. Med. 120*: 569–76 (1964).

3. Central Lymphoid Organs

Immunocompetent cells are formed in such "central" lymphoid organs as the *thymus*, the avian *bursa of Fabricius*, and possibly the mammalian *appendix* (Figs. 2.1; 3.1). These organs lack an afferent pathway and antigen-trapping mechanism that might permit immunization, and the cells which they contain are not capable of an immune response. However, hematogenous antigen may penetrate their parenchyma and play a role in the induction of tolerance (Section 2), and they possess a pathway for the entry of stem cells and departure of cells which have completed or are about to complete their maturation to immunocompetence. Of these organs, the thymus has been studied in the greatest detail.

Both in embryonic and adult life, cells that mature in the thymus are derived from the bone marrow. *Bone marrow lymphocytes* (Figs. 3.2,3) have a distinctive morphology and make up an independent, rapidly replicating cell population. These are probably *stem cells*, which can act as precursors of the erythrocytic, myelocytic, thrombocytic, or monocytic cell lines, as well as of immunocompetent lymphoid cells, but this has not been firmly established. They appear to leave the marrow by way of fenestrated sinusoids (Fig. 3.4), and *travel to the thymus* by the hematogenous route (Fig. 3.9). In early development and in adults depleted of thymocytes and lymphocytes by irradiation or treatment with corticosteroids (Fig. 5.13), population of the thymus by marrow-derived cells can readily be demonstrated. With such techniques as the use of chromosomal markers (Fig. 4.7), labeling with tritiated thymidine, genetic experiments, and immunofluorescent identification of cells with defined histocompatibility antigens (Fig. 3.13), it can be shown that *these cells are* subsequently *seeded into the peripheral pool* of immunocompetent small lymphocytes, which recirculates between the blood and the peripheral lymphoid organs. Their departure from the thymus takes place by active immigration into the large thymus blood vessels (Figs. 3.9,10) and in particular into lymph vessels that accompany them (Figs. 3.10,12).

During their sojourn in the thymus, the cells coming from the marrow apparently acquire immunologic specificity; i.e. they undergo a change that endows them with the genetic information for production of a single, specified immunoglobulin, as shown by the fact that they become amenable to the induction of specific immunologic tolerance by antigen which enters the thymus. They do not acquire immunologic competence, however, since they fail to give significant immune responses, either when stimulated *in situ*, when used in attempts to restore thymectomized animals to immunologic competence, or when used in an attempt to produce graft-vs.-host lesions in suitable recipients. The plasma cells and occasional germinal centers formed in the thymus after local injection of antigen (Figs. 3.5,6) appear to be derived from small numbers of immunocompetent cells present in the vascular sheaths and the interlobular connective tissue septa rather than from the thymocytes themselves.

The development of specificity in lymphocytes maturing within the thymus has been referred to as the *generation of diversity*. It is accompanied by a progressive decrease in the size of these cells (Figs. 3.11,12,15) and repeated cell division (Fig. 3.14). It is also manifested by striking changes in their surface properties, notably a reduction in the concentration of histocompatibility antigens (Fig. 3.13) and the appearance of characteristic new antigens such as the TL and θ-antigens of the mouse thymus. The TL antigen is not present in peripheral lymphocytes which are the progeny of thymus cells. The maturation of thymus lymphocytes occurs under the inductive influence of mesenchymal cells and may require the action of a hormone produced within the thymus. Several cell types have been suggested as possible sources of such a hormone, but an active substance has yet to be clearly identified as promoting lymphopoiesis (within or without the thymus) and/or the genetic change in question. The inductive process can be studied in organ culture (Figs. 3.16,17).

The experimental production of tolerance within the thymus suggests the possibility that this is the site at which *tolerance to host antigens* normally *is induced*, with the consequent ability to distinguish self from nonself. The barrier to penetration of host antigen into the thymus (Fig. 3.15), as noted earlier, is relatively slight early in ontogeny. A very high proportion of cells maturing in the thymus die there. The generation of diversity depends on a genetic mechanism, analogous to mutation, which may result in many "lethal mutant" cells. Alternatively, the induction of tolerance to host antigens with consequent killing of many thymocyte clones may be responsible for the high level of cell death seen in the thymus. In spite of the resulting slow output of surviving cells, more than half the small lymphocytes in the peripheral pool are of thymic origin.

Thymic neoplasia, whether induced by virus infection or chemical or physical carcinogenesis, gives rise to a characteristic lymphoma or chronic lymphocytic leukemia. In general, the neoplastic cells are not immuno-competent. However, in the NZB/Bl mouse, a viral neoplasm of the thymus (Fig. 3.7) is accompanied by leukemia in which the neoplastic cells show an apparent inability to develop specific immunologic tolerance while retaining immunologic competence. These animals show a corresponding failure of self-recognition (failure to develop tolerance to autoantigens) and form multiple autoantibodies with the development of acquired hemolytic anemia, wire-loop lesions of the glomeruli, etc., a picture much like that seen in systemic lupus erythematosus in man. It is possible that generation of diversity continues in the neoplastic lymphocytes as they enter the peripheral circulation, permitting them to be immunized before they have had an opportunity to be rendered tolerant. Neoplastic changes of the thymus such as "germinal centers" (Fig. 13.8) and thymoma are frequently found in myasthenia gravis and in systemic lupus as well.

Hypoplasia or aplasia of the thymus results in varying degrees of immunological deficit (Section 8). There are several well-recognized syndromes in man. The best characterized are *ataxia telangiectasia*, in which there is a striking deficiency of both γA-immunoglobulin antibody formation and development of the cellular type of hypersensitivity, and *thymic alymphoplasia* (Swiss-type agammaglobulinemia), in which there is a marked deficiency in all immune responses, usually with early death. Surgical *thymectomy* of the newborn animal or adult thymectomy accompanied by treatment with an agent that destroys peripheral lymphocytes (X ray, corticosteroids, antilymphocyte serum) is followed by persistent lymphopenia and an immunologic deficit comparable to that seen in human subjects lacking a thymus: complete failure of γA-immunoglobulin synthesis and cellular sensitization (e.g. tuberculin sensitization, experimental autoallergic disease, homograft rejection), together with a partial deficiency in γG synthesis and slight reduction in γM formation. Thymectomized animals show striking deficits in their resistance to infection and in their ability to reject various types of tumors. They are permanently restored to normal function by grafts of thymus and temporarily restored by infusions of sufficient numbers of competent peripheral lymphocytes.

In birds it is quite clear that there are two central lymphoid organs in which lymphocytes competent for different classes of immune response mature. The thymus controls only reactions of cellular hypersensitivity, whereas the bursa of Fabricius controls all types of immunoglobulin synthesis. Bursal lymphocytes are somewhat larger than thymus-derived lymphocytes, and each recirculates through a different anatomic element of the lymph nodes and spleen (Section 4). The bursa develops in a manner much like the thymus (Fig. 7.7), and there is some evidence that its development may be under thymic control (Fig. 3.18). Many of the experimental findings described for the mammalian thymus can be duplicated in experiments on the bursa. Viral neoplasia of the bursa (fowl leukosis) leads to a type of lymphoma resembling giant follicular lymphoma in man. Bursal agenesis, hormonally induced, and bursectomy at an early age lead to varying degrees of hypogammaglobulin-emia or even agammaglobulinemia.

In mammals there is no exact homologue of the bursa of Fabricius. Recent evidence suggests that the appendix and Peyer's patches (Fig. 5.14) may be the source of a population of cells competent to produce γM-immuno-globulin antibodies. On present evidence, these lymphoid organs possess both central and peripheral functions. Removal, combined with ablation of the peripheral lymphocyte pool, results in selective loss of the individual's ability to make γM. Conversely, administration of antigen directly to these organs results in both local and systemic γM-antibody synthesis.

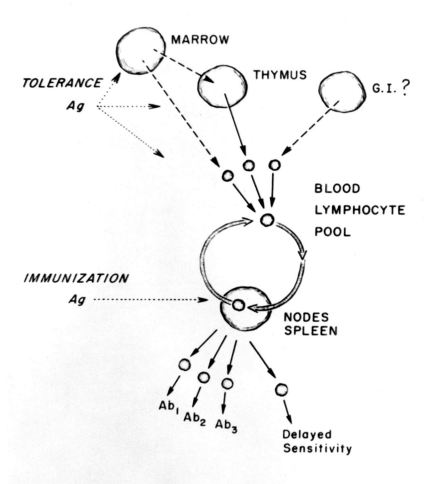

Fig. 3.1. Diagram showing the relation of central and peripheral lymphoid organs in adult mammals such as the rat and the life history of cells participating in immune reactions. Proliferating stem cells in the bone marrow give rise to progeny which undergo, in the thymus and possibly in such other organs as the appendix and Peyer's patches, further proliferation and differentiation to become nondividing, immunocompetent cells of the peripheral pool of small lymphocytes. These recirculate between the blood and the parenchyma of spleen and lymph nodes and, when exposed to antigen which has been processed by suitable phagocytic cells, are triggered to further proliferation and differentiation to become memory cells, "sensitized cells" of delayed hypersensitivity, or end cells, such as plasma cells, forming specific antibody. If directly exposed to unprocessed antigen, these cells can be blocked in some yet undefined way and become unreactive (tolerant) toward that specific antigen.

From Isaković, Smith, and Waksman, *J. Exp. Med. 122*: 1103–23 (1965).

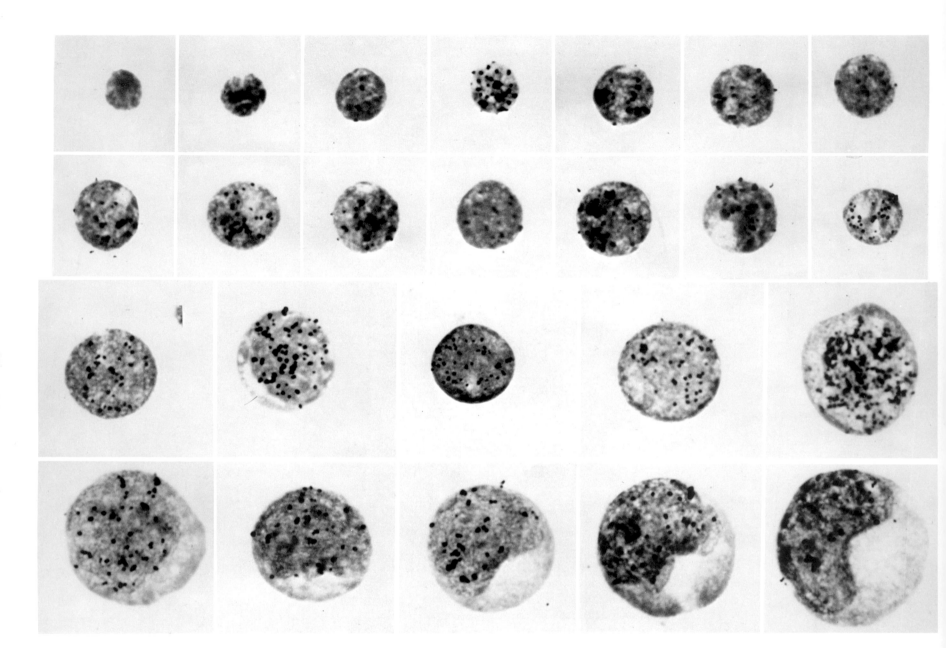

Fig. 3.2. Precursor cells of the bone marrow. Autoradiographs of adult guinea pig bone marrow cells, taken 1 hour after pulse of H³-thymidine (1 μC/g body weight). The first two cells in the upper row are typical pachychromatic small lymphocytes; these do not incorporate labeled thymidine. The remaining cells of the upper two rows are the dividing lymphoid cells, which Yoffey calls "transitional" cells. Blast cells of various sizes, also dividing, are illustrated in the lower two rows. These three cell types are present in a ratio of 10:1:1. Labeling studies show that the majority of marrow lymphocytes are formed *in situ*, the entire marrow small lymphocyte population being renewed in 3 days or less. Quantitative data suggest that the small lymphocytes may be derived from the larger cell types, but are as yet not completely convincing.

Humeral marrow smear, dipped in Kodak NTB-3 emulsion, exposed, developed, and stained with MacNeal's tetrachrome stain; ×2,100. From Yoffey, Hudson, and Osmond (The lymphocyte in guinea pig bone marrow), *J. Anat. 99*: 841–60 (1965). By permission of Cambridge Univ. Press.

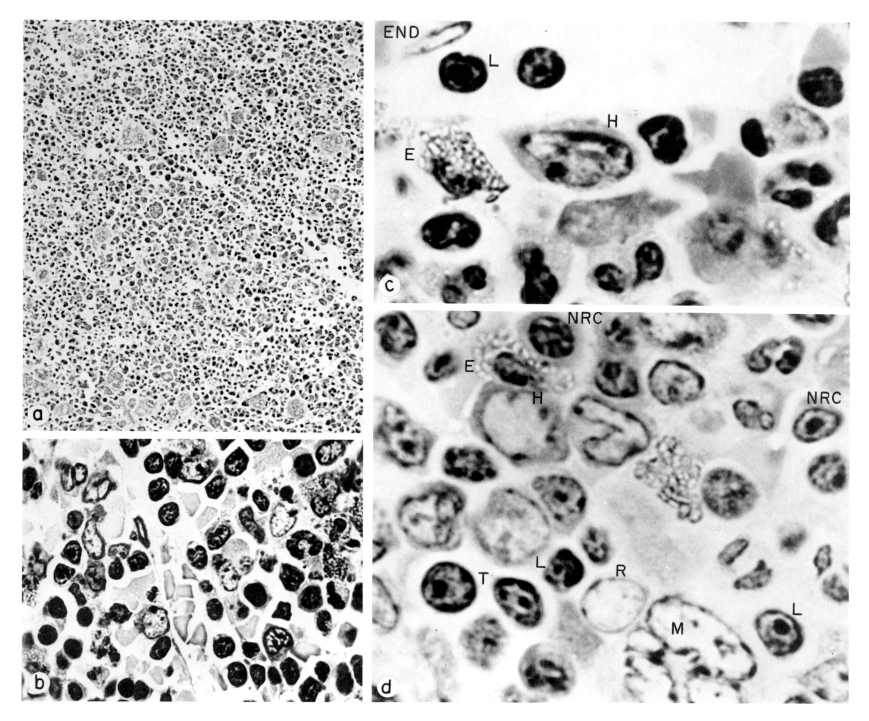

Fig. 3.3. Precursor cells of the bone marrow. Femoral marrow of adult guinea pig. (a) Low-power view, showing absence of lymphoid nodules; ×300. (b) Higher power, showing the phenomenon of "lymphocyte loading"; ×975. Scattered lymphocytes are shown in marrow parenchyma and a number, presumably passing from the marrow into the blood stream, are seen in the sinusoid. The interrupted sinusoidal endothelium is well shown. (c, d) Still higher power, showing cells in parenchyma and in the sinusoids; ×3,000. These include reticulum cells (R), hemocytoblasts (H), transitional cells (T), and small lymphocytes (L); also nucleated red cells (NRC), megakaryocytes (M), eosinophil myelocytes (E), and endothelium (END).

Zenker-formol fixation; 2μ sections stained with Dominici's eosin–orange G–toluidine blue. (a, c, d) From Yoffey, Hudson, and Osmond (The lymphocyte in guinea pig bone marrow), *J. Anat. 99*: 841–60 (1965). By permission of Cambridge Univ. Press. (b) From Yoffey, *Bibl. Anat. 7*: 298–303 (1965).

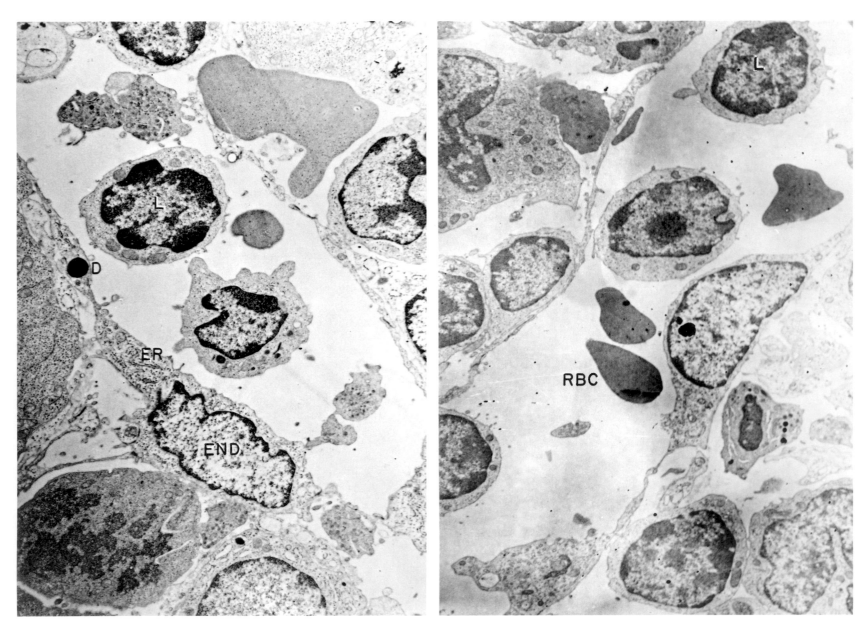

Fig. 3.4. Precursor cells of the bone marrow. Electron micrographs of femoral marrow in the adult guinea pig. (Left) Marrow sinusoid, containing two cells, one of which (L) shows the features of a lymphocyte; ×6,000. Endothelial cell (END) contains a few profiles of endoplasmic reticulum (ER), some free ribosomes, and a dense inclusion (D). (Right) "Lymphocyte loading." The marrow sinusoid contains typical lymphocytes (L) and red cells (RBC) in approximately equal numbers; ×4,400.

Araldite embedding. From Hudson and Yoffey, *Proc. Roy. Soc. B. 165*: 486–96 (1966).

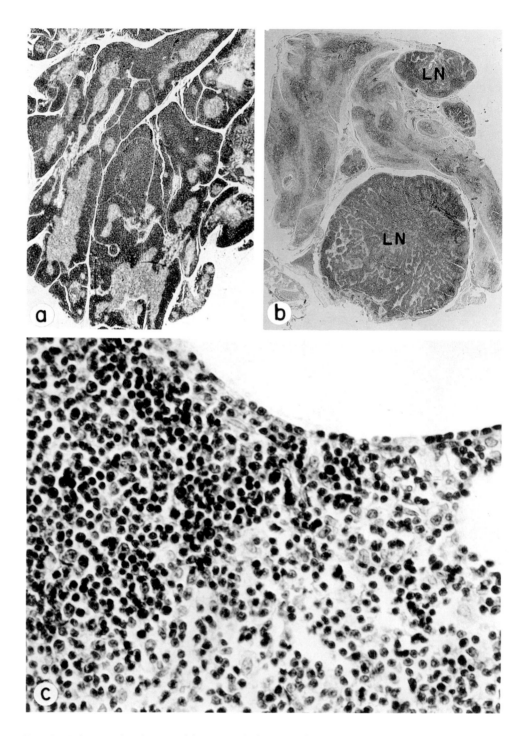

Fig. 3.5 Thymus in the rat. (a) Normal thymus: lobular structure and separation of each lobule into cortex and medulla are clearly seen. (b) Thymus depleted by stress: lobules are collapsed, and cortex is pale and empty of lymphocytes. Two lymph nodes (LN) embedded in thymus show normal germinal centers and medulla but minimal cortex. (c) Normal structure of cortex (left) and medulla immediately adjacent to droplets of injected adjuvant mixture, seen here as empty vacuoles (above and right). Dense population of cortex with lymphocytes of different sizes is well shown.

All hematoxylin-eosin; (a, b) ×10, (c) ×400. From Blau and Waksman, *Immunology* 7: 332–41 (1964), and unpublished.

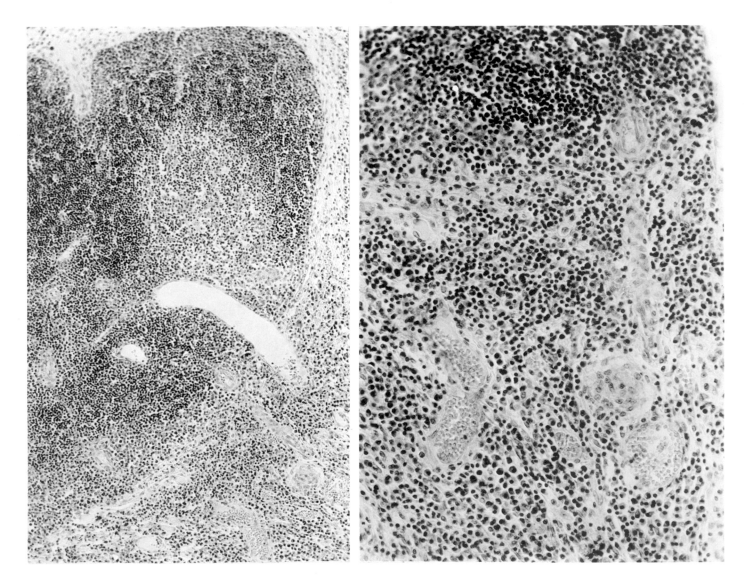

Fig. 3.6. Rat thymus injected with BSA in complete Freund's adjuvant. (Left) Formation of massive plasma cell infiltrates about vessels at surface of lobule (to right) and invasion of lobule by the infiltrate; ×120. (Right) Higher power of same field showing character of cells in the infiltrate and disappearance of surface membrane of thymus lobule in zone of invasion; ×240

Hematoxylin-eosin. From Blau and Waksman, *Immunology* 7: 332–41 (1964).

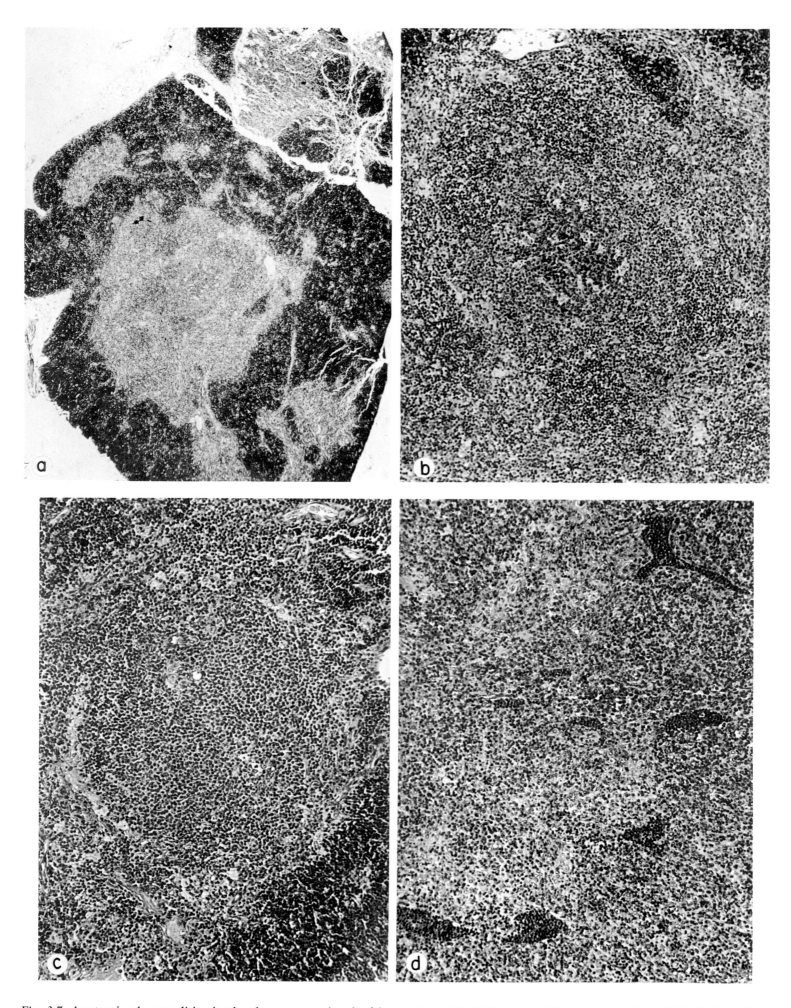

Fig. 3.7. Anatomic abnormalities in the thymus associated with "autoimmunization" in NZB mice. This process is associated in an as yet unknown manner with a characteristic viral infection, and is thought to provide a model for changes observed in the human disease, systemic lupus erythematosus. (a, b) Proliferative centers in the medulla under low and higher magnifications; ×54, ×169. (c) Lymphoid focus in medulla; ×215. (d) Medullary lymphatic vessels choked with lymphocytes, resembling the efferent lymphatic sinuses of lymph nodes during an active immune response; ×215.

Hematoxylin-eosin. Courtesy of Drs. B. J. Helyer and J. B. Howie.

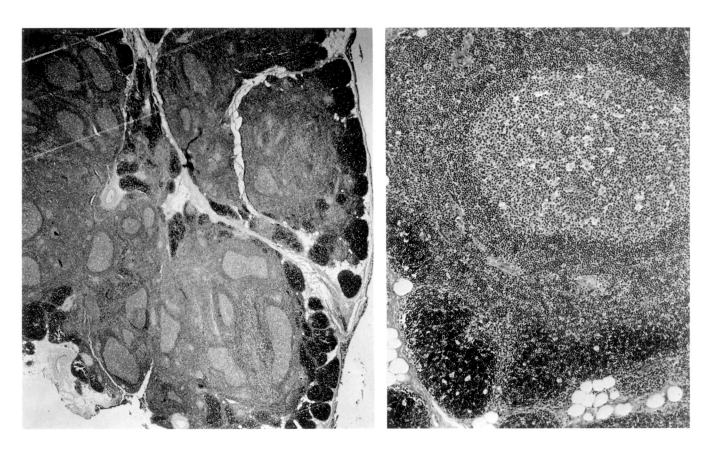

Fig. 3.8. Thymic abnormality in myasthenia gravis. Human thymus, showing hyperplasia with formation of "germinal centers" in medulla.

Hematoxylin-eosin; magnifications not given. Courtesy of Dr. B. Castleman.

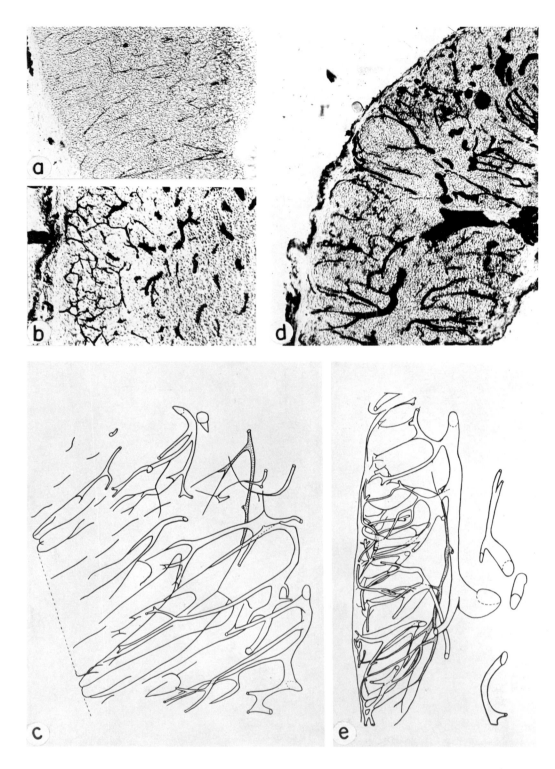

Fig. 3.9. Vasculature of mouse thymus. (a) Normal 20–30-day mouse. Cortex shows fine parallel capillaries. (b) Same, 18 hours after 410 r whole-body irradiation. Thymus involution with collapse and thickening of cortical vessels and distention of those in medulla. (c) Reconstruction of cortical vessels in normal 31-day thymus from eleven sections. Arteries and arterial capillaries stippled; veins clear. (d) Normal 80–100-day mouse. Cortical capillaries and medullary vessels are larger and more crowded than in thymus of younger animal. (e) Reconstruction of cortical vessels in 77-day thymus from study of eleven sections.

(a, b, d) India ink injection; 30 μ frozen sections; ×100. (c, e) Original drawings; ×100. (a, b, d) From E. Holst: Honor paper, Mt. Holyoke College, 1952. (c, e) From Figs. 11 and 17, pp. 213, 217, in C. Smith, E. C. Thatcher, D. Z. Kraemer, and E. S. Holt (Studies on the thymus of the mammal. VI. The vascular pattern of the thymus of the mouse and its changes during aging), *J. Morph. 91*: 199–220 (1952).

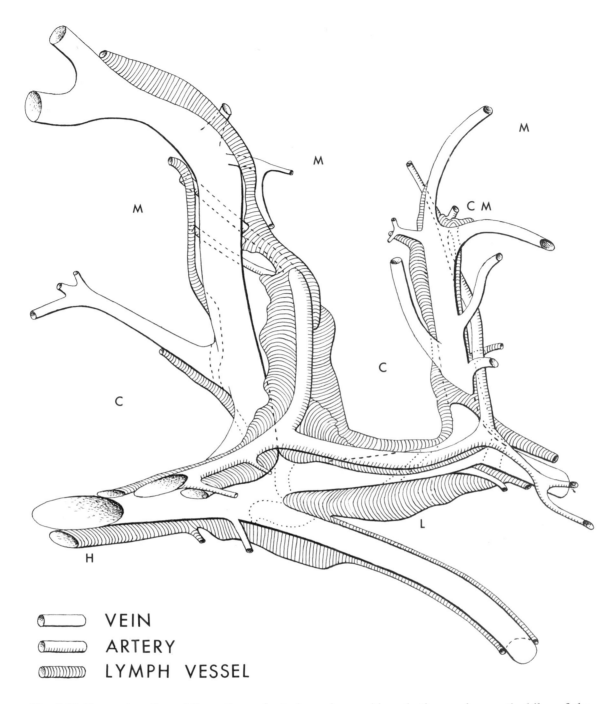

VEIN

ARTERY

LYMPH VESSEL

Fig. 3.10. Reconstruction of the pattern of arteries, veins, and lymphatic vessels near the hilus of the thymus in a 96-day-old mouse. The blood vessels were injected with India ink, the lymph vessels were packed with lymphocytes. C, cortex; CM, corticomedullary line; H, region of the hilus; L, lymph vessel external to vein at base of septum.

Original drawing; ×100. From Fig. 1, C. Smith, *Anat. Rec. 122*: 173–80 (1955).

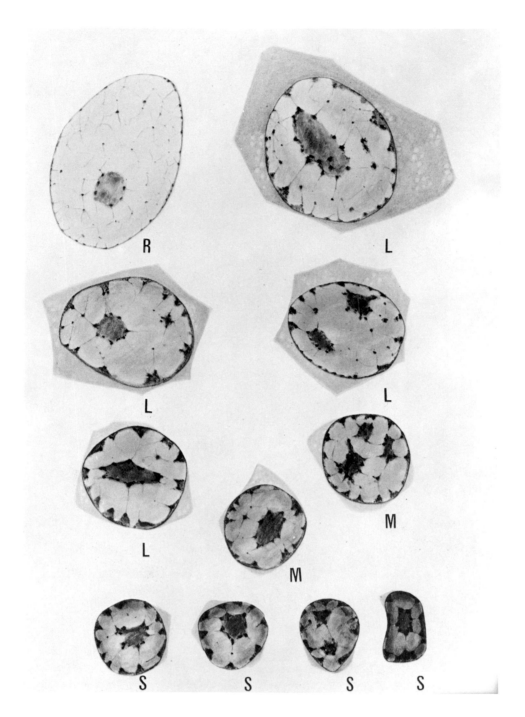

Fig. 3.11. Drawings of cell types in the cortex of normal rat thymus after sections of tissue fixed in Bouin-Hollande and stained with Dominici. Only the nucleus of the reticular cell (R) is represented, since its cytoplasm is hardly visible in tissue sections. The letters L, M, and S refer to large, medium, and small lymphocytes. Several specific points are illustrated: (a) the nuclei vary markedly in size, from that of the reticular cell to that of the smallest lymphocyte; (b) in the lymphocytes, the amount of cytoplasm and of nuclear sap is proportional to nuclear size; (c) the staining intensity of the nuclear sap, the nucleoli, and the chromatin masses is inversely proportional to nuclear size.

From Sainte-Marie, *Proceedings, Third Canadian Cancer Conference*, Academic Press, New York, 1959.

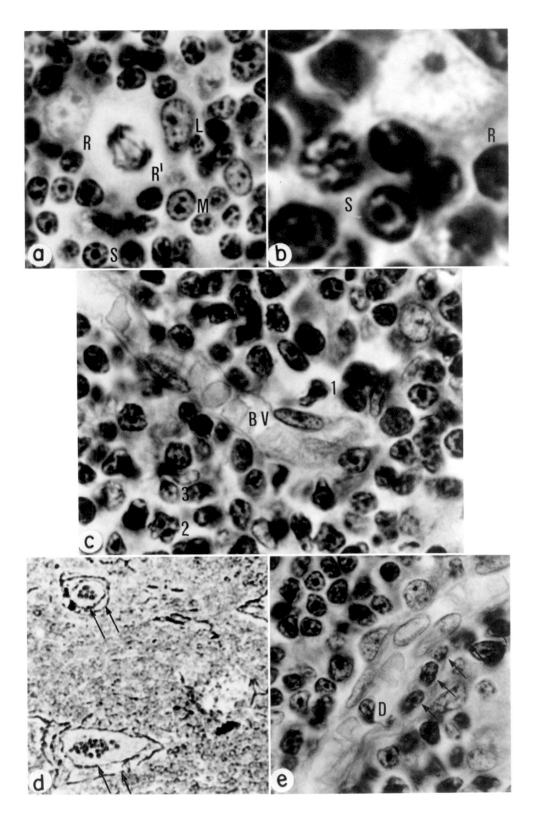

Fig. 3.12. Cell types, their proliferation, and movement in the normal rat thymus. (a, b) Photographs of cortex, showing reticulum cells (R, R′) and large, medium, and small lymphocytes (L, M, S). A reticulum cell (R′) is shown in the anaphase stage of mitosis and a small lymphocyte (S, in b) in prophase. Note that the cell size does not change during mitosis and that almost all the nuclei are round or oval; ×1,750, ×4,000. (c–e) Photographs of the medulla, showing blood vessels (BV) and "perivascular lymphatic channels"; ×1,750, ×230, ×1,450. The nuclei of small lymphocytes in (c) show a much greater degree of deformation that those of cortical lymphocytes (note particularly cells numbered 1, 2, and 3). This finding suggests a high degree of motility in this thymic area. "Perivascular lymphatic channels" are outlined by reticulum and surround the blood vessels partially or completely (d). Flattened small lymphocytes moving in this channel are indicated by arrows (e), and one is shown during diapedesis, D, in the blood vessel.

All except (d) Bouin-Hollande fixation, paraffin sections, Dominici stain; (d) silver impregnation for reticulum. From Sainte Marie, *Proc. Soc. Exp. Biol. Med.* **98**: 909–15 (1958).

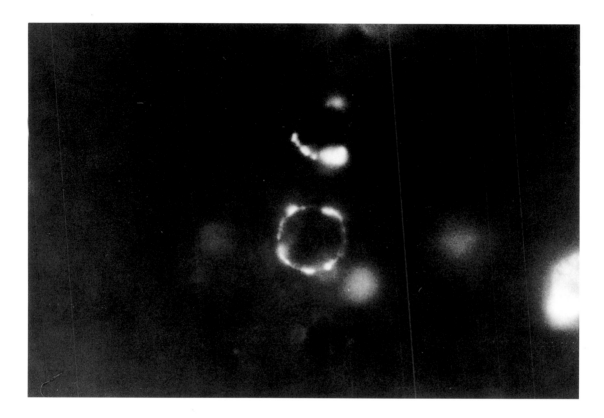

Fig. 3.13. Technique used to demonstrate metamorphosis in surface properties of thymic lymphocytes. Suspension of living normal rat (BN strain) thymus cells, stained with iso-antiserum (Lewis) against strong histocompatibility antigen of BN rats and fluorescein-labeled rabbit antibody against rat γ-globulin. Location of antigen in cell membrane of two medium-large lymphocytes is clearly shown by chains of fluorescent spots. Unstained smaller cells are seen dimly in background. Cells of the type shown here retain the ability to return to the bone marrow but do not act as stem cells. In small thymocytes the histocompatibility antigen in the cell membrane is largely or entirely replaced by a thymus-specific antigen, and these cells have lost their ability to colonize the marrow.

   × 2,000 Courtesy of Dr. S. Order.

Fig. 3.14. Pattern proposed for the mode of lymphocyte formation in the cortex of rat thymus. R refers to reticular cells, L, M, S to large, medium, and small lymphocytes. Each generation of a given type of lymphocyte is indicated by the corresponding letter. Each letter is followed by a small numeral referring the generation under consideration and is preceded by the number of cells involved. The small circles symbolize mitoses. The dimension is so divided that each generation time is proportionally represented. This diagram indicates that, on the average, with the occurrence of each reticular cell mitosis another reticular cell and a large lymphocyte of first generation (L1) are formed. Before the new reticular cell in turn enters mitosis, the large lymphocyte passes through four generations. Large lymphocytes of the fourth generation (L4 cells) transform by mitosis into medium lymphocytes of which there are two generations. The medium lymphocytes of second generation (M2) cells give rise to small lymphocytes which divide to yield 128 end product small lymphocytes of second generation (S2 cells). These do not divide, but after a certain time leave the cortex (arrow) by migrating into the medulla. This cycle is repeated indefinitely. Note that this scheme takes no account of migration of cells into the thymus from the blood stream.

From Sainte-Marie and Leblond, *Proc. Soc. Exp. Biol. Med. 97*: 263–70 (1958).

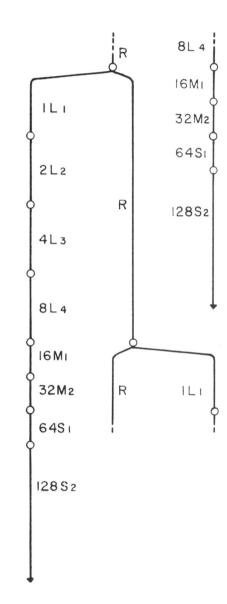

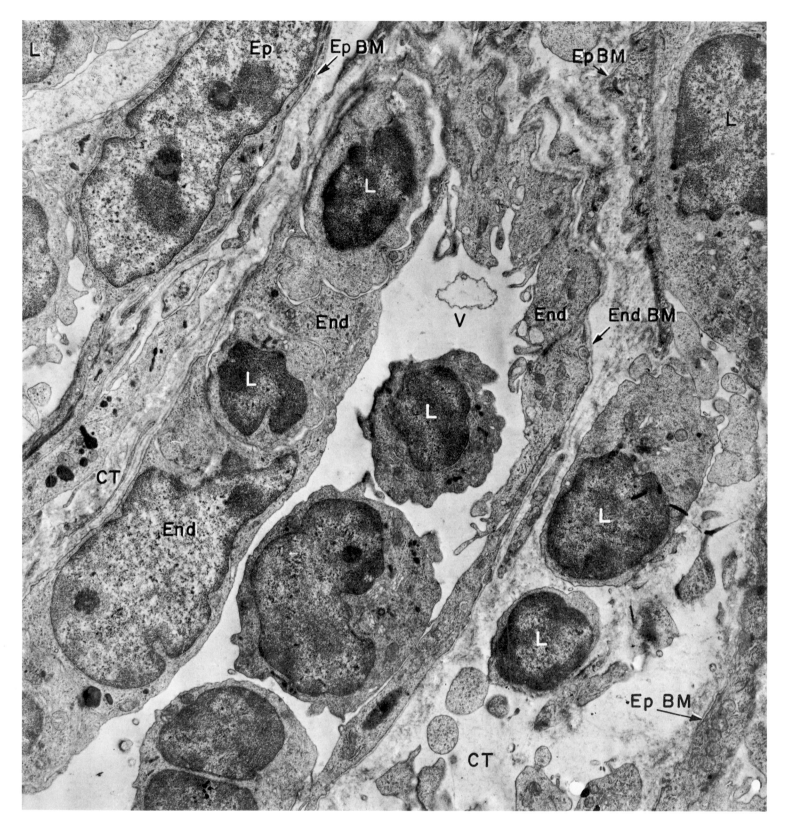

Fig. 3.15. Venule and "perivascular lymphatic channel" in cortex of normal mouse thymus; V, lumen of venule; End, venular endothelium; Ep, thymic epithelial cells; L, lymphocytes; End BM and Ep BM, endothelial and epithelial basement membranes delimiting lymphatic channel; CT, perivascular connective tissue. Lymphocytes are present in the thymic parenchyma (upper left), the perivascular lymphatic channel, and within the lumen of the venule. Two are seen apparently passing through the endothelium.

Electron micrograph; ×7,000. From Fig. 22, S. L. Clark, Jr., *Am. J. Anat. 112*: 1–33 (1963).

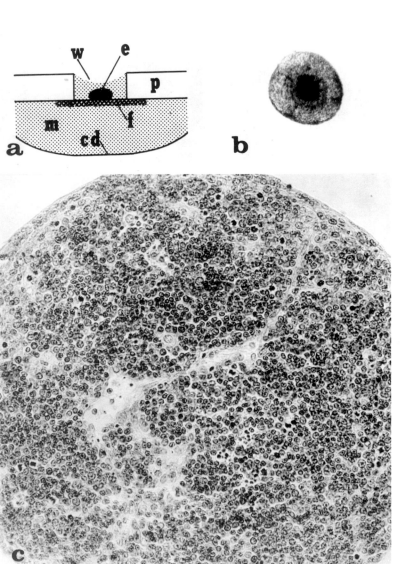

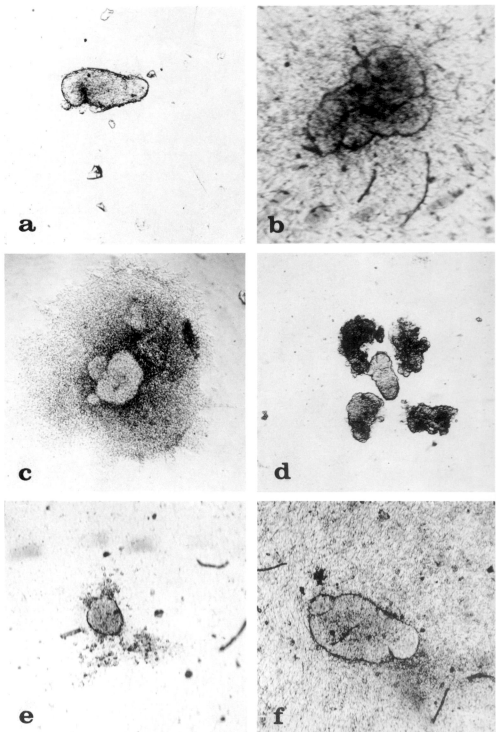

Fig. 3.16. Thymus morphogenesis in tissue culture. (a) Filter well culture assembly: w, well; e, explant; p, plastic mount; f, millipore TH filter; m, medium; cd, culture dish. (b) Culture of 12-day mouse thymus after 1 week in filter well. (c) Histological detail of (b). Note lymphoid organization of explant.

From Auerbach, in *The Thymus in Immunobiology*, R. A. Good and A. E. Gabrielson, eds., Harper and Row, New York, 1964, pp. 95–113.

Fig. 3.17. Morphogenesis of 12-day-mouse thymus epithelium in presence or absence of mesenchyme. (a) Twelve-day thymus at time of explantation. (b) Same after 4 days in culture, growing at glass-clot interface. (c) Culture of thymus epithelium with lung mesenchyme, 4 days. (d) Thymus epithelium surrounded by four pieces of mesenchyme, immediately after explantation. (e) Culture of thymus epithelium without mesenchyme, 4 days. (f) Culture of thymus epithelium with salivary gland mesenchyme, 4 days. Inductive stimulus of mesenchyme leads to normal development of epithelium which in turn determines normal differentiation of lymphocytic stem cells coming from bone marrow.

From Auerbach, in *The Thymus in Immunobiology*, R. A. Good and A. E. Gabrielson, eds., Harper and Row, New York, 1964, pp. 95–113.

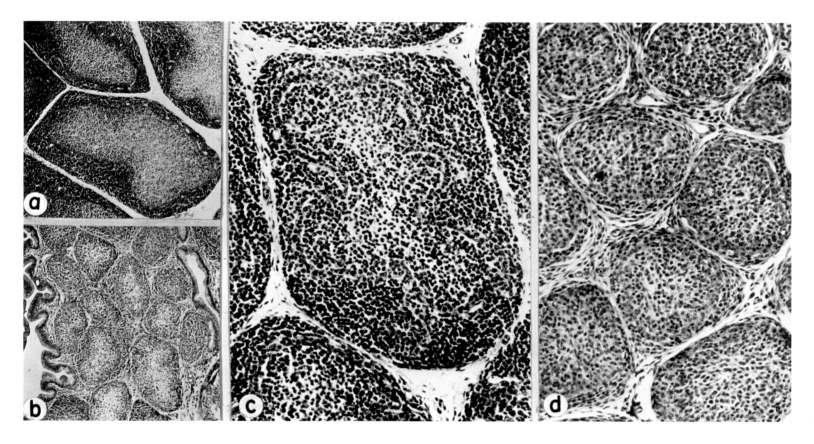

Fig. 3.18. Effect of neonatal thymectomy on function of bursa of Fabricius in Rhode Island Red chickens, 8–9 weeks old. (a, c) Normal. (b, d) Thymectomized immediately after hatching. Note small size of bursal follicles and absence of lymphocytes in thymecto-mized bird.

Hematoxylin-eosin; (a, b) ×30, (c, d) ×120. From Janković and Isaković, *Int. Arch. Allergy 24*: 278–95 (1964).

4. Lymphocytes and Their Recirculation

Several distinct cell types, present in the central and peripheral lymphoid organs and traveling in the blood and lymph, have the morphology of small lymphocytes and are difficult to distinguish by light microscopy (Fig. 4.1). They differ nonetheless both in ultrastructure and in their functional attributes. They include the following types.

Stem cells, continuously formed in the bone marrow (Figs. 3.2–4), pass by way of the blood stream to the thymus, where they act as precursors of thymocytes. They may also enter other central lymphoid organs, such as the bursa of Fabricius and the appendix. They are thought to be the same as hematopoietic stem cells which give rise within the marrow to erythrocytic, myelocytic, and other blood cell lines and which, on infusion into irradiated animals, produce individual colonies of the corresponding cell types in the spleen. Those which enter the thymus are, however, already committed to a lymphocytic line of differentiation. Additional "bone marrow-derived" lymphocytes enter the peripheral pool directly.

Thymus lymphocytes (Figs. 3.12,13,15) are derived from bone marrow stem cells. They go through a phase of replication and differentiation within the thymus, finally becoming precursors of immunocompetent cells in the peripheral pool of small lymphocytes. They appear to possess immunological specificity and can be made tolerant but are not immunocompetent. Similar precursor cells may be formed in other central lymphoid organs.

"Uncommitted" *immunocompetent small lymphocytes* make up the major element in the recirculating peripheral pool of these cells (Figs. 4.3,6; 6.16). These are nondividing cells with a very *long life span*, months in the rat and several years in man. They follow a *complex route of recirculation*, passing from the blood into the parenchyma of peripheral lymphoid organs, specifically the white pulp of spleen and the diffuse cortex of lymph nodes, and returning again within a few hours to the blood (from spleen) or efferent lymph (from nodes) (Fig. 4.4). They enter the white pulp through fenestrated arteriolar capillaries, which branch directly from the white pulp arteriole, and leave by way of the marginal sinus around the white pulp. In the lymph node, they pass from the blood through the cytoplasm of endothelial cells lining specialized postcapillary venules of the lymph node cortex (Figs. 4.5,6). Their passage through the postcapillary venules is determined by polysaccharides in the lymphocyte cell membrane and, presumably, corresponding specific receptor sites on the surface of the endothelial cells. This recirculation mechanism guarantees that in the course of a few days most of the competent cells in the body will enter any lymph node subjected to an antigenic stimulus and be given an opportunity to respond to the stimulus. It is not known at present how many functionally distinct populations of cells follow the pathways described here. Most or all of these cells appear to be thymus-dependent or actually derived from precursors in the thymus. Lymphocytes in the lymph node follicles and Malpighian bodies of the spleen represent, on the other hand, a distinct, nonthymus-dependent population of immunocompetent cells, apparently following a different route of recirculation. The former are depleted in neonatally thymectomized animals, the latter in bursectomized birds and appendectomized mammals (rabbits). Their pathways of recirculation have been established by ablation of organs or depletion (e.g. thoracic duct drainage) and replacement experiments with the use of purified cell populations and of cells labeled with histocompatibility or chromosomal markers (Figs. 3.13; 4.7) or isotopically, as with tritiated thymidine or adenosine (Figs. 4.4,5).

The recirculating small lymphocytes include the *precursors* of several types *of immunological end cells*, which make different immunoglobulins. The thymus-dependent lymphocytes are responsible for cellular hypersensitivity and probably become the specific effector cells (see below). They are essential for γA-antibody formation and probably for some γG. In this case, however, the antibody-forming cells are the progeny of bone marrow-derived cells which have not passed through the thymus. The thymus-derived cells may play their role by facilitating the interaction of antigen with the latter. They may at the same time, after undergoing replication, serve as memory cells. Appendix-derived cells appear responsible for γM-immunoglobulin formation. In birds, thymus-derived cells are responsible for cellular hypersensitivity alone and bursa-derived cells for all types of circulating immunoglobulins. All, while still "uncommitted," have begun the synthesis of specific immuno-globulins, which appear in low concentration in their surface. These provide receptor sites that permit interaction with antigen and the production of tolerance or triggering of transformation of the uncommitted lymphocyte to a memory cell or effector cell. Tolerance may represent nothing more than the blocking of specific immuno-globulin receptor sites by antigen or fragments of antigen. Alternatively, it may represent cell lysis or an aberrant type of transformation. The triggering of an immune response appears to follow interaction of the lymphocyte with antigen which has been processed by a phagocytic cell (Section 6).

The recirculating peripheral lymphocyte pool includes two closely similar types of "committed" cells. *Memory cells* are produced after a single antigenic stimulus and respond to a secondary (anamnestic) stimulus with rapid proliferation. They may interact in an unknown manner with bone marrow-derived cells and promote the transformation of the latter into end cells such as plasma cells, which synthesize and release immunoglobulin. They are nondividing cells with a long life span ($\geqslant$ 15 months in the rat) and follow a pathway of recirculation like that of uncommitted cells. The *effector cells of cellular hypersensitivity* have similar properties, though they have been reported to have a shorter life span ($\leqslant$ 6 months in human subjects). This cell type must be regarded as a memory cell as well, its secondary response being elicited by the re-exposure to antigen at a local test site, e.g. with tuberculoprotein (Section 18). There is much evidence to suggest that memory cells and the effector cells of delayed or cellular hypersensitivity do not differ qualitatively from their precursors, the so-called uncommitted cells, but represent an enrichment of precursor cells of a given specificity, i.e. an increase in their numbers by several orders of magnitude. Not only do uncommitted and committed cells recirculate in an apparently identical manner, but their radiosensitivity is the same, as are other functional attributes which have been examined.

The term *lymphon* has been coined to describe the lymphocyte which synthesizes small amounts of immuno-globulin and can be rendered tolerant by antigen or stimulated by processed antigen to an immune response. It includes both uncommitted and committed cells, which are in the majority in the peripheral small lymphocyte pool.

Various agents which act on lymphocytes affect immune responses profoundly. Inadequate production of these cells, as in pyridoxine deficiency, or their removal, as by thoracic duct drainage, lead to marked deficiency of immune responsiveness. X-Irradiation, radiomimetic drugs (e.g. nitrogen mustard and cyclophosphamide), and steroids all destroy peripheral lymphocytes and are highly immunosuppressive. In general, cellular hyper-sensitivity and the production of γM-antibody are less readily inhibited by this means than formation of other classes of immunoglobulin. Milder agents, such as antilymphocyte sera which act at the cell membrane and *in vitro* induce lymphocytes to undergo transformation to primitive, rapidly replicating cells (the "blast" trans-formation), produce immunosuppression *in vivo*. In this case cellular hypersensitivity is affected more than other forms of response. Other substances active at the cell surface and perhaps on lysosomal membranes, among them phytohemagglutinin, pokeweed mitogen, streptolysin S, and staphylococcal alpha toxin, also induce a very high proportion of lymphocytes to undergo blast transformation (Fig. 4.2) and act *in vivo* as immunosup-pressants.

More selective forms of immunologic deficit are produced by agents which selectively affect defined popula-tions of lymphocytes. Heteroantibody against a specific class of immunoglobulin induces blast transformation in lymphocytes which are producing small amounts of this molecule and may be able, in the intact animal, to suppress for a longer or shorter period synthesis of the corresponding immunoglobulin. An even more limited deficit is produced by isoantibody against a particular allotype of γG-immunoglobulin, for example, which suppresses formation of this allotype in the intact animal and produces a corresponding blast transformation in a small proportion of peripheral lymphocytes *in vitro*.

Finally, specific antigen affects too few uncommitted cells to give countable numbers of transformed cells *in vitro*, yet by inhibiting the function of specific clones it renders the animal tolerant, i.e. unable subsequently to produce antibody specific for that antigen. In the case of primed animals, which have memory or delayed hypersensitivity, antigen added to cells *in vitro* gives blast transformation of a small proportion (Fig. 4.2) which presumably are specific committed cells (Fig. 18.1). *In vivo* it produces desensitization, a specific state of non-reactivity, more transient than tolerance simply because of the increased rate of formation of new reactive cells of a given specificity in the primed animal.

The action of these various agencies in the intact animal is limited to some extent by their molecular size and by barriers they may have to cross. Thus in adult animals, large molecular or particulate antigens may enter the parenchyma of thymus, spleen, and lymph nodes with difficulty and thus be ineffectual in producing tolerance. Antilymphocyte antibody, which also penetrates these organs slowly, principally affects cells in the circulation. X ray, on the other hand, and small molecules like nitrogen mustard may be expected to reach all lymphocytes with equal intensity.

A third type of committed cell, which by light microscopy has the aspect of a small lymphocyte, is the antibody-forming *lymphokinecyte* (Figs. 6.13,17). Such cells are found in the circulation and in the peripheral lymphoid organs of immunized animals, but it is not known whether they recirculate in the same manner as the uncommitted cells and memory cells.

A final cell type which must be listed here is the small *monocyte* (Fig. 2.13) (called by some a prehistiocyte), which not only looks like a small or medium-sized lymphocyte but shares some of its functional attributes, such as lack of ability to stick to glass and absence of phagocytic activity. These are short-lived cells, derived from rapidly dividing precursors in the bone marrow. They contain the lysosomal enzymes characteristic of reticulo-endothelial cells, notably esterase, peroxidase, etc., and are direct precursors of histiocytes and macrophages appearing in various specific and nonspecific inflammatory reactions (Figs. 2.3; 16.9,18,19).

Although the various cells described thus far all resemble small lymphocytes in conventional light microscopic preparations, they possess distinctive ultrastructural attributes—for example, multiple nucleoli, high ribosome content, and well-developed Golgi system of stem cells; the presence of rough endoplasmic reticulum in lympho-kinecytes, and lysosomes and phagocytic vacuoles in monocytes. Uncommitted small lymphocytes are almost devoid of significant structural features. Further structural details are not given here.

Larger lymphocytes are in most instances *replicative* and/or differentiating *forms* of the small cells listed above. In particular, large and medium cells within the thymus develop after many cell divisions into the small thymocytes. The germinal centers of lymph nodes and spleen are foci of replicating large cells whose progeny apparently are the small recirculating memory cells. Lymphoblasts of the diffuse lymph node cortex are replicating precursors of the effector cells of cellular hypersensitivity. Some larger lymphoid cells, both in the tissues and the blood stream, are themselves antibody-forming cells (see the next sections).

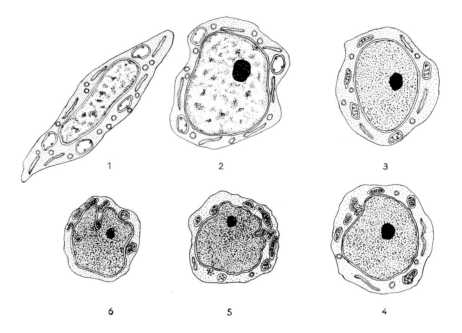

Fig. 4.1. The principal ultrastructural features of cells in the lymphocyte series. Derivation of lymphoblasts and large, medium, and small lymphocytes (3–6) from fixed and activated reticular cells (1, 2) was widely accepted for several years, but is now regarded as improbable.

From Bernhard and Granboulan, *CIBA Symposium on Cellular Aspects of Immunity*, G. E. W. Wolstenholme and M. O'Connor, eds., Churchill, London, 1960, pp. 92–121.

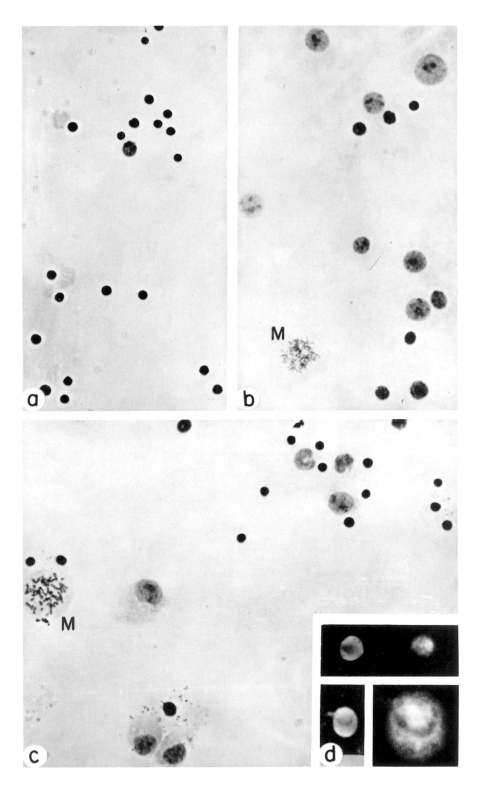

Fig. 4.2. Specific and nonspecific stimulation of lymphocytes in peripheral blood. Culture of lymphocytes from human subject with elevated antistreptolysin-O titer. (a) Without stimulation (negative control). (b) Nonspecific stimulation by phytohemagglutinin: smear shows preponderance of large cells and one mitosis (M). (c) Stimulation by specific antigen, streptolysin O: over one third of the cells are large, and mitosis is seen. In both (b) and (c), some of the larger cells are "early forms."

All are stained with orcein and photographed under phase contrast; × 350. Insert shows cells after stimulation with phytohemagglutinin stained with a fluorescent antiserum specific for human γ-globulin; × 500 and × 2,000. Courtesy of Dr. K. Hirschhorn.

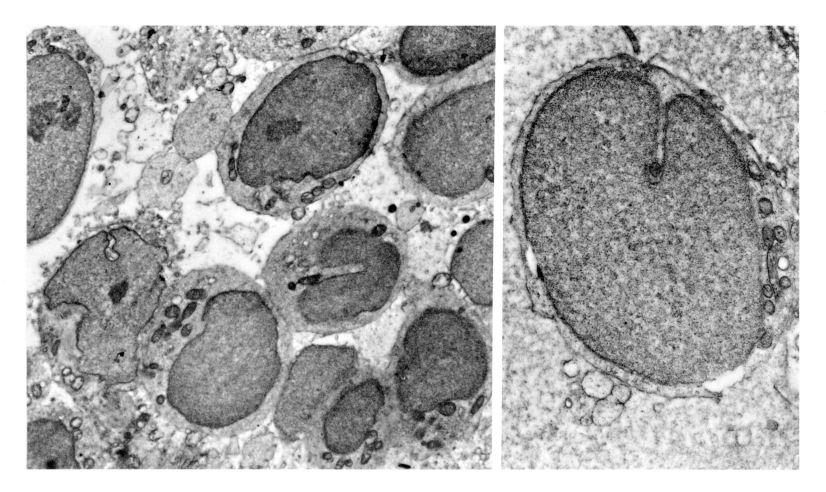

Fig. 4.3. (Left) Lymphocyte population of cortex in normal human lymph node. (Right) Higher power of small lymphocyte. Note paucity of cell organelles and variable presence of nucleolus.

Electron micrograph; magnifications not given. From Bernhard and Granboulan, in CIBA *Symposium on Cellular Aspects of Immunity*, G. E. W. Wolstenholme and M. O'Connor, eds., Churchill, London, 1960, pp. 92–121.

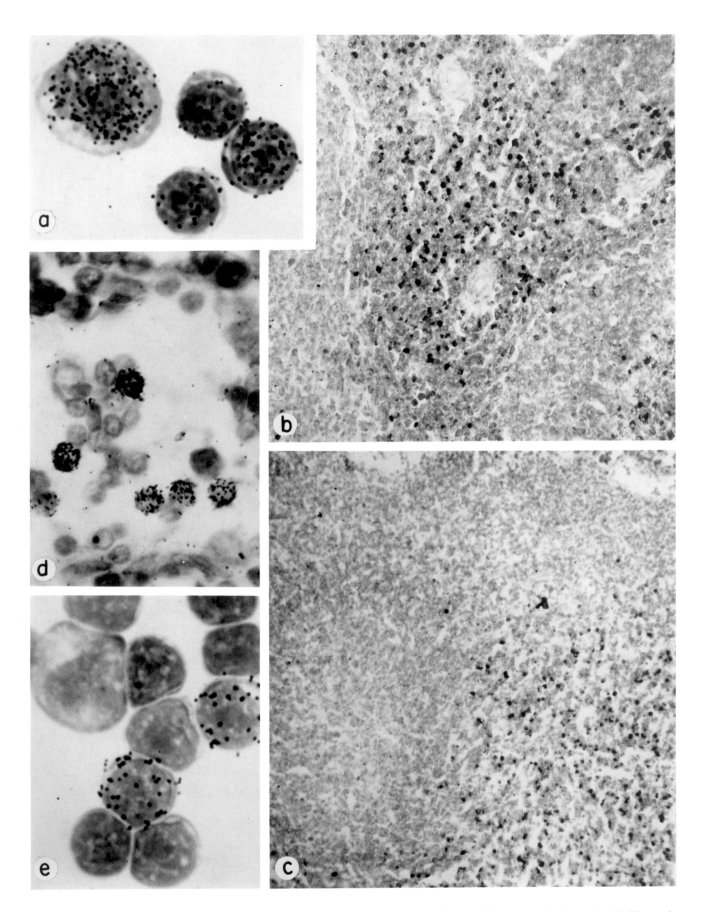

Fig. 4.4. Recirculation of lymphocytes from blood to parenchyma of lymphoid organs in the rat. (a) Thoracic duct (TD) cells after incubation for 1 hour *in vitro* with H³-adenosine; ×2,250. Small and large lymphocytes, labeled in RNA and in RNA and DNA respectively. (b) Spleen 24 hours after iv tranfusion of H³-adenosine-labeled TD cells; ×210. Localization to white pulp. (c) Bronchial node of similar rat; ×180. Localization to cortex. There is no localization of labeled cells in germinal center (at left) or in zone between marginal sinus (at top) and cortex. (d) Cervical node of similar rat; ×1,200. Medullary sinus contains labeled small lymphocytes, which have passed from blood to efferent lymph. (e) Cells in thoracic duct at same time include labeled small lympho-cytes which have completed cycle of recirculation; ×2,250. Large lymphocytes are unlabeled.

All figures are radioautographs on stripping film, exposed 7 or 14 days before developing and staining. (a, c) From Gowans and Knight, *Proc. Roy. Soc. B. 159*: 257–82 (1964). (b, d, e) From Gowans, unpublished.

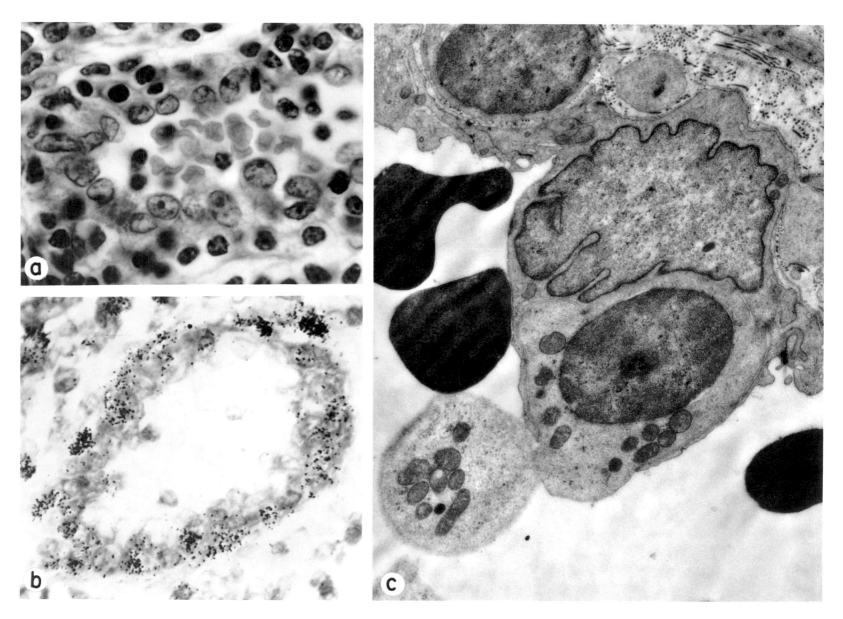

Fig. 4.5. Function of postcapillary venule in normal rat lymph node. (a) Cervical node; hematoxylin-eosin, ×1,050. Pale endothelial nuclei making up venule are surrounded by small lymphocytes. Venule contains red blood cells. (b) Cervical node 30 minutes after continuous 8-hour infusion of labeled thoracic duct cells; radioautograph, ×1,200. Venule is ringed with labeled lymphocytes, most of which are under the endothelium. The cortex of this node is packed with labeled cells. (c) Electron micrograph of venule in similar node; ×13,500. Small lymphocyte penetrating cytoplasm of an endothelial cell. Nucleus of endothelial cell is above lymphocyte. A second lymphocyte (cytoplasm and mitochondria only) lies in the lumen.

(a, b) From Gowans and Knight, *Proc. Roy. Soc. B. 159*: 257–82 (1964). (c) From Marchesi and Gowans, ibid., pp. 283–90.

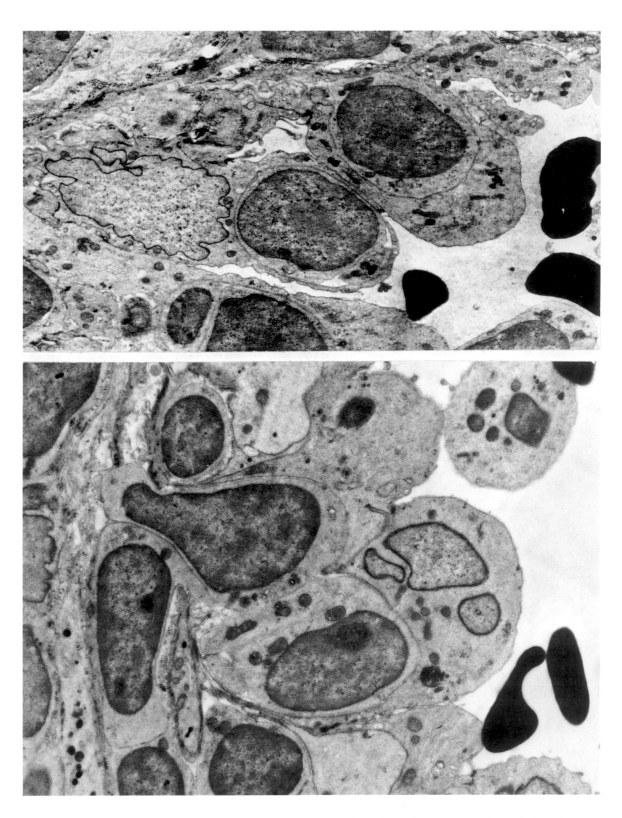

Fig. 4.6. Function of postcapillary venule in normal rat lymph node. Passage of small lymphocytes through cytoplasm of endothelial cells. (Above) The lower of the two lymphocytes appears to be completely enclosed within an endothelial cell. Endothelial nucleus is to left; × 5,700. (Below) Penetration of pseudopod of a similar lymphocyte into deepest layers of periendothelial connective tissue; × 7,500.

Electron micrographs. From Marchesi and Gowans, *Proc. Roy. Soc. B. 159*: 283–90 (1964).

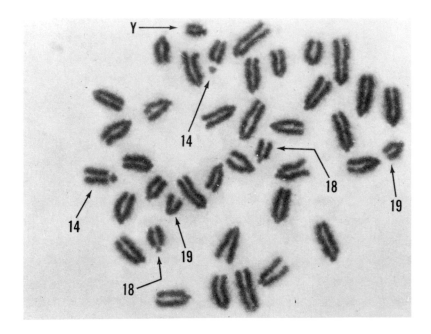

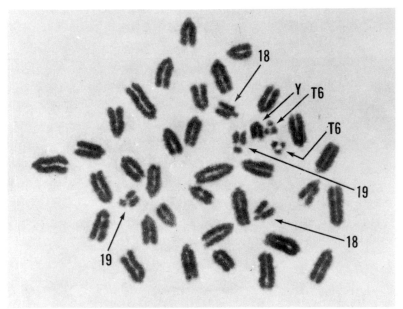

Fig. 4.7. Karotypic analysis as a technique of cell labeling. (Above) Spleen cell of male CBA mouse. Smaller chromosomes are identified by number. Secondary constrictions usually seen in pair 19 are not visible in this cell. (Below) Lymph node cell of male CBA-T6T6 mouse. The characteristic T6 chromosomes are readily identified. The development of these two completely histocompatible strains of mouse has permitted extensive studies of lymphoid cell migration by cell and tissue grafting, with the use of T6 as a marker.

Air-dried preparations, stained with lactic-acetic orcein. Preparations of Dr. C. E. Ford. From Micklem and Loutit, *Tissue Grafting and Radiation*, Academic Press, New York, 1966, pp. 67–68.

5. Peripheral Lymphoid Organs

Organs in which immune responses occur (antibody formation, production of memory cells and effector cells of the cellular type of sensitization) were first identified by ablation and cellular transfer experiments and more recently by measurement of antibody formation by tissue slices or in culture. The fluorescence technique and electron microscopy have been used for the morphologic localization of antibody-forming cells and *in vitro* methods for identifying and counting these cells, as discussed in the next section.

The principal organs involved in antibody synthesis (Fig. 2.1) are the *spleen* and *hemolymph nodes*, the peripheral *lymph nodes*, and *surface lymphoid tissues* in the respiratory and gastrointestinal tracts, each with a different afferent pathway of immunization, as noted earlier. A small intravenous immunizing dose of antigen will tend to induce a response only in the spleen, and this limitation applies particularly to colloidal or particulate antigens. With larger doses and especially with soluble antigens, the other peripheral lymphoid organs may be involved in the primary response. Similarly, small doses of antigen given at a local site will immunize only the regional lymph nodes while larger doses, especially of soluble materials, will spill over into the systemic circulation and reach the spleen and remote nodes. Antigen entering mucosal surfaces will affect primarily the surface organs, but excess material may reach regional nodes or the circulation. With large doses of antigen and with prolonged antigenic stimulation, antibody formation occurs in lymphoid organs remote from the primary locus of immunization and antibody-producing cells also appear in the *bone marrow, lung*, and *liver* and in *sites of metastatic antibody formation* throughout the body. Finally, when colloidal or particulate antigens are given locally or antigens are administered in an adjuvant vehicle which forms a local depot, a *local focus* ("granuloma") will develop *of antibody-forming cells*. Local antibody formation also is prominent when antigen is introduced into a site (eye, joint) from which it cannot escape freely.

The anatomy of the peripheral lymphoid organs is complex since it provides simultaneously for uptake and processing of antigen, recirculation of lymphocytes, and production of end cells and antibody. The spleen has a further order of complexity, since it also plays a role in erythrocyte homeostasis, serving as a site both of red cell destruction and at times of hemopoiesis. Thus in transfer experiments or *in vitro* experiments involving the use of cell suspensions, spleen cells must be viewed as containing lymphocytes like those of lymph node, plus some or all of the cell populations usually found in the bone marrow.

The essential immunologic elements of the *spleen* (Fig. 5.1) are a sheath of small lymphocytes which accompanies the branching splenic arterioles (*white pulp*) and follicular masses of small lymphocytes occurring at random locations in the white pulp and containing dendritic, nonphagocytic reticulum cells and often a rounded collection of dividing medium and large lymphocytes (germinal center)—the latter structure is known as a *Malpighian corpuscle* (Figs. 5.6–8). The white pulp and Malpighian bodies are surrounded by a marginal zone of highly phagocytic histiocytes (reticulum cells). The remainder of the spleen is known as the *red pulp*, made up of cords of blood cells and other cells alternating with thin-walled venous sinusoids lined with a phagocytic reticulum. The *vascular arrangements* of the spleen have been elucidated by dye injections and by study of the splenic architecture with reticulum stains (Figs. 5.2,3). The white pulp arterioles are continued as straight penicilli arterioles which either terminate in the cords of the red pulp or curve back to end in the vicinity of the white pulp. The white pulp and Malpighian corpuscles are surrounded by a marginal venous sinus, from which originate the multiple sinusoids of the red pulp. The major zone of antigen or particle uptake is the histiocytic marginal zone, through which these sinusoids pass before entering the red pulp. In the presence of specific antibody, antigen uptake also occurs, however, on the surface of dendritic reticulum cells in the Malphighian follicles. The white pulp is apparently drained by a *system of lymphatics* (Fig. 5.4), which may simply provide a means of returning intercellular fluid to the blood stream or another route whereby lymphocytes leave the spleen.

Thymectomy at birth (or thymectomy followed by irradiation in older animals) leads to depletion of white pulp lymphocytes and to a lesser degree follicular lymphocytes (Figs. 5.6,9,12) but does not affect the development of the normal reticular framework of the white pulp and Malpighian bodies or the germinal center and plasma cell responses (Fig. 5.9). Conversely, bursectomy of chickens at hatching leads to loss of germinal centers and plasma cells with retention of the thymus-dependent white pulp lymphocytes (Fig. 5.12).

The response of the spleen to blood-borne antigen involves a characteristic sequence, over a few days, of blast formation in the white pulp and evolution of these blasts to more or less mature plasma cells (Figs. 5.15,16). Shortly after, there is active germinal center formation, which may be strikingly enhanced by such agents as endotoxin (Gram-negative bacterial cell wall lipopolysaccharide) (Figs. 5.15,17). Plasma cells, which arise in the white pulp, move down the white pulp arterioles and are found in nests along the penicilli arterioles (Figs. 5.7,15,16). They also move directly to the periphery of the white pulp and thence into the red pulp (Figs. 5.15,16). The lymphocytes which arise by the replication of germinal center cells appear to leave by way of the marginal sinus.

The *lymph node* is made up of elements which are homologues of those in the spleen (Figs. 5.1,18). The thymus-dependent small lymphocytes form large, *diffuse cortical (paracortical) masses* comparable to the white pulp. These are strikingly depleted after neonatal thymectomy (Figs. 5.10,11) or treatment of the adult with antilymphocyte serum (Fig. 5.13). The *follicles and germinal centers*, unlike the Malpighian bodies of the spleen, are quite separate from the diffuse cortex. These are affected slightly if at all by thymectomy (Fig. 5.11). Recirculation of long-lived small lymphocytes by way of the postcapillary venules, through the paracortical masses, and back to the blood stream by way of medullary sinuses, has been mentioned (Section 4). The *medulla* of the node is made up of cords of cells containing arterioles and venules and tortuous lymph sinuses lined with highly phagocytic reticulum cells. Antigen is taken up primarily in the latter as well as in the closely similar subcapsular sinus and the intermediate sinuses which pass between the follicles and paracortical masses of lymphocytes. The response to antigen involves several distinct elements (Figs. 5.18,19). The first is the formation of large pyroninophilic blast-like cells in the paracortical masses (Section 6). These are related to cellular hypersensitivity, and mature to small lymphocytes which enter the blood stream by way of the medullary sinuses and the efferent lymph. Secondly, plasma cells arise at the medullary border of the paracortical tissue and migrate along the vessels of the medullary cords as they mature. Finally, the germinal centers increase in size and numbers. The route followed by cells leaving these is as yet unclear.

Surface lymphoid organs, such as the tonsil, may have essentially all the same anatomic elements as lymph nodes. However, individual lymph node elements may also appear alone. One finds, in the intestinal mucosa for example, poorly defined aggregates of lymphocytes, apparently similar to the paracortical tissue of lymph nodes, and organized groups of follicles containing germinal centers but lacking paracortical or medullary elements (the Peyer's patches, Fig. 5.14). Plasma cell aggregates are also found in the absence of other lymphoid elements.

Local introduction of antigen anywhere in the body results in a local immune response (the "progressive immunization reaction") with re-creation of one or another of the anatomic elements discussed above at the particular site affected. This process has been best studied in special organs such as the eye (Figs. 5.20–24) or joint, after injection of exogenous antigen, but may occur anywhere. An almost identical cell sequence is observed, for example, in kidney homografts, as immunization is initiated. One can distinguish early a local lymphocytic infiltrate which appears to correspond to the process of cellular sensitization, beginning within a day or two and maximal by 5–7 days (Figs. 5.20,21,24), and a later plasma cell infiltrate associated with humoral antibody formation (Figs. 5.22–24; 7.8). Germinal centers are seen only in situations providing for long-continued local stimulation (not illustrated here). The "progressive immunization reaction" commonly occurs at the site of elicitation of a local Arthus or delayed reaction (Figs. 16.11–14) and complicates the interpretation of late cellular events in such reaction sites. Some of the experimental autoallergies (Section 21), notably auto-allergic thyroiditis, in which there is a continuing supply of eliciting local antigen, may be characterized by massive plasma cell accumulations and germinal center formation after the initial cellular hypersensitivity lesion.

Fig. 5.1. Rat spleen. Normal anatomic relations. (a) White pulp arteriole. (b) Sheath of small lymphocytes (white pulp). (c) Marginal zone of phagocytic RE cells and venous sinuses. (d) White pulp lacking marginal zone. (e) "Malpighian corpuscle," consisting of germinal center surrounded by zone of small lymphocytes and marginal zone. (f) Germinal center on surface of white pulp. (g) Similar germinal center, cut tangentially so that white pulp is not seen. (h) Penicilli arteriole, beyond region sheathed with lymphocytes, surrounded by irregular aggregate of plasma cells. (i) Red pulp.

From Waksman, Arnason, and Janković, *J. Exp. Med. 116*: 187–206 (1962).

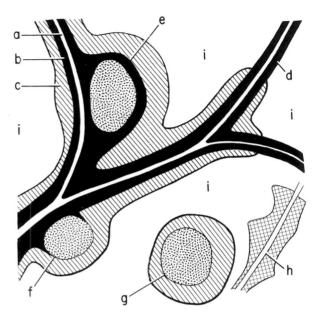

Fig. 5.2. Rat lymph node. Normal anatomic relations in period of activity. (a) Diffuse cortex (paracortical tissue), consisting of more or less densely packed small lymphocytes with moderate numbers of other types of cells. (b) Tongues of lymphocytes extending from cortex into medullary sinuses, from which individual lymphocytes escape into the efferent lymph and ultimately the blood stream. (c) "Postcapillary venules" with cuboidal endothelium, through which lymphocytes pass from blood stream into the lymph node cortex. (d) Follicle containing germinal center ("secondary nodule" of certain authors). (e) Follicle not containing germinal center. (f) Subcapsular and intermediate sinuses, containing afferent lymph. (g) Medulla, consisting of cords of plasma cells and sinuses containing efferent lymph.

From Waksman, Arnason, and Janković, ibid.

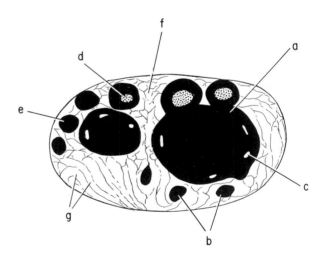

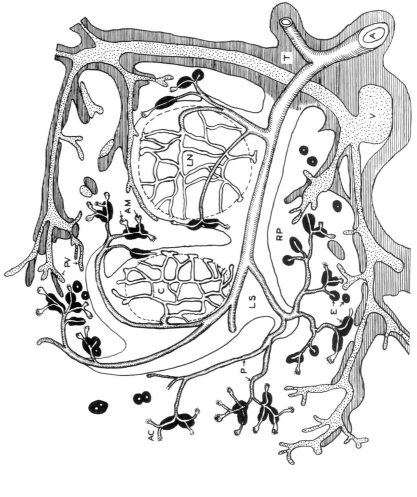

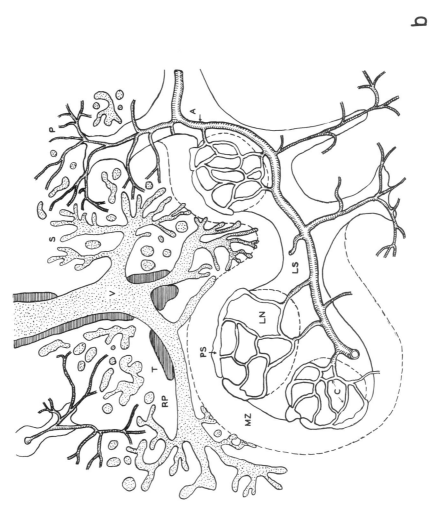

Fig. 5.3. Vascular architecture of the spleen in man and several commonly studied experimental animals. (a) Rat; ×90. (b) Cat; ×90. (c) Man; ×95. (d) Horse; ×66. (e, f) Dog; ×90, ×260. A, white pulp artery; AC, arterial capillary; ACT, arterial capillary termination; AM, ampulla; C, capillary; CA, capsule; E, ellipsoid sheath; HA, "Hof" artery; L, Lymphatic vessel; LN, lymphoid nodule; LS, lymphoid sheath; MZ, marginal zone; P, penicillus; PS, perifollicular spaces; PV, primordial vein (capillary venule); RP, red pulp; S, sinus; T, trabecula; V, vein.

From Figs. 2, 4, 6, 7, 8, 10 on pp. 38, 42, 45, 46, 48, 52 in Snook, *Am. J. Anat. 87*: 31–78 (1950).

b

a

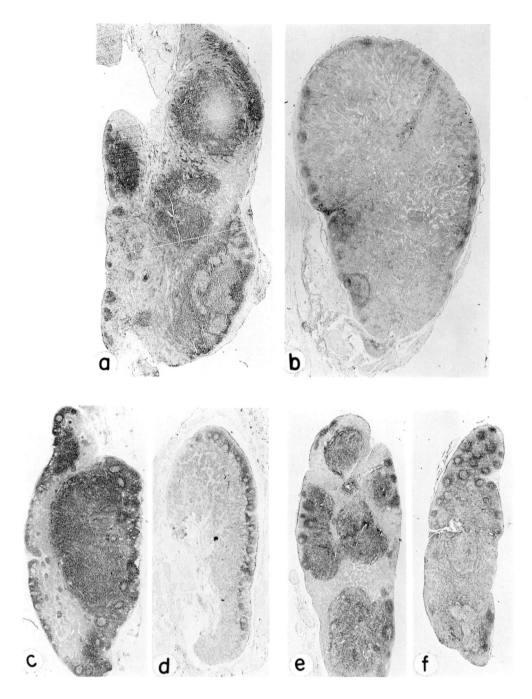

Fig. 5.10. Lymph nodes. (a, b) Left axillary (draining) nodes from control and thymectomized rats given spinal cord and adjuvant. (c, d) Left inguinal (draining) nodes from control and thymectomized rats given adjuvant without incorporated antigen. (e, f) Right axillary (nondraining) nodes from grafted control and thymectomized rats. Diffuse cortex in thymectomized rats is completely lacking in small lymphocytes, but germinal centers and surrounding zone of small lymphocytes are normal in appearance. Pale area in node shown in (a) is mass of epitheloid cells surrounding injected adjuvant mixture.

Hematoxylin-eosin; × 10.

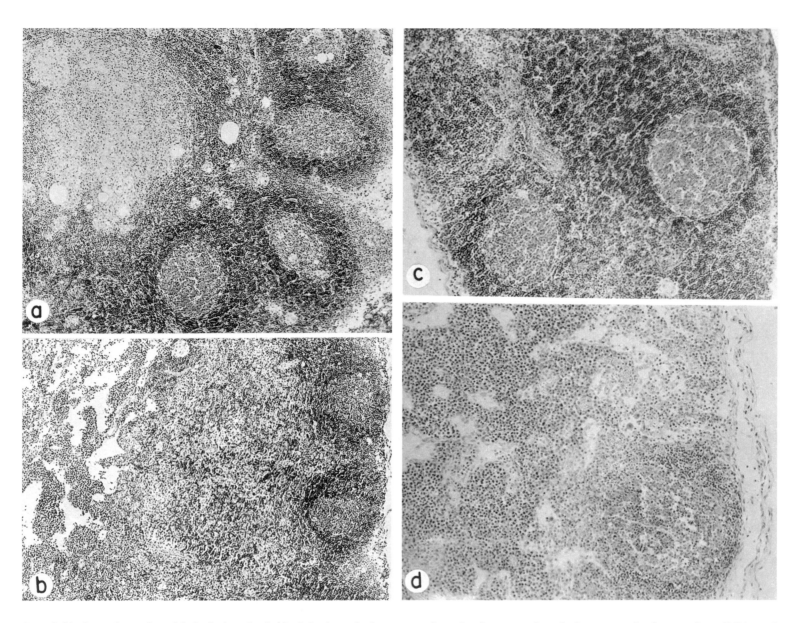

Fig. 5.11. Lymph nodes. (a) Left inguinal (draining) node in control rat given BSA and adjuvant; ×90. (b) Left axillary node in thymectomized rat given adjuvant; ×90. (c, d) Mediasti-nal nodes in control and thymectomized rats given BSA and adjuvant; ×120.

Hematoxylin-eosin.

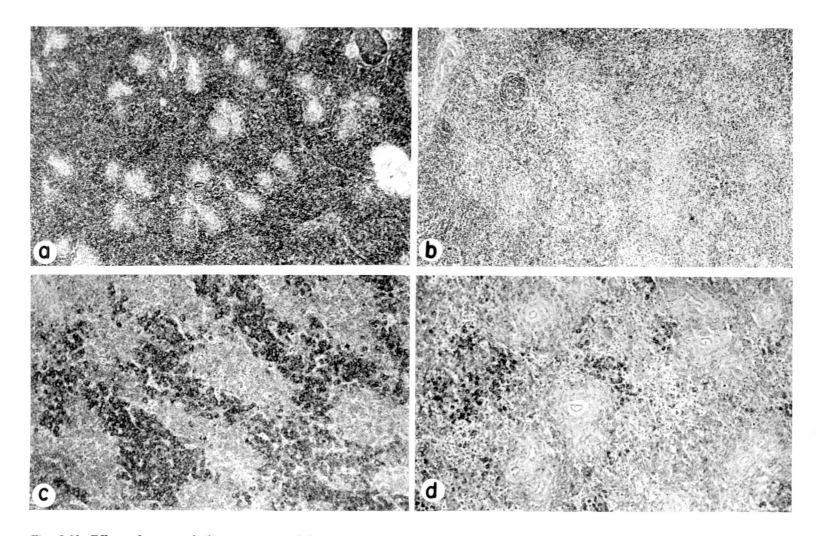

Fig. 5.12. Effect of neonatal thymectomy and bursectomy on function of spleen in 8-week-old chickens. (a) Normal. (b) Thymectomized at hatching. (c) Normal, 6 days after injection of heterologous erythrocytes. (d) Bursectomized at hatching, similarly injected. Spleen of thymectomized bird shows marked depletion of small lymphocytes, while bursectomy results in deficit of pyroninophilic plasma cells and absence of germinal centers.

(a, b) Hematoxylin-eosin; ×30. (c, d) Methyl green–pyronine; ×100. From Isaković and Janković, *Int. Arch. Allergy 24*: 296–310 (1964)., S. Karger, Basel, New York.

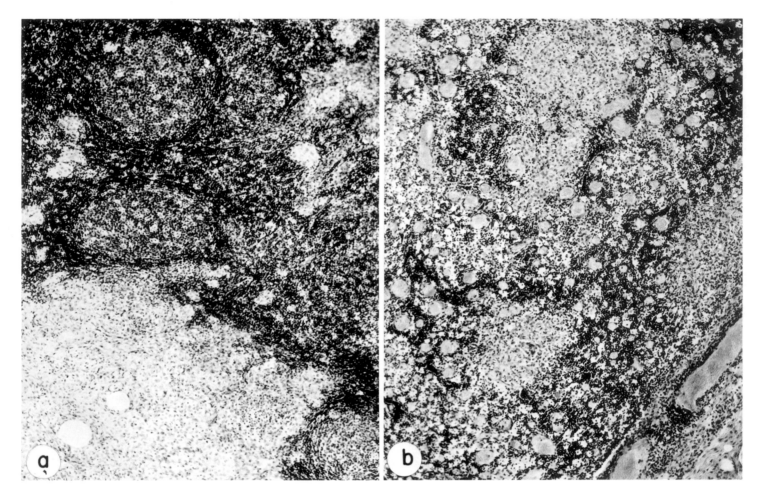

Fig. 5.13. Lymphopenic effect of antilymphocyte serum (rabbit) in guinea pig. Lymph nodes draining site of inoculation with nervous tissue and adjuvant, in animals treated with normal serum (a) and antilymphocyte serum (b) over several days during latent period following inoculation and sacrificed at 14 days. Control animal developed allergic encephalomyelitis; treated animal failed to do so. Control node shows cortical lymphocyte aggregates and normal follicular structure with germinal centers, as well as vacuoles, representing injected adjuvant and epithelioid cell masses. Treated node shows depletion of lymphocytes and loss of normal architecture.

Hematoxylin-eosin; ×80. From Waksman et al., *J. Exp. Med. 114*: 997–1022 (1961).

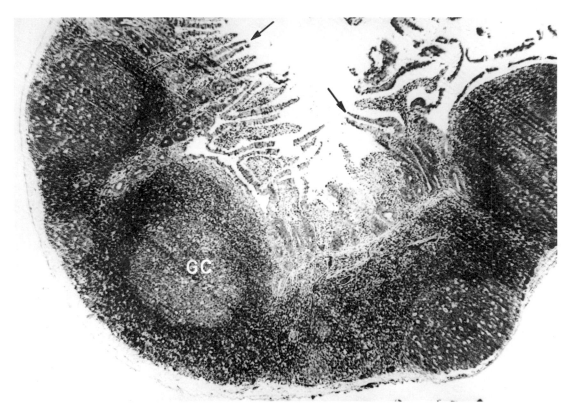

Fig. 5.14. Normal rat Peyer's patch. Organ consists entirely of large follicles containing characteristic germinal centers (GC), placed just beneath the intestinal mucosa (arrows). There is no structure clearly corresponding to diffuse cortical tissue or medulla of normal lymph nodes.

Giemsa; ×80. Courtesy of Dr. S. Order.

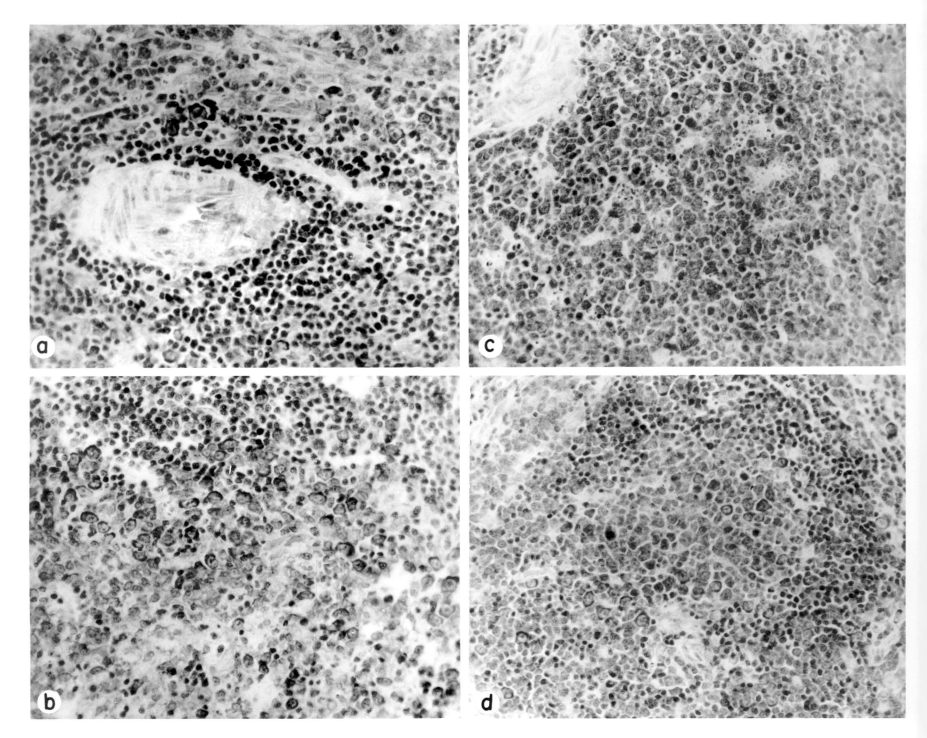

Fig. 5.15. Primary response to iv bovine γ-globulin in rabbit spleen. (a) Two days after antigen, more than 24 hours before antibody production is detectable, even *in vitro*. White pulp, showing slight increase in number of large blast cells, as compared with earlier biopsy of same spleen and other normal spleens from clean animals. (b) Same, 4 days after BGG. Antibody production high. Blast cells and immature plasma cells now at border between white pulp (above) and red pulp. (c, d) Same, 7 days after BGG. Antibody production low. Two views showing germinal centers (secondary nodules) with "starry sky" appearance and tingible bodies (c), and predominance of medium lymphocytes (d).

Methyl green–pyronine; all ×500. Courtesy of Dr. G. J. Thorbecke (see Langevoort et al., *J. Immunol. 90*: 60–71, 1963).

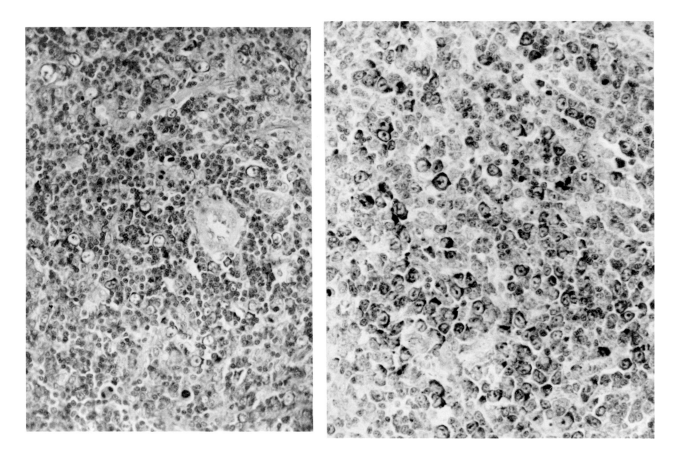

Fig. 5.16. Rabbit spleen changes during secondary response 2 days after iv BGG, 4 weeks after primary. Antibody response already high. (Left) Large blast cells in white pulp, many more than in primary response. (Right) Blast cells and immature plasma cells in red pulp.

Methyl green–pyronine; ×470. From Thorbecke, Asofsky, Hochwald, and Siskind, *J. Exp. Med. 116*: 295–310 (1962).

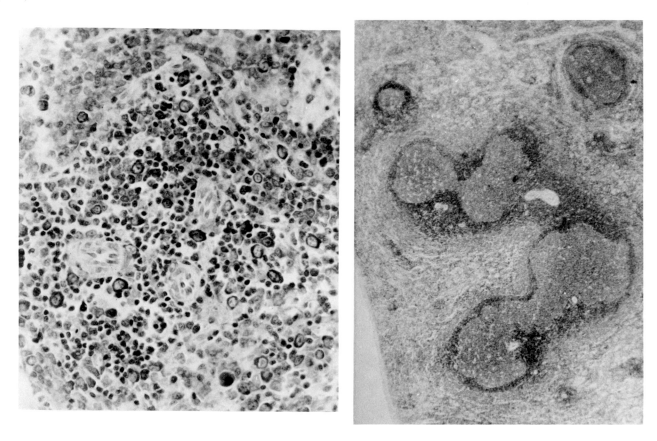

Fig. 5.17. Primary response to BGG and endotoxin in rabbit spleen. (Left) Four days after stimulus. Antibody production high. Blast cells in and around white pulp, and immature plasma cells in red pulp ; ×475. (Right) Ten days. Low-power view, showing enormous confluent germinal centers (secondary nodules). Antibody formation absent; ×57.

Methyl green–pyronine. Courtesy of Dr. G. J. Thorbecke.

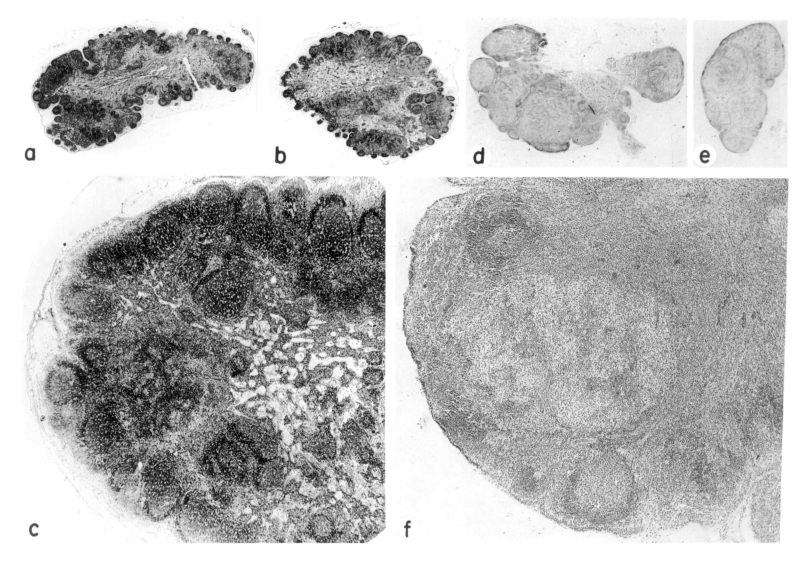

Fig. 5.18. Rabbit popliteal lymph nodes after footpad injection of washed typhoid vaccine. (a–c) Normal nodes showing usual proportion between diffuse cortex and follicles. There is active germinal center formation. (d–f) Immunized nodes showing formation of large "tertiary nodules" full of reticulum cells after repeated stimulation.

Azure II-eosin; (a, b, d, e) ×8, (c, f) ×60. From Ehrich and Harris, *J. Exp. Med. 76*: 335–48 (1942), and Ehrich, *J. Exp. Med. 49*: 347–60 (1929), and unpublished.

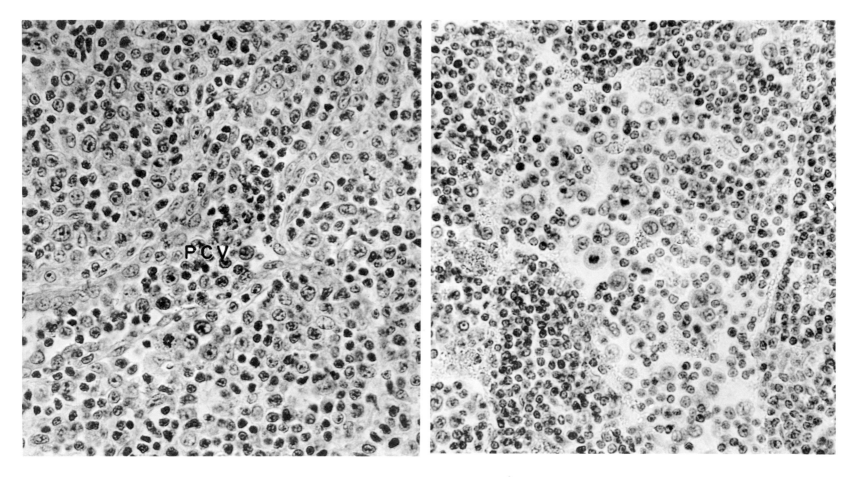

Fig. 5.19. Rabbit mesenteric node after similar stimulation. (Left) Cortex, showing postcapillary venule (PCV) and numerous lymphocytes entering parenchyma; ×570. (Right) Medullary sinus filled with variety of cell types, predominantly small lymphocytes. Some large cells are dividing. There is a good deal of free pigment; ×595.

Methylene blue–eosin. From Ehrich and Harris, *J. Exp. Med.* *76*: 335–48 (1942), and Ehrich, *Am. J. Anat. 43*: 347–401 (1929), and *J. Exp. Med. 49*: 347–60 (1929).

FIGURES 5.20–5.23
Local immune response in rabbit cornea. From Parks, Leibowitz, and Maumenee, *J. Exp. Med. 115*: 867–80 (1962).

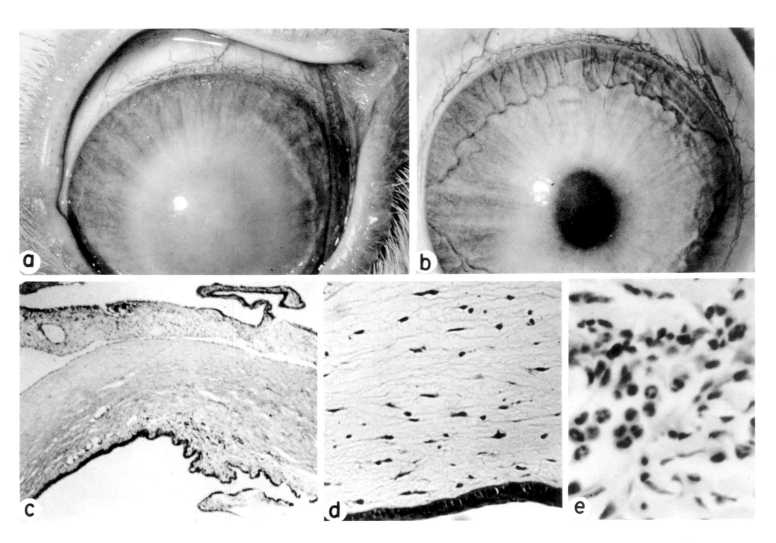

Fig. 5.20. Rabbit cornea after intracorneal inoculation of 4 mg BSA. (a) Immediately after: central cloud represents injected material. (b) At onset of primary, delayed-phase reaction: circumlimbal flare—cornea still relatively clear. (c)

Normal cornea and limbus. (d) Normal cornea. (e) Limbus 2 days post inoculation: infiltration by pseudoeosinophils. (c–e) Hematoxylin-eosin, × 60, × 220, × 450.

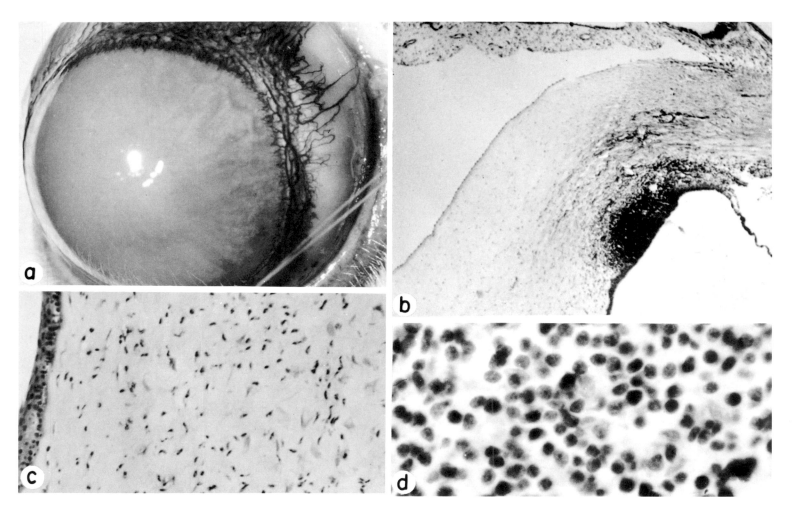

Fig. 5.21. Rabbit cornea 5 days after inoculation of 4 mg BSA: primary, delayed-phase reactions. (a) Marked circumlimbal flare and dense, diffuse corneal clouding. (b) Corneal and limbal infiltrates. (c) Cornea: infiltration by pseudo eosinophils. (d) Limbus: focal infiltration by lymphoid elements.

(b–d) Hematoxylin-eosin, × 80, × 220, × 480.

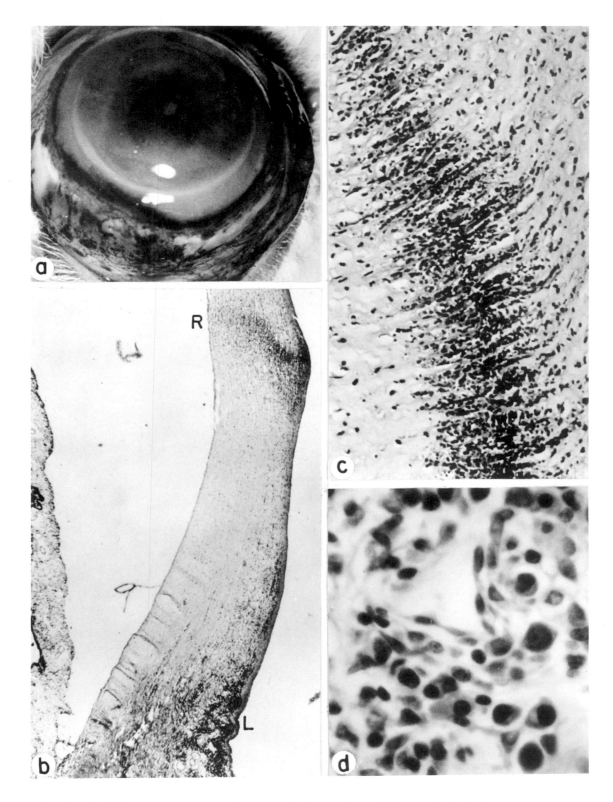

Fig. 5.22. Rabbit cornea 14 days after inoculation of 4 mg BSA: peak of Arthus-type response. (a) Wessely ring and marked circumlimbal flare. (b) Ring (R) and limbal infiltrate (L). (c) Higher-power view of Wessely ring: antigen–antibody precipitate, damaged corneal cells, infiltrating cells, and debris. (d) Limbus at 8 days: lymphocytes and immature and mature plasma cells—first antibody detectable in these cells by Coons technique.

(b–d) Hematoxylin-eosin; ×60, ×180, ×480.

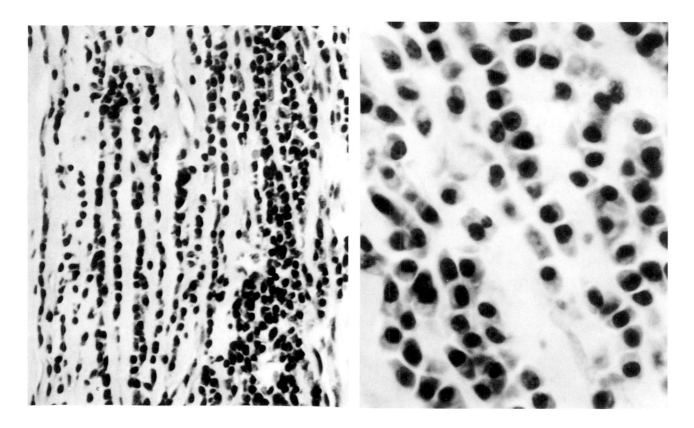

Fig. 5.23. Rabbit cornea after inoculation of 4 mg BSA. (Left) Rows of plasma cells "migrating" into cornea stroma at 18 days; × 240. (Right) Plasma cell infiltrate of limbus at 16 days; × 480. Hematoxylin-eosin.

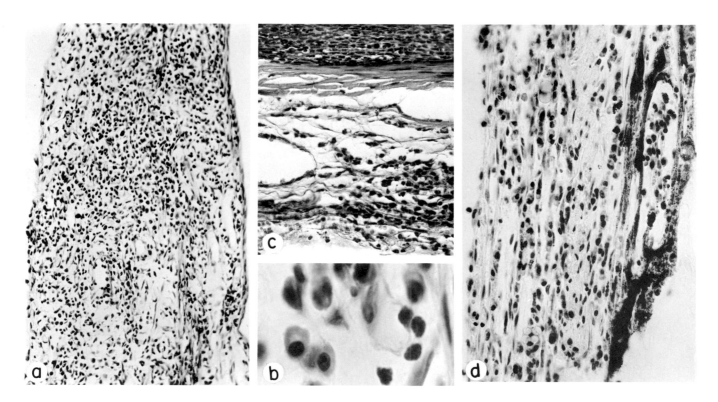

Fig. 5.24. Local immune response in rabbit eye. (a) Rabbit iris, 7 days after inoculation of 1 mg ovalbumin into the vitreous: developing anterior uveitis with diffuse infiltration of lymphocytes and histiocytes; × 175. (b) Same reaction 6 days later: inflammation has subsided and diffuse mononuclear infiltrate has given way to foci of plasma cells at all stages of maturity; × 935. (c) Same eye as in (b): infiltrate in choroid, sclera, and episclera is mononuclear in character; × 280. (d) Human nongranulomatous uveitis for comparison. Resolving iris lesion, with diffuse infiltrates of lymphocytes and large numbers of plasma cells, some containing Russell bodies; × 280.

(a–d) Hematoxylin-eosin (AFIP negs. 60–812, 60–809, 59–3172, 56–4820). From Silverstein, Walter, and Zimmerman, *J. Immunol.* 86: 312–23 (1961).

6. Cells Making the Immune Response

The identity of antibody-forming cells was first established by showing a correlation between antibody formation in, e.g., the splenic red pulp and the presence of a particular cell type, in this case plasmablasts and immature plasmacytes. However, the direct demonstration and identification of these cells could be achieved only after the introduction of the immunofluorescence technique (Figs. 6.10–13) and its electron microscopic equivalent, with the use of ferritin- or peroxidase-labeled antibody as a specific stain. Simple numerative techniques have been recently developed, notably the counting of plaque-forming cells (Fig. 6.14) (this method has been adapted for systems involving various protein and polysaccharide antigens, and for both γM- and γG-antibody responses), of cells giving rosettes of adherent red cells or bacteria bearing specific antigen (Fig. 6.8), and of cells releasing antibody in microdroplet cultures of single cells. Morphologic study in conventional stained preparations (Figs. 5.15,16; 6.6) or by electron microscopy (Figs. 6.7; 8.6–8) has been combined effectively with immunofluorescence (Fig. 6.13), with the use of tritiated thymidine incorporation as a measure of DNA synthesis (Figs. 6.9,13), and with the plaque-formation technique (Figs. 6.15–17). Early correlative studies frequently made use of neoplasms of immunoglobulin-forming cells (myeloma, Waldenström's macroglobulinemia) (Figs. 6.11; 8.6–8). The newer methods permit characterization and quantitation of individual cell types making well-defined specific antibodies in normal and immunized subjects.

A gamut of cell types has been found to make antibody in the tissues (Figs. 6.1,3; 4.1). In general γG-globulin is formed by *plasma cells* of varying degrees of maturity (Figs. 6.2,6,7; 8.6), containing more or less well-elaborated endoplasmic reticulum in laminar array; γM by *large lymphocytes* (lymphogonia, lymphocytoid plasma cells), containing free ribosomes and in some instances a few isolated loops of ergastoplasm (Fig. 8.8); and γA by mature plasma cells or *Russell body plasma cells* (Mott cells, thesaurocytes) (Fig. 8.7), in which the endoplasmic reticulum is dilated to form large sacs filled with antibody (the "constipated cell"). However, any type of immunoglobulin may be formed by cells of any of these morphological types (Figs. 6.10,11) in addition to cells described as reticular cells and cells resembling small lymphocytes by light microscopy, so-called *lymphokinecytes* (Fig. 6.13). Cells of the plasma cell series are found principally in the red pulp of the spleen and medulla of lymph nodes, while lymphogonia and lymphokinecytes are located in the splenic white pulp and diffuse cortex of nodes. Plasma cells forming γA-globulin are, however, most numerous in the lamina propria of the respiratory and gastrointestinal mucosa rather than in the peripheral lymphoid organs. Antibody-forming cells are also found in thoracic duct lymph and blood, and these also may be of any morphologic type (Figs. 6.15–17).

After a primary immunizing stimulus, in general, only scattered cells are found to form antibody, whereas after secondary immunization there will be large nests of dividing antibody-forming cells (Fig. 6.10) in the appropriate lymphoid organs. *Germinal centers*, which are round masses of rapidly dividing cells probably derived from single precursors, appear late in the primary response (Figs. 6.10,11). These may form any type of immunoglobulin and are thought to be related to the development of immunologic memory (see below). There may be extensive multiplication of antibody-forming cells in locations outside the lymphoid organs in cases of long-continued immunization or local immunization (Fig. 6.12). Needless to say, neoplasia results in large masses of immunoglobulin-forming cells (Fig. 6.11), the location varying with the cell type.

The use of immunofluorescence with specific staining for individual polypeptide chains and the use of double labeling have shown that a single cell makes only a single antibody. A whole germinal center may make a single homogeneous immunoglobulin. In a heterozygous animal, different plasma cells may make different products, e.g. different allotypes coded for by different alleles at a single gene locus. One plasma cell may however contain products of different loci, i.e. both an H and an L chain; but a single cell never contains both κ and λ or α and γ chains (some neoplastic cells are exceptions to this rule). The proportion of cells making a particular product is closely parallel to the plasma level of that product and to the frequency with which neoplasms of corresponding type arise.

The problem of immunological memory has not been fully resolved in cytological terms since no technique has been devised for identifying individual cells of this functional type. During the first weeks following an antigenic stimulus, X-irradiation has little suppressive effect on the development of immunologic memory, manifested by the ability to give an anamnestic response to a secondary dose of antigens. Later, however, memory is quite radiosensitive. Correspondingly, in the first weeks memory is unaffected by thoracic duct drainage, whereas later the memory cells are found to be part of the recirculating lymphocyte pool and to share most or all the properties of uncommitted small lymphocytes except for their greater number. Immunofluorescence and tissue culture studies suggest strongly that the lymphoid follicles and perhaps the germinal centers of spleen and lymph node are the site of formation of memory cells, some of which are discharged into the circulation as lymphocytes. Stimulation of those cells remaining in the follicle may lead to formation of a germinal center of antibody-forming cells (Figs. 6.10,11). Their stimulation elsewhere in the individual may give rise to the plasma cells appearing in the splenic red pulp and lymph node medulla. Circulating memory cells are ablated by treatment with antilymphocyte serum, with a corresponding loss of ability to give a secondary response.

A similar problem is presented by the effector cells of cellular (delayed) hypersensitivity. Indirect evidence suggests very strongly that large, dividing, blast-like (pyroninophilic) cells in the paracortical tissue of lymph nodes draining a site of immunization (Figs. 6.18–20) are responsible for this class of responses. Their progeny appear to be circulating small to medium-sized lymphocytes (committed cells, effector cells), which are capable of reacting with antigen at the site where a lesion is elicited (Section 16). These too are radiosensitive and easily destroyed by antilymphocyte serum (Fig. 16.5), and indeed are formally parallel to memory cells in many of their properties. Accordingly, the large pyroninophilic cells of the diffuse cortex may be morphologically indistinguishable from germinal center cells found in the follicles. However, the former are thymus-dependent and probably thymus-derived, whereas the origin of the latter is as yet unclear. The specificity requirements for molecules capable of eliciting an anamnestic response, on the one hand, or a delayed skin reaction on the other, in appropriately sensitized animals are closely comparable, and there appears to be a processing step (see below) in both cases.

An essential part of immunization is the processing of antigen in cells by which it is first taken up. An increasing mass of evidence suggests that for some (and possibly all) immune responses two cells are involved, a phagocytic cell and an immunocompetent lymphocyte. The most convincing studies concern interactions of cells in *in vitro* systems (Fig. 6.4). The morphologic equivalent of the immunization process may be the formation of reticulolymphocytic or reticuloplasmacytic islands commonly observed in cultures of spleen (Fig. 6.5) or lymph nodes. It can be shown that material (as large as ribosomes) can pass through cytoplasmic bridges between the cells of these islands. Various functional experiments show that lymphocytes are stimulated to form antibody after their contact with macrophages which have taken up antigen. The material that passes appears to be a special RNA moiety with attached antigen or an antigen fragment. It has been suggested that the RNA is thus brought to (or into) lymphocytes which possess specific combining sites for the antigen in question, i.e. are precoded to form antibody of appropriate specificity. It has also been suggested that the reaction of antigen (without attached RNA) with lymphocytes of appropriate specificity, with blocking of the specific sites or possibly lysis of the cells, results in tolerance. To avoid confusion, attention should be called to numerous experiments, involving both antibody formation and delayed hypersensitivity, in which specific reactivity is apparently conferred on normal lymphocytes treated with RNA extracted from already sensitized cells. Here one may be dealing with transfer of m-RNA; the significance of such experiments for events *in vivo* remains unknown. Recent findings suggest, however, that the immunization process, for some antigens, involves three cells rather than two. In mice immunized with sheep erythrocyte, the immune response (formation of

γM-antibody) is thymus-dependent and is characterized by a wave of replication in thymus-derived cells (these are large, pyroninophilic cells); yet the cells which finally make antibody come directly from the bone marrow. It is also suggested by recent work that the antigen–RNA complex may be an experimental artefact and that the antigen effective in immunization is that which remains attached to the surface membrane of the macrophage.

There have been extensive kinetic studies of primary and secondary immune responses *in vitro* or in diffusion chambers *in vivo* and of the biochemical and genetic events underlying antibody synthesis. These are of necessity nonmorphologic in character. Kinetic studies *in vivo* have almost all involved use of tritiated thymidine uptake, usually in conjunction with some method of identifying antibody-forming cells (Figs. 6.9,13,18), or the plaque-formation (Fig. 6.14) or rosette (Fig. 6.8) techniques. Heavy and light chains appear to be synthesized as single biosynthetic units on different polysomes. The heavy chains are not released from their polysomes until light chains, present in excess, combine with them to form complete dimers or possibly the complete antibody molecule. The carbohydrate component of the molecule is added, one sugar at a time, as part of the process of excretion of the antibody from the cell. At the height of the primary γM response or the secondary formation γG-globulin, more than 95 per cent of the antibody-forming cells divide. Cell-doubling times are often less than 12 hours, and the doubling time for RNA may be as low as 4 hours. Thus antibody formation is inhibited by inhibitors of DNA synthesis (bromouridine deoxyriboside, H^3-thymidine of high activity) or RNA synthesis (actinomycin D). The rate of protein formation is determined by both processes, being logarithmic at first and arithmetic after cell division stops. Synthesis is inhibited by amino acid analogues, chloroamphenicol, puromycin, etc.

With regard to the relationship of precursor cells to memory cells to end cells actually synthesizing antibody, variously described as $PC_1 \rightarrow PC_2 \rightarrow P$ or $X \rightarrow Y \rightarrow Z$, there has been a good deal of speculation concerning the cell number and proliferation in each compartment, cell generation time, uni- or multipotentiality, antigen concentration required to paralyze or to stimulate transformation to the next cell type, type of immunoglobulin formed, etc. The existing theories are not consistent as yet. Attempts to study successive steps of this process *in vivo* have been only partially successful, as a result of the problem of H^3-thymidine reutilization (Fig. 6.9) and our inability to identify precursor or memory cells morphologically. Cell multiplication in germinal centers occurs at a rate comparable to that of plasma cell division in the secondary response.

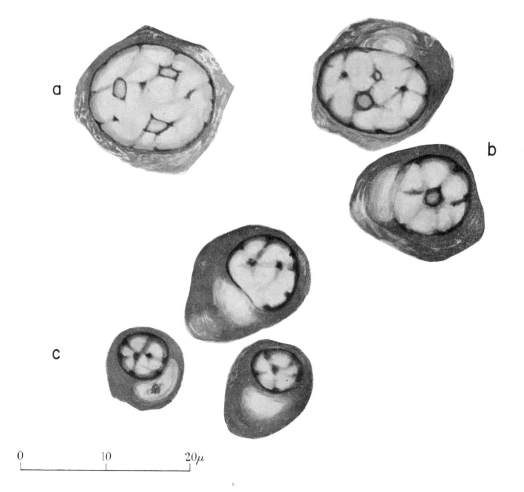

Fig. 6.1. Sequence of cell forms in the plasmacyte series, as described by Fagraeus and later by Coons and his collaborators and by Marshall and White, showing appearance of cells in sections stained with methyl green–pyronine and illustrating progressive decrease in size and in nucleocytoplasmic ratio, condensation of nuclear chromatin, increase in pyroninophilia, and development of cytoplasmic "Hof" representing the Golgi body. (a) Earliest form in the series, variously referred to as activated reticulum cell, large lymphocyte, splenic tumor cell, transitional cell, hemocytoblast, immunoblast, or simply blast. (b) Plasmablasts. (c) Immature and mature plasmacytes.

From Marshall and White, *Brit. J. Exp. Path. 31*: 157–74 (1950).

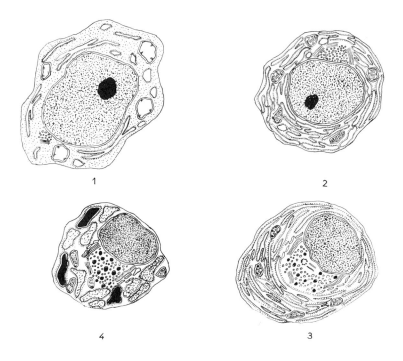

Fig. 6.2. Principal ultrastructural features of cells in the plasma cells series. In mature cell (3), note well-elaborated rough endoplasmic reticulum and prominent Golgi apparatus, both essential elements of cell which synthesizes and secretes protein. In degenerating cell (4), there are dilated cisternae of endoplasmic reticulum, filled with antibody. These correspond to Russell bodies.

From Bernhard and Granboulan, in CIBA *Symposium on Cellular Aspects of Immunity*, G. E. W. Wolstenholme and M. O'Connor, eds., Churchill, London, 1960, pp. 92–121.

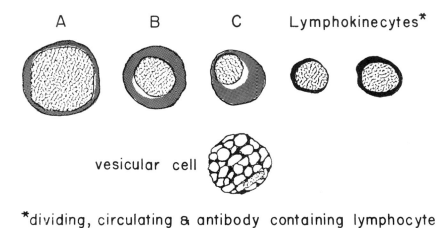

Fig. 6.3. Types of antibody-forming cells. The lymphokinecytes are dividing, circulating, and antibody-containing lymphocytes.

From Vazquez, in *The Thymus in Immunobiology*, R. A. Good and A. E. Gabrielson, eds., Harper and Row, New York, 1964, pp. 298–316.

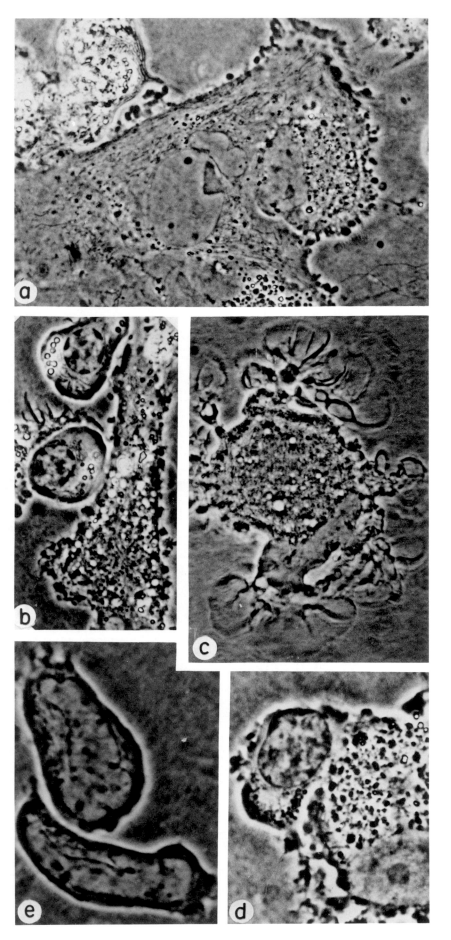

Fig. 6.4. Cells types seen in living cultures (9–12 days) of guinea pig spleen in the presence of homologous serum and chick embryo extract. (a) Nonphagocytic reticulum cell. Note pale nucleus with moderate-sized nucleolus, mitochondria, and granular cytoplasm. This may be type of cell primarily involved in uptake of antigen at surface membrane, as in follicles (Figs. 2.4, 5, 7). (b–d) Phagocytic reticulum cells. All show inclusions of various sizes, and cell illustrated in (c) shows active pinocytosis. Plasma cells with clock-face nuclei are adherent in (b), and a small lymphocyte in (d). (e) Histiocytes, actively motile and with few inclusions. These appear to correspond to the blood-borne, marrow-derived cells which participate secondarily in nonspecific inflammation and in reactions of delayed hypersensitivity. They are designated monocytes or prehistiocytes while they remain in the circulation.

Phase contrast; (a–c) ×1,265, (d, e) ×1,900. Courtesy of Drs. R. Robineaux and J. Pinet.

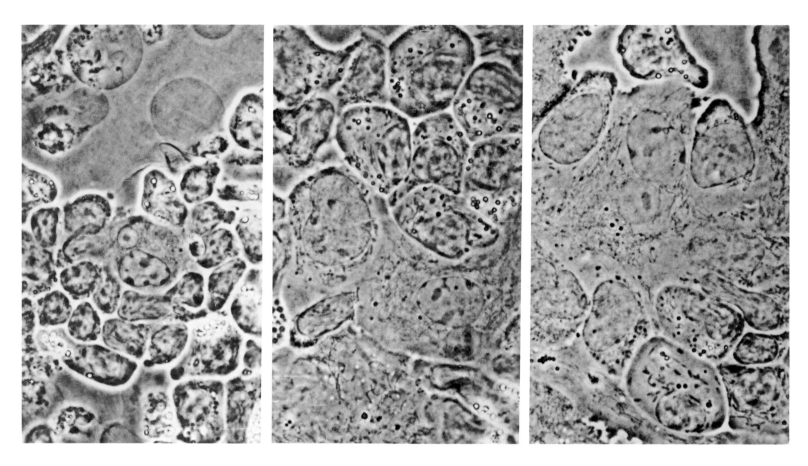

Fig. 6.5. Formation of islands or clusters of lymphocytes or plasma cells about reticular cells in long-term cultures of chicken spleen. Culture medium contains foreign serum. Clustering permits cell-cell interaction and initiation of an immune response. Left to right: 11-, 13-, and 15-day cultures. (Left) Satellite cells are small lymphocytes; (center and right) predominantly plasma cells.

Phase contrast; ×1,250. From Robineaux, Pinet, and Kourilsky, *Compt. rend. Soc. Biol. 156*: 1025–34 (1962).

Fig. 6.6 Mediastinal lymph node of young adult rat. Portion of a medullary cord showing the cells that fill it. L, M, and S indicate large, medium, and small plasmocytes respectively. Note that (1) all gradations of size exist between the largest and the smallest nuclei; (2) cells have a well-outlined, deeply basophilic, and usually pentagonal cytoplasm showing, in several cells, a pale Golgi zone; (3) the nucleolar apparatus may vary in appearance even in nuclei, of similar size, although the two largest plasmocytes seen here have a single large nucleolus.

Bouin-Hollande fixation, Dominici stain; × 2,433. Courtesy of Dr. G. Sainte Marie.

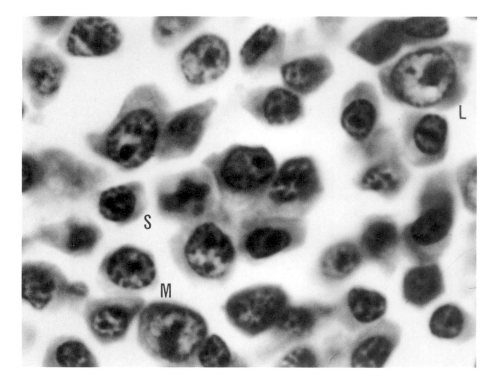

Fig. 6.7. Normal plasma cell from lymph node medulla. Cytoplasm is filled with rough endoplasmic reticulum (ergastoplasm) (ER) and there is a prominent nucleolus. Chromatin condensations along the nuclear membrane, forming the clock-face pattern common in conventional histologic preparations, are not seen with this type of fixation and embedding.

Electron micrograph; × 12,000. From Bessis, in *Electron Microscopic Anatomy*, S. M. Kurtz, ed., Academic Press, New York, 1964.

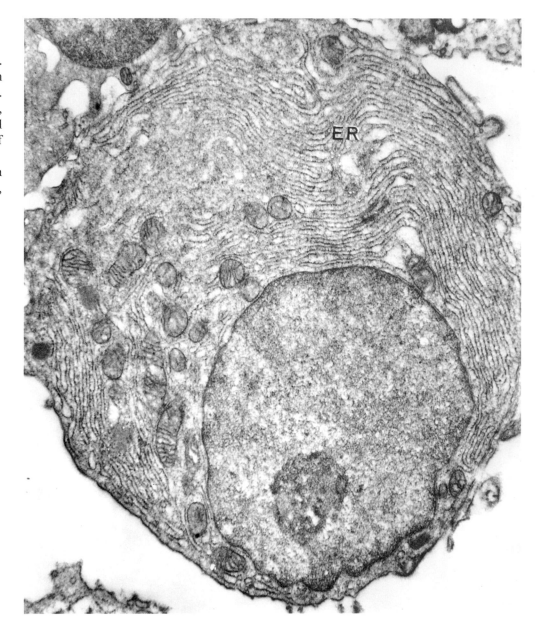

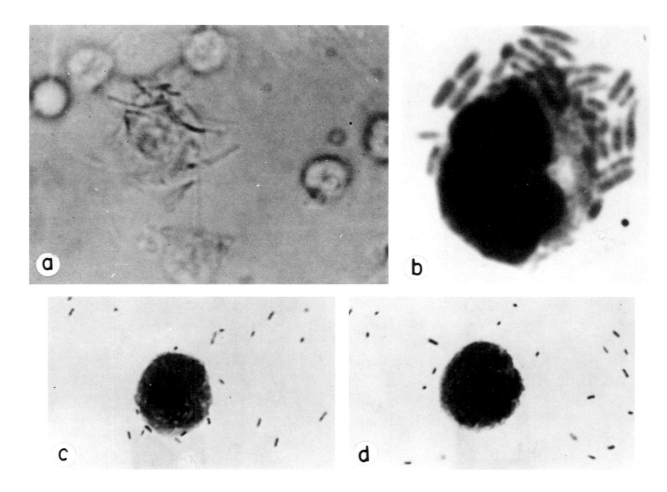

Fig. 6.8. Adherence of antigen-containing bacteria to antibody-forming cells. (a) Cell suspension from popliteal lymph node of rabbit inoculated 5 days earlier in footpad of same extremity with typhoid bacilli. Note adherence of bacteria to single antibody-forming plasma cell. (b) *Salmonella adelaide* adhering to antibody-forming cell isolated by micromanipulation from a rat popliteal lymph node cell suspension. (c) Round cell in rat peripheral blood 5 days after iv injection of typhoid bacilli. (d) Control cell showing absence of adherence. (a) Living Janus-green preparation; × 1,250; (b) orcein-light green; × 2,500. (c, d) Wright's stain; × 1,250. (a) From Reiss, Mertens, and Ehrich, *Proc. Soc. Exp. Biol. Med. 74*: 732–35 (1950). (b) Courtesy of Dr. G. J. V. Nossal. (c, d) From Gunderson, Juras, LaVia, and Wissler, *J. Am. Med. Assoc. 180*: 1038–47 (1962).

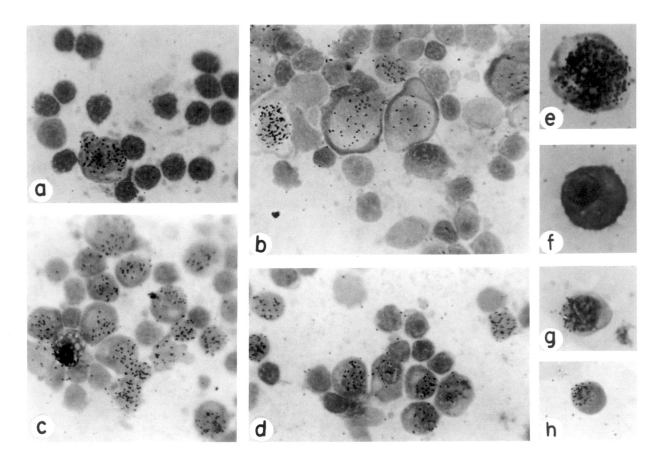

Fig. 6.9. (a–d) Autoradiographs of rat lymph node smears prepared at various times after a single brief pulse of H³-thymidine. Two hours after the isotope, a secondary antigenic stimulus (*Salmonella adelaide* flagellin) was given. Rats were killed at intervals. The times cited below refer to the period allowed to elapse between isotope injection and killing. (a) Two hours; note the labeled large lymphocyte and unlabeled small lymphocytes. (b) Two days; note the labeled plasmablasts, an unlabeled mature plasma cell, and an occasional labeled small lymphocyte. (c) Four days; note the many labeled cells, including immature and mature plasma cells and small lymphocytes. A Russell-body plasma cell is very heavily labeled. (d) Six days; the plasma cells now look quite mature and are all labeled. Some labeled small lymphocytes are also present. In experiments done in this manner, there is extensive reutilization of thymidine.

(e–h) Individual cells taken from lymph nodes of similar rats at various intervals after secondary stimulus and after a pulse of H³-thymidine. Each cell was tested for its antibody-forming activity in microdroplet culture and then used to prepare the autoradiograph. (e) Two days after antigen, 1 hour after label; blast cell, which formed antibody weakly takes up thymidine, i.e. is dividing. (f) Five days after antigen, 1 hour after label; mature plasma cell, forming antibody strongly, is apparently nondividing. (g, h) Five days after antigen, 12 and 48 hours after label; immature and mature plasma cells, forming antibody and labeled.

All are stripping film autoradiographs, stained with Giemsa; ×2,400. From Nossal and Mäkelä, *J. Exp. Med. 115*: 209–44 (1962).

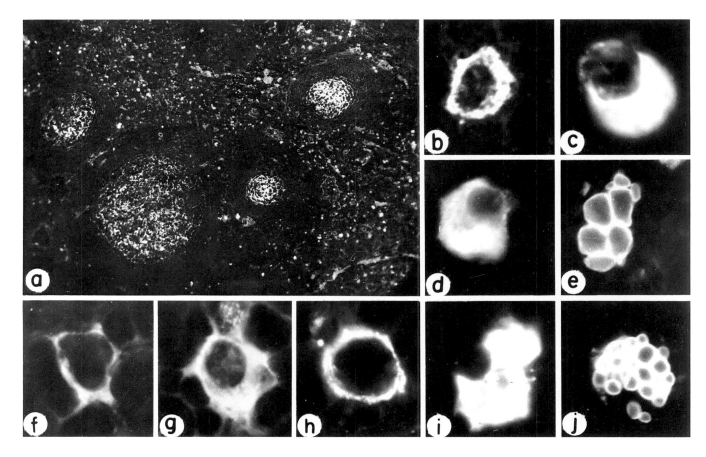

Fig. 6.10. Cellular origin of human immunoglobins, in biopsy specimens of lymph nodes and other tissues from subjects with various non-neoplastic diseases. (a) Four germinal centers forming γG-globulin. (b) Primitive (reticular) cell forming mouse γG-globulin in thymus gland of 6-week-old mouse. (c) Mature plasma cell forming γG-globulin. (d) Mature plasma cell forming γA-globulin. (e) Russel body plasma cell forming γA-globulin. (f) Large primitive (reticular) cell forming γM-globulin. (g) Primitive (reticular) cell forming γM-globulin. (h) Plasmablast forming γM-globulin. (i) Mature plasma cell forming γM-globulin. (j) Russel body plasma cell forming γM-globulin in spleen.

Frozen sections, fluorescence technique; (a) $\times 100$, others $\times 1,500$. From Mellors and Korngold, *J. Exp. Med. 118*: 387–96 (1963).

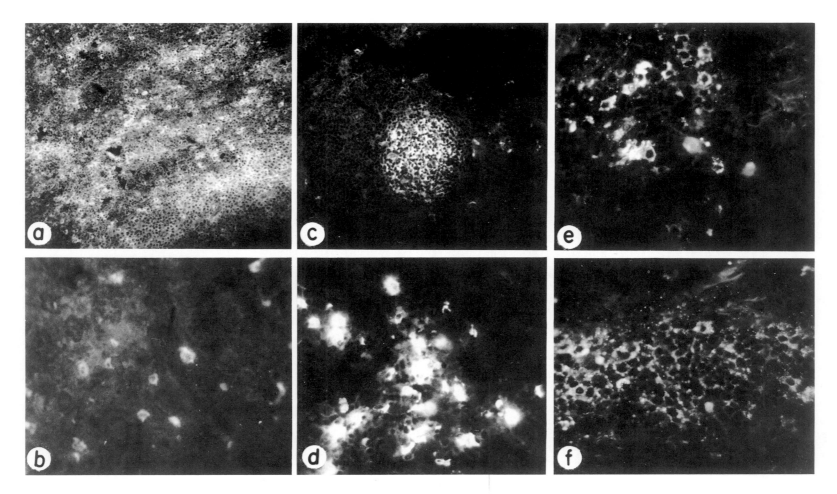

Fig. 6.11. Cells forming γM-globulin. (a) Localization of γM in lymph node of patient with Waldenström's macroglobulinemia. (b) Localization in isolated plasma cells in node of patient with cholecystitis. (c, d) Localization in germinal center and medullary plasma cells of lymph nodes in patient with rheumatoid arthritis.

(e, f) Localization of rheumatoid factor, by the use of aggregated fluorescent fraction II, in germinal center and medullary cords of epitrochlear nodes in rheumatoid arthritis.

Fluorescence technique. Courtesy of Dr. M. H. Kaplan.

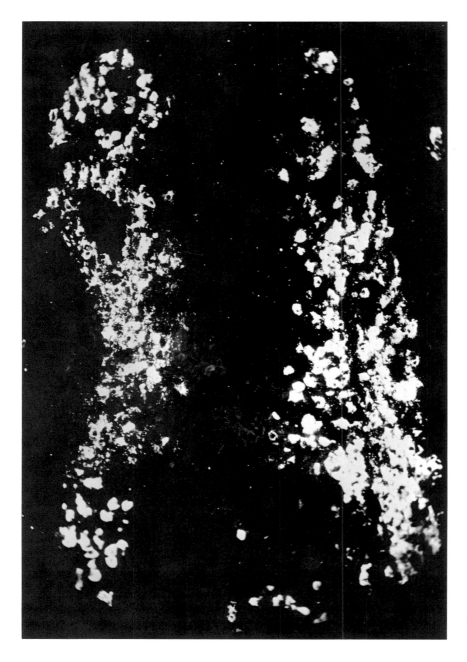

Fig. 6.12. Synovial membrane of patient with rheumatoid arthritis, stained by fluorescence method for cellular origin of rheumatoid factor. Two hypertrophic villi, vertically oriented with their submesothelial inflammatory cores rich in plasma cells containing rheumatoid factor.

×245. From Mellors, Heimer, Corcos, and Korngold, *J. Exp. Med. 110*: 875–86 (1959).

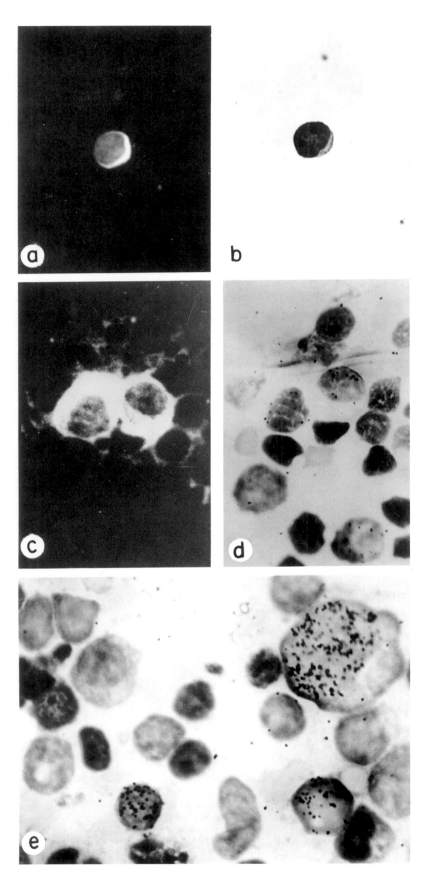

Fig. 6.13. Different types of antibody-forming cells from spleens of immunized rabbits. (a, b) Immunization with BSA. Lympho-kinecytes stained for antibody by fluorescence technique and later restained with Giemsa. (c, d) Spleen cells 4 days after secondary stimulus with BGG in rabbit receiving primary immunization 4 weeks earlier. Pair of immature plasma cells (type B) stained for antibody (fluorescence) and corresponding autoradiograph, counter-stained with Wright's stain (H³-thymidine 0.25 mC/g given at 6-hour intervals from time of secondary stimulus). One non-fluorescent cell also shows nuclear grains. (e) Autoradiograph, showing blast cell and small lymphoid cell (lymphokinecyte) labeled by single pulse of H³-thymidine given 2 hours earlier. Giemsa.

All are brush smear preparations; various magnifications. From Vazquez: (a, b) in *The Thymus in Immunobiology*, R. A. Good and A. E. Gabrielson, eds., Harper and Row, New York, 1964, pp. 298–316; (c, d) *Proc. Soc. Exp. Biol. Med. 109*: 1–4 (1962); (e) unpublished.

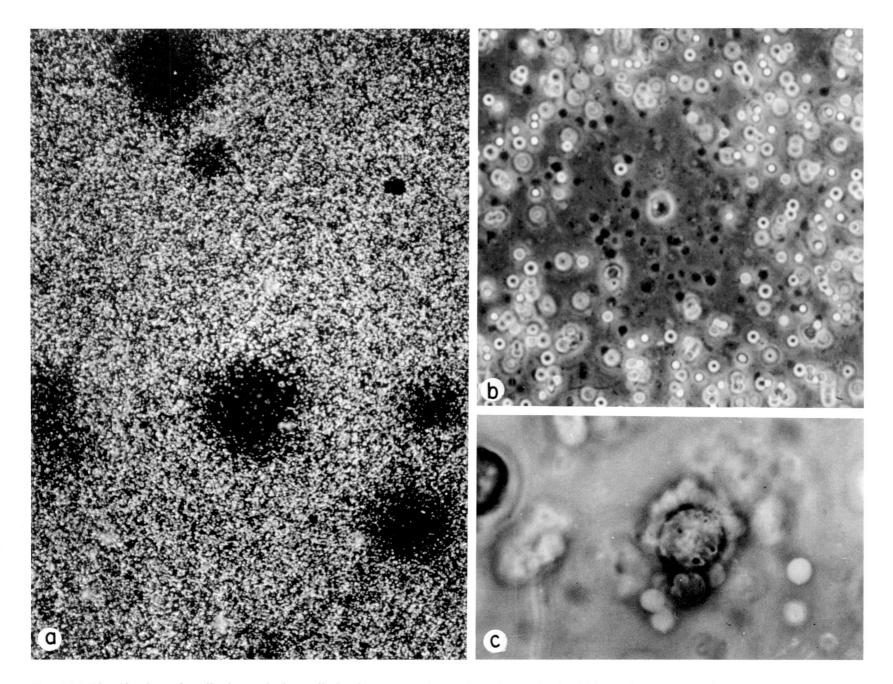

Fig. 6.14. Identification of antibody-producing cells by formation of plaques of lysis in suspension of red cells in agar gel after incubation and addition of complement. (a) Mouse peritoneal exudate cells incubated for 24 hours with sheep erythrocytes and showing primary (?) antibody response. Several large and small plaques are seen in test suspension. (b) Single plaque-forming cell in suspension of spleen cells from immunized rabbit, maintained in culture with erythrocytes for 4 hours. (c) Higher-power view of "normal" mouse peritoneal cell in center of plaque of lysis.

Phase contrast. (a) ×40, (b) ×320, (c) ×800. Courtesy of Dr. A. E. Bussard.

Antibody-producing cells in rabbit lymph and blood. Plaque-forming cells (forming 19S γM antibody) in efferent lymph from the draining popliteal node, 4 days after footpad injection of sheep red blood cells (Figs. 6.15, 6.16) and in the blood 3 days after secondary stimulation with the same antigen iv (Fig. 6.17). Cells picked from each plaque and examined by electron microscopy. N, nucleus; M, mitochondria; ER, endoplasmic reticulum; G, Golgi complex.

From Hummeler, Harris, Tomassini, Hechtel, and Farber, *J. Exp. Med. 124*: 255–62 (1966).

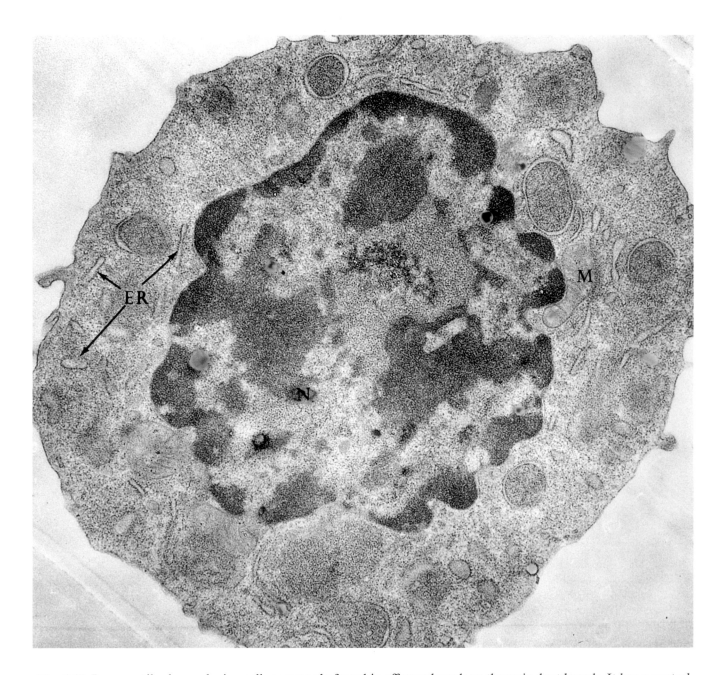

Fig. 6.15. Large antibody-producing cell, commonly found in efferent lymph or thoracic duct lymph. It has a central, irregular nucleus with condensed chromatin; short, wide endoplasmic reticulum channels; and many free ribosomes. ×24,000.

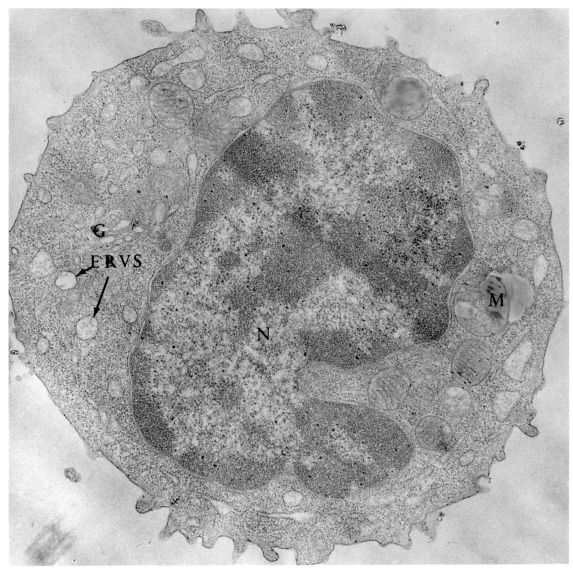

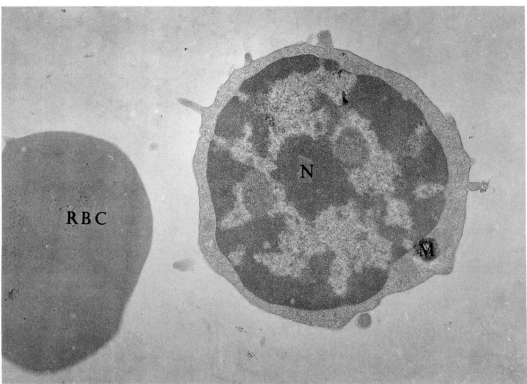

Fig. 6.16. (Above) Smaller cell of same type, with slightly eccentric, indented nucleus having condensed chromatin. This cell has well-developed Golgi complex, with many smooth vesicles. The endoplasmic reticulum is widened in places to give appearance of vesicles (ERVS); ×24,000. (Below) Small lymphocyte outside plaque. This cell is not forming antibody and adjacent red cell is not lysed. Minimal cytoplasm with few mitochondria and no endoplasmic reticulum; ×16,000.

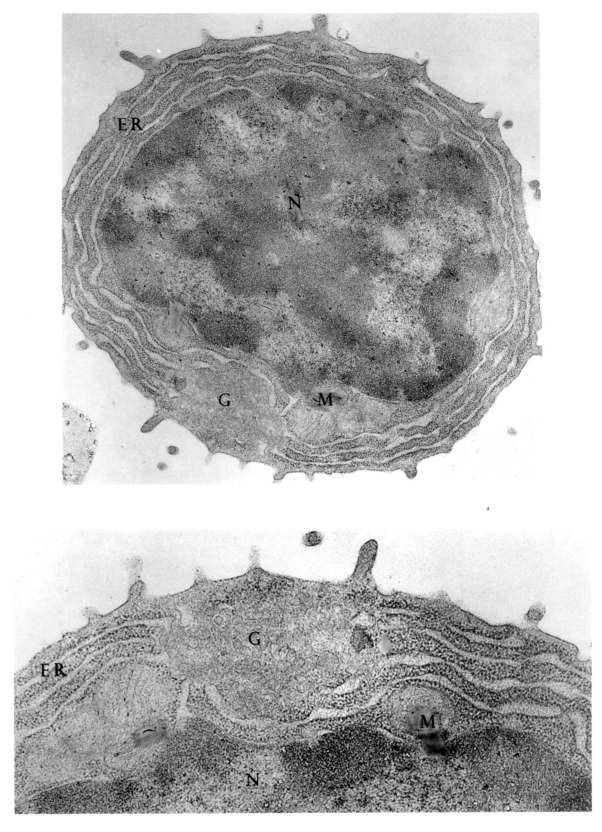

Fig. 6.17. Small antibody-forming lymphocyte. This cell has central irregular nucleus with condensed chromatin. Limited cytoplasm contains a few mitochondria, a large, well-developed Golgi zone, and parallel lamellae of widened endoplasmic reticulum; ×24,000. Higher-power view (below) shows direct connections between channels of ER and smooth vesicles of Golgi apparatus; ×40,000.

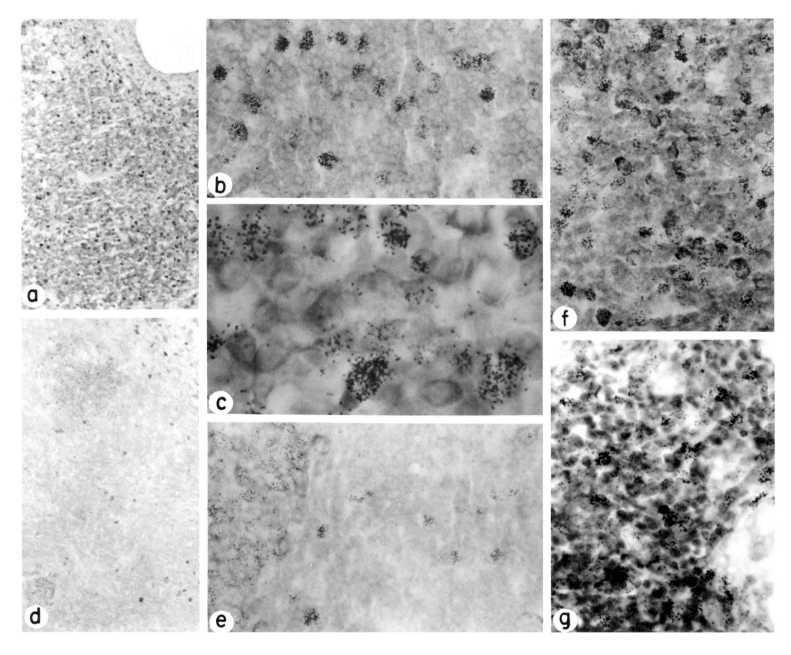

Fig. 6.18. Dividing lymphoblasts (lymphogonia) in lymph nodes of rats injected in left hind footpad with rat spinal cord and adjuvant. (a–c) Draining (left inguinal) node at 5 days, 1 hour after pulse of H³-thymidine. Large numbers of medium and large, more or less basophilic, cells synthesizing DNA are seen throughout cortex. Oil droplet is seen at upper right in (a). (d, e) Nondraining (contralateral) node of same rat showing two germinal centers. In higher-power view, incorporation of thymidine is seen in germinal center cells. There are almost no dividing cells in cortex. (f, g) Draining nodes in rats given repeated doses of H³-thymidine on days 4 and 5 and sacrificed on days 7 and 10 respectively. At 7 days there are large numbers of labeled cortical lymphoblasts, somewhat smaller than cells initially labeled (compare b). By 10 days, remaining labeled cells are almost all small or medium sized and few are basophilic.

Stripping-film autoradiographs, stained with Giemsa; (a, d) ×80, (b, e–g) ×240, (c) ×500. Unpublished data of T. U. Kosunen and B. H. Waksman.

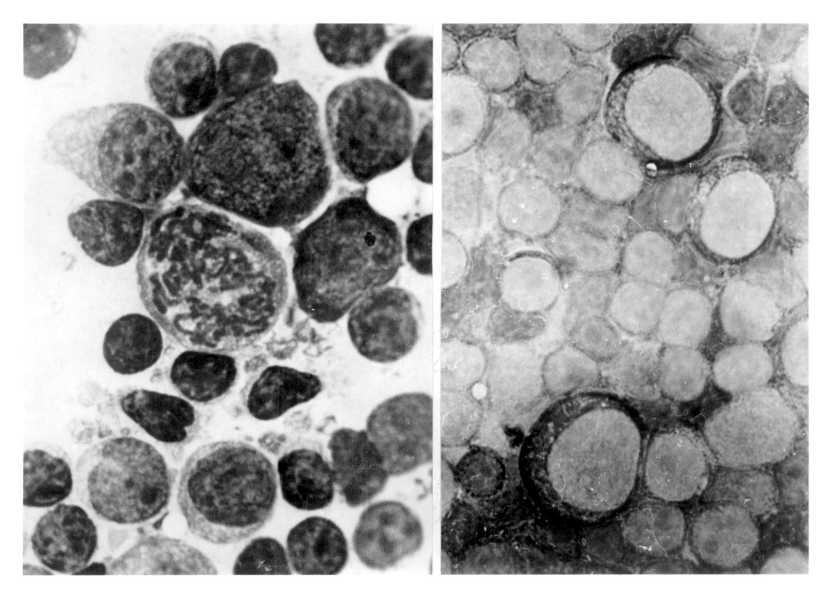

Fig. 6.19. Large pyroninophilic cells in prints of rabbit lymph nodes draining sites of implantation of skin homografts. These lymphoblasts or "lymphogonia" (Amano) characteristically proliferate in the cortex during responses involving cellular sensitization. They are indistinguishable from large germinal center cells and the earliest blasts of the plasma cell series, which form antibody. (Left) First-set graft, 6 days. Cells are stained with con-

ventional Romanowsky stain. Of the two lymphogonia, one is in mitosis and the other has two very prominent nucleoli. (Right) Second-set graft, 4 days. Methyl green–pyronine, which brings out intense cytoplasmic basophilia, corresponding to the large number of free ribosomes seen in electron micrographs of these cells.

×2,000. From André and Schwartz, *Blood 19*: 313–33 (1962).

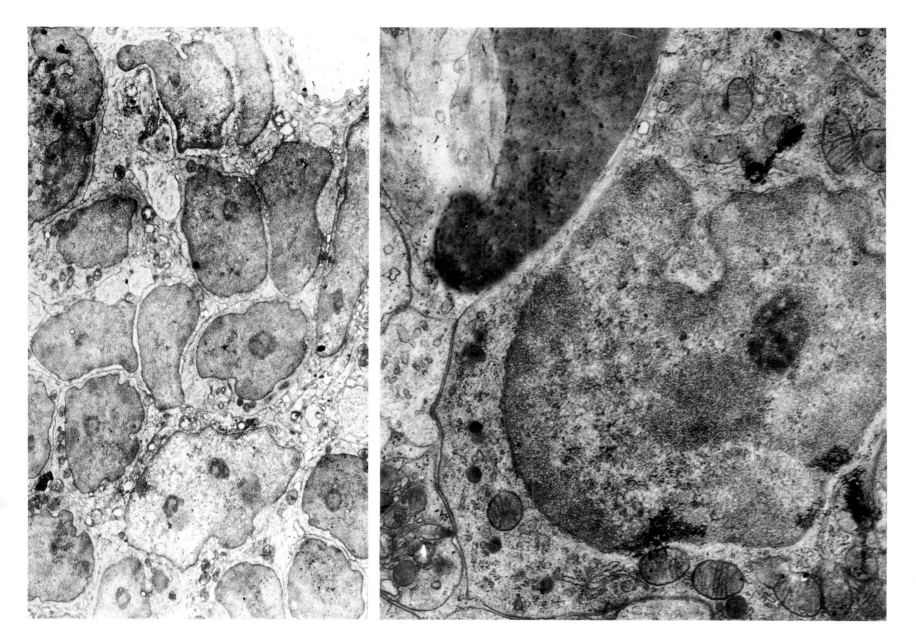

Fig. 6.20. Large pyroninophilic cells (lymphoblasts, "lymphogonia"). (Left) Cortex of regional lymph node in C57B1 mouse, 7 days after receiving a first-set graft from DBA/2 donor. (Right) Rat splenic white pulp, 30 days after first-set skin homograft. Note large centrally placed nuclei, prominent nucleoli, absence of endoplasmic reticulum, and numerous free ribosomes.

Electron micrographs; ×2,800 and ×28,000. (a) Courtesy of Dr. J.-L. Binet. (b) Courtesy of Dr. J. André-Schwartz (see André and Schwartz *Blood 24*: 113–33, 1964).

7. Phylogeny and Ontogeny of Lymphoid Organs

Adaptive immune responses have not been clearly identified in *invertebrates*. Nonspecific agglutinating and lytic "antibodies" are formed rapidly after a variety of stimuli, and each species has an elaborate array of phagocytic cell types which also respond rapidly to foreign bodies entering their tissues or fluids. Current research on tissue grafting suggests the possibility that specific responses may yet be discovered.

In *poikilothermic vertebrates*, all the characteristic adaptive immune responses are found, except that γG-antibody is not formed by elasmobranchs and holosteans. Antibody formation and the cellular type of sensitization are as intense and specific as in birds and mammals, the *rate* being *controlled by temperature* (in hibernating mammals the rate is also controlled by temperature). Antibody formation is correlated with the presence of a thymus and a system of lymphocytes in the blood and tissues, and with pyroninophilic cells in lymphoid organs and immunoglobulins in the blood stream (Fig. 7.1). In cyclostomes, responses and the corresponding blood and tissue elements are lacking (hagfish) or minimal (lamprey). In urodeles, responses have been regarded as weak, resembling those in immature anurans. However, recent work shows that these weak responses are the result of widespread sharing of histocompatibility antigens rather than an actual deficiency in immune responsiveness.

In lower poikilotherms, the *thymus* placode has a structure indistinguishable from that of the mammalian and avian thymus (Fig. 7.1). The peripheral lymphoid organs also contain familiar parts, but often in unfamiliar arrangements. The development of the *spleen* may be traced from fusion of gut-associated masses of lymphoid tissue (Fig. 7.1). In the toad, the spleen already possesses an antigen-trapping mechanism while the *jugular bodies*, presumed precursors of lymph nodes, lack follicles, cortex, medulla, or antigen-trapping reticulum (Fig. 7.2). In monotremes such as the echidna, in addition to the thymus, appendix, and spleen one finds *vascular lymphoid nodules* intermediate in character between the jugular bodies and true lymph nodes (Figs. 7.3–6); each is a follicle surrounded by a circular sinus and containing a germinal center. They possess an antigen-retaining reticulum and look like lymph node follicles without accompanying cortex or medulla. In birds the bursa of Fabricius functions as a separate and important central lymphoid organ.

The synthesis of all immunoglobulins begins during fetal life in various mammalian species, including man. The sequence following an antigenic stimulus resembles that in the adult, but the levels attained are very low. Ontogeny appears to recapitulate phylogeny, in that the capacity to form γM- and γA-immunoglobulins and to develop the cellular type of sensitization, e.g. rejection of skin homografts, appear earlier in gestation than the formation of γG-immunoglobulin. Indeed, the latter cannot be detected in the circulation until after birth in many cases (4–6 weeks in man). All systems mature slowly; adult levels are reached over months or in some instances years.

The *ability to respond* has been specifically *related to the presence of lymphocytes in peripheral lymphatic tissue* (spleen, lymph nodes, gastrointestinal mucosa). Thus in the chicken, lymphopoiesis is seen in the embryonic thymus by 11 days and in the bursa of Fabricius a day or two later (Fig. 5.2), but lymphocytes appear in the spleen only at 15 days, in the gut at 19 days, and in the circulation at about the time of hatching. Immune reactivity appears only after 15 days. Similarly in the opossum, which is born 12–13 days after conception, thymus lymphopoiesis begins 2–5 days after birth and lymphocytes appear in the lymph nodes and spleen at 6–10 and 17–25 days respectively; antibody responses can first be elicited after 8 days. Antigen introduced at a time when the preponderant lymphocyte population is in the thymus (and bursa) will induce tolerance in these cells, and the immune response of lymphocytes already present in the periphery may be so small as to require special means of detection. The formation of "natural" antibodies against various bacteria and heterologous erythrocytes, generally thought to be induced by immunization against the gastrointestinal flora and other common antigenic stimuli, parallels the development of immunologic competence.

The actual induction of cellular sensitization and formation of γM and γA types of antibody are associated with the development of large lymphocytes and cells of the lymphogonia type (lymphocytoid plasma cells). The later maturation of the γG function parallels the maturation of the germinal center and plasma cell system, and the intensity of the response is related to the presence of a follicular antigen-trapping mechanism. In rats an antigen-trapping reticulum is first seen 10–14 days postnatally and the adult follicular structure at about 3 weeks. The maturation of peripheral lymphoid elements may be accelerated under intensive antigenic stimulation such as infection (Fig. 7.8). Conversely, if antigenic stimuli are reduced postnatally, as in *germ-free* (axenic, gnotobiotic) *animals*, large lymphocytoid elements, germinal centers, and plasma cells do not develop in the peripheral lymphoid organs and "natural" antibodies fail to make their appearance. Ablation of central lymphoid organs early in development leads to later deficits in the corresponding lymphocyte populations of the peripheral lymphoid organs and of end cells derived from these (Sections 3–5).

It is of interest that the *ability to respond to antigens of different specificity* matures at widely different times. It is thought that this facet of immune responsiveness is determined by qualitative changes in antigen-processing cells, either with regard to "receptor" sites on their surface or their complement of enzymes. Indirect support for the former is derived from study of the responses of different inbred mouse strains, whose ability to respond to specific antigenic molecules is found to be linked genetically to histocompatibility antigens, i.e. cell membrane characteristics. Passive transfer studies between animals genetically able and unable to respond to a particular antigen have shown that the defect in "nonresponders" depends on specific characteristics of the processing system.

The fetal and newborn animals' weak immunologic defenses are supplemented by *antibody transferred passively from the mother*, either prior to birth (rabbit, guinea pig, man), after birth (ruminants, horse, pig), or both (chicken, rat, mouse, carnivores). In the chicken, antibody passes through the yolk sac entoderm into the vitelline circulation, and this absorption from the yolk sac continues after hatching. In the rabbit and guinea pig also, maternal antibody passes only by way of the yolk sac entoderm and vitelline vessels. In the rat and mouse this mechanism is the same, but there is also absorption of antibody from the amniotic fluid in the fetal stomach and similar absorption from the gut continues 18–20 days postnatally. In ruminants, the only antibody to pass at any time is taken up from the colostrum in the first day or two after birth. In each case, only γG-immunoglobulin passes the yolk sac or gastrointestinal entoderm. In man, γG may pass directly through the placenta and there is evidence that the placenta itself, in the last trimester of pregnancy, may become an antibody-forming organ.

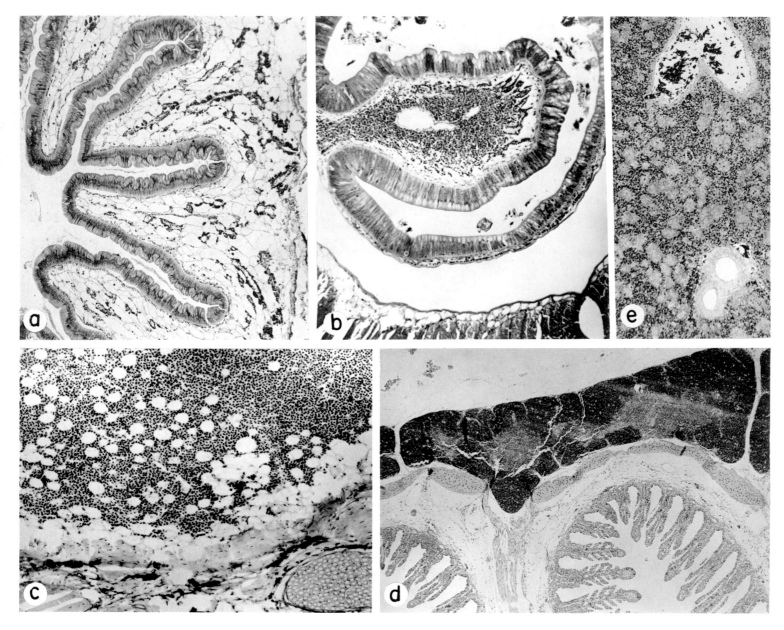

Fig. 7.1. Phylogeny of central and peripheral lymphoid organs. (a) Cross section of the gut tract of the hagfish showing primitive blood islands in the submucosa. The hagfish has no spleen. (b) Ammocete larva of the lamprey, *Petromyzon marinus:* section through the gut tract showing accumulation of hematopoietic tissue. A true spleen is not found until the higher fishes, elasmobranchs and teleosts. (c) Hematopoietic tissue in the cartilaginous vertebral arch of the lamprey. This tissue reacts to antigenic stimulation with cell proliferation. This is the most primitive form of intramedullary hematopoiesis. (d) Thymus of a newborn guitarfish, *Rhinobatos productus,* located above the gill arches. Note cortical and medullary areas already developed in this newborn elasmobranch. (e) Spleen section from *Amia calva,* the Mississippi bowfin, a holostean fish. This animal has complete immunological competence, including ability to give delayed reactions, produce circulating antibody, and reject homografts. From Finstad, Papermaster, and Good, *Lab. Invest.* 13: 490–512 (1964).

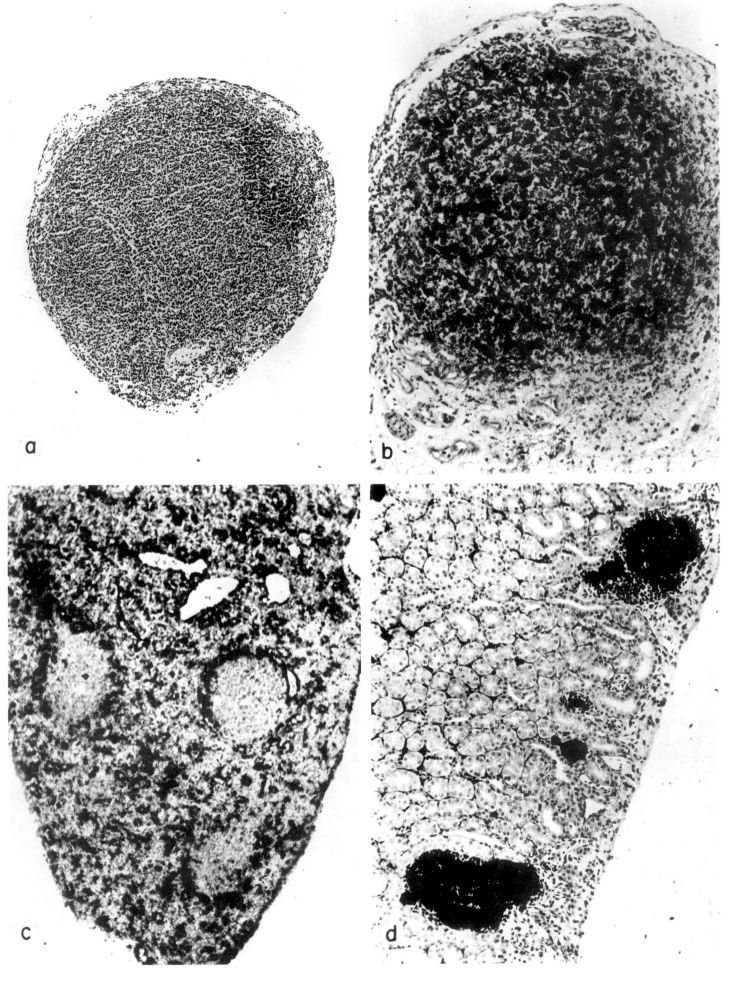

Fig. 7.2. Principal lymphoid organs of the toad, *Bufo marinus*. (a, b) Jugular bodies, small yellow-brown nodules attached to the main vessels close to the pericardium at each side of the heart. In conventional cell stain (a) note absence of circular sinus, germinal centers, or differentiation into cortex and medulla. In autoradiograph, prepared 1 day after footpad injection of 50 μg I^{125}-flagella (b), antigen is seen to be randomly scattered throughout the nodule. (c) Spleen in similar animal shows uptake of labeled flagella at scattered points in red pulp and selective accumulation around the borders of white pulp islands. (d) Uptake of colloidal carbon 24 hours after injection, in lymphoid foci of kidney. The absence of a follicular antigen-trapping reticulum and of germinal centers in these organs may be related to the absence of immunological memory.

(a) Toluidine blue; $\times 80$. (b, c) Methyl green-pyronine; $\times 150$, $\times 100$. (d) Hematoxylin-eosin; $\times 200$. From Diener and Nossal, *Immunology 10*: 535–42 (1966).

FIGURES 7.3–7.6
Lymphoid organs of a monotreme, the Australian echidna, *Tachyglossus aculeatus*.
From Diener, Ealey, and Legge, *Immunology 13*: 339–47 (1967).

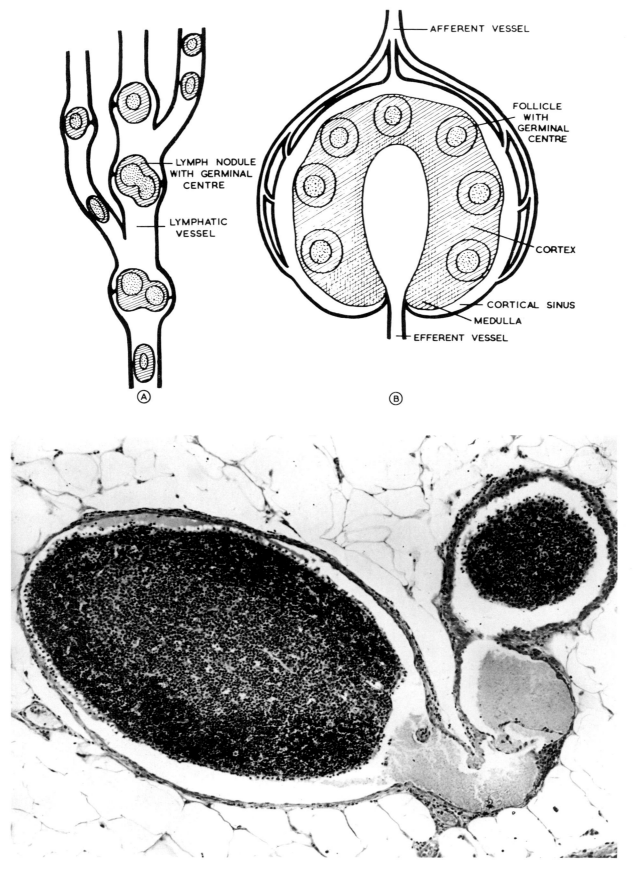

Fig. 7.3. (Above) Comparison of lymph nodules of the echidna within lymphatic vessels, A, and the lymph node of the rat, B. (Below) Typical lymph nodules. The "circular sinus" is defined by the interspace between the periphery of the nodule and the wall of the lymphatic vessel. These lymph nodules seem closely comparable, in their histologic character and functional attributes, to the cortical follicles in lymph nodes of higher mammals.

Hematoxylin-eosin; ×140.

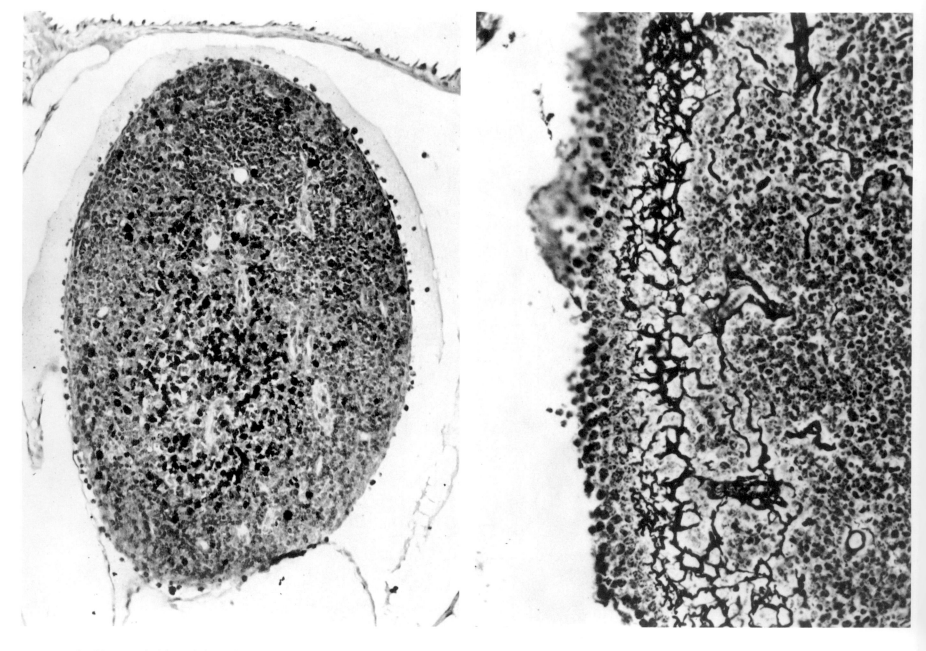

Fig. 7.4. (Left) Lymphoid nodule, 3 hours after injection of H³-thymidine. High labeling of germinal center area represents rapid cell proliferation, comparable to that seen in germinal centers of lymph nodes in placental mammals. (Right) Periphery of nodule, stained for reticulum, shows web-like processes of reticulum cells which take up labeled antigen or carbon.

(Left) Methyl green–pyronine; × 200. (Right) Silver impregnation technique of Gordon and Sweets; × 600.

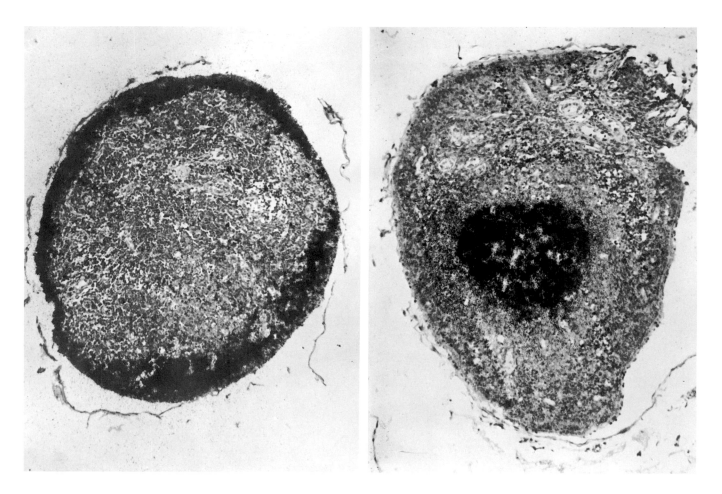

Fig. 7.5. Autoradiographs of lymph nodules, 24 hours (left) and 5 days (right) after subcutaneous and intravenous injection of I¹²⁵-labeled flagella. Uptake of antigen is seen first in periphery of nodule, in close relation to dendritic reticulum. Later it is concentrated in central, proliferative zone of nodule. This sequence is closely similar to that observed in primary follicles of placental mammalian lymph node. Methyl green–pyronine; × 112, × 156.

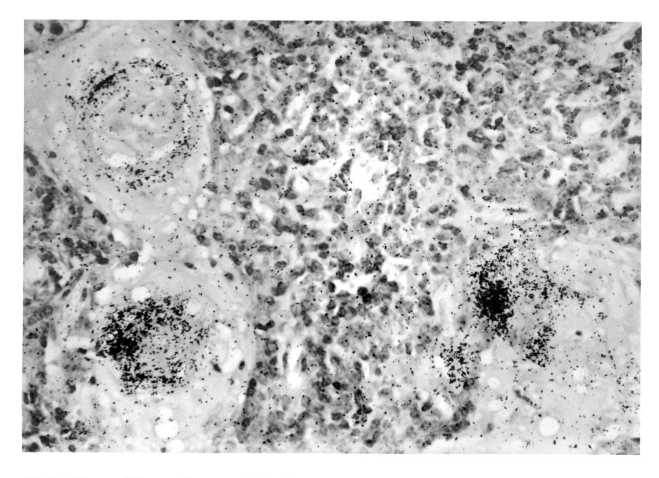

Fig. 7.6. Thymus, 24 hours after systemic injection of I¹²⁵-labeled flagella. Antigen is selectively taken up by the Hassall's corpuscles. (Grains visible outside the Hassall's corpuscles are background label.)
Methyl green–pyronine; × 840.

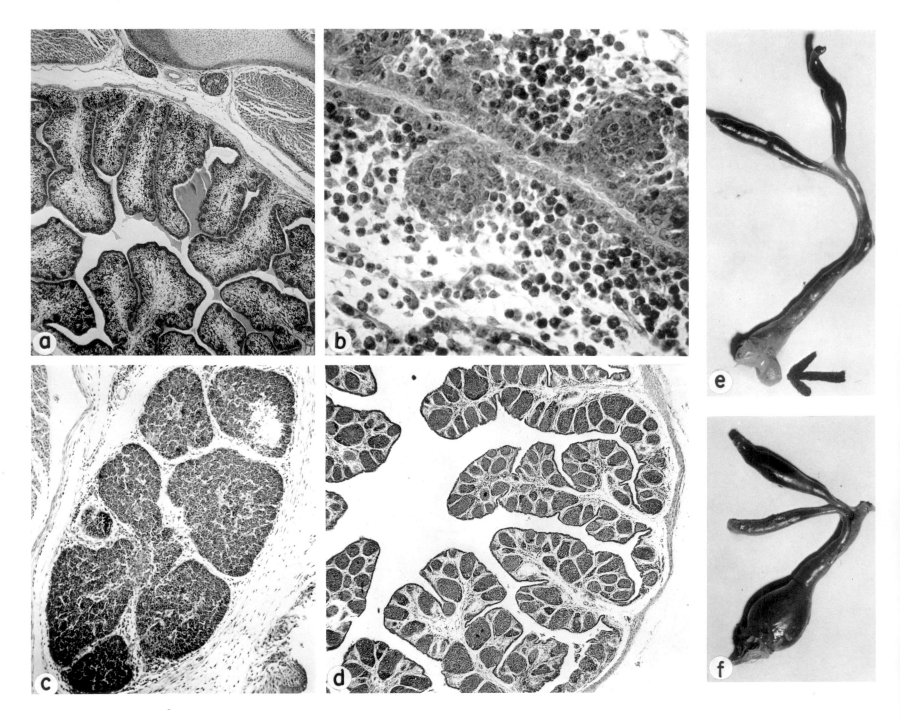

Fig. 7.7. Development of the bursa of Fabricius in the chicken. (a) Low-power view of cross section of the bursa from 14-day embryo. (b) High-power view of the same, showing lymphoepithelial buds. (c) Thymus of the 14-day chick embryo. Lymphoid development in the thymus precedes that of the bursa. (d) Bursa at 17 days. (e) Cloacal region of the normal, newly hatched chick with arrow pointing to the bursa of Fabricius. (f) Cloacal region of newly hatched chick treated with 19-nortestosterone on the fifth day of incubation, with resulting absence of the bursa.

Courtesy of Drs. B. Papermaster and R. A. Good.

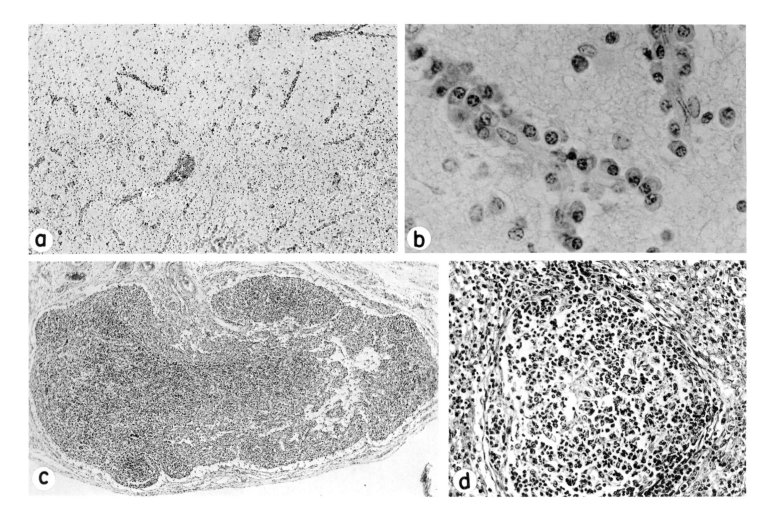

Fig. 7.8. Fetal response to antigenic stimulus. (a) Cerebral cortex in congenital toxoplasmosis. Radiating capillaries with numerous adherent plasma cells adjacent to an infected area; × 55. (b) Higher-power view of the same area. Clusters of Marschalko plasma cells, intermingled with plasmacytoid mononuclear cells, are adherent to vessel walls; × 630. (c) Precocious development of a lymph node in congenital syphilis. Several discrete lymphoid nodules are seen in irregularly thickened cortex. One contains a small early germinal center; × 50. (d) Early germinal center in the spleen in congenital syphilis. This early center, consisting of widely separated small and large mononuclear cells and a few cytoplasmic reticulum cells that contain basophilic debris, lacks a lymphocytic mantle. The center is in striking contrast to the closely packed lymphocytic primary nodule of the uninfected fetus and the typical well-demarcated and mantled germinal center in the adult; × 200.

Hematoxylin-eosin (AFIP negs. 62–3195, 62–3193, 62–2442, 62–2454). Courtesy of Dr. A. M. Silverstein (see Silverstein and Lukes, *Lab. Invest. 11*: 918–32, 1962).

8. Deficiency States and Neoplasms of Lymphoid Organs

A variety of immunological deficiency states is recognized. The most extreme condition is *agammaglobulinemia with alymphocytosis* (thymic alymphoplasia, the Swiss type of agammaglobulinemia), in which there is a total absence of both humoral antibody formation and the cellular type of sensitization. As the name implies, there is complete atrophy of the thymus and absence of all functional cells from the peripheral lymphoid organs (spleen, lymph nodes, gastrointestinal mucosa, bone marrow) (Figs. 8.1–3). Patients with this disease die early of overwhelming infection.

Various partial deficiency states are commonly found. The best known is hypogammaglobulinemia or *agammaglobulinemia* (congenital or acquired), in which there is a decrease in all the recognized immunoglobulins and of humoral antibody formation against all antigens tested, with a relative preservation of cellular types of sensitization. Patients with this illness have a marked deficit of defense against pyogenic bacteria but show almost normal immune responses to tuberculosis and similar chronic bacterial agents, to fungi, and to most viruses. Various forms of the illness appear to be familial, frequently showing an overlap with the connective tissue diseases. Accordingly, thymus abnormalities such as thymoma are commonly present. There is at the same time a more or less complete absence of germinal centers and plasma cells from the various peripheral lymphoid organs (spleen, lymph nodes, gastrointestinal mucosa, bone marrow) (Figs. 8.1–3).

In so-called *dysgammaglobulinemia* there is a deficit in formation of γG- and γA-immunoglobulins and normal or increased γM-formation, for example antibody against erythrocyte antigens or against the typhoid "O" antigen. A similar condition exists in which depressed formation of all the immunoglobulins is seen except for γE; the patients develop normal reaginic allergies. In *ataxia telangiectasia*, a disease dependent on a single Mendelian recessive allele, mesenchymal and vascular developmental abnormalities are observed together with a combined deficiency in γA-immunoglobulin and cellular hypersensitivity. Finally *isolated defects* are seen in one or another form of response. These may be common (γA deficiency) or relatively rare (γM deficiency, isolated deficiency of cellular hypersensitivity). In each of these cases, abnormal patterns of cellular development in central and peripheral lymphoid tissues are seen which correspond to the character of the defect (Figs. 8.1–3). Similarly, the immunologic abnormality determines the nature of the subject's response to infection. Patients with γA deficiency suffer repeated sinopulmonary infection and may show malabsorption. Patients with isolated deficiency of cellular hypersensitivity may die of overwhelming virus infection (vaccinia gangrenosum).

The basic abnormality in the more global deficiency syndromes appears to be determined by agenesis or functional failure of one or more of the central lymphoid organs. The defect in ataxia telangiectasia, for example, resembles the defect in neonatally thymectomized animals very closely. That in agammaglobulinemia suggests the consequences of early bursectomy in birds. Thymic alymphoplasia may depend on developmental abnormality at a more fundamental level or possibly earlier in ontogeny. Isolated defects, on the other hand, must depend on a late anomaly affecting a single circumscribed family of precursor cells. The observation that peripheral lymphocytes in agammaglobulinemia respond abnormally to agents such as phytohemagglutinin has been interpreted as defining a functional abnormality of these cells, but it may rather show the absence of certain populations from the peripheral pool of lymphocytes.

An acquired defect of the cellular type of sensitization is seen in *Boeck's sarcoid* and in *Hodgkin's disease*, antibody formation remaining normal. These are diseases, possibly allergic in character, which directly affect some or all of the peripheral lymphoid organs. In Hodgkin's disease the immunologic deficiency has been related clearly to the characteristic lymphopenia rather than the extent of involvement of lymphoid organs. Lymphocytes of the peripheral pool are not only decreased but are abnormal in response to phytohemagglutinin;

again this may represent absence of certain specific populations of lymphocytes rather than a true abnormality of those remaining. This possibility is supported by the fact that transfer of delayed sensitivity, e.g., tuberculin sensitivity, to the Hodgkin's patient with cell extracts, a process which requires participation of the recipient's own cells, is unsuccessful. These patients have lowered resistance to tuberculosis, mycotic agents, and most viruses and usually die of one of these infections.

In *measles* and to a lesser extent in certain other infections, existing cellular hypersensitivity is temporarily abolished. This effect must be related to the direct destruction of cells in lymphoid organs caused by the measles virus, but it is not known which cells in particular are affected.

In *lymphoma* patients there is a general and progressive diminution in immune responsiveness, related to the gradual replacement of the peripheral pool of immunocompetent lymphocytes by neoplastic cells (see below). Much more limited degrees of immunologic deficiency may be seen in *myeloma and macroglobulinemia*, as a result of the progressive replacement of functional peripheral lymphoid tissue by tumor.

Overproduction of immunoglobulins has two aspects. First, overproduction is a characteristic feature of *chronic infections* such as tuberculosis, *Nocardia* infection, and kala azar; of *granulomatous diseases* like sarcoid; and of "*autoimmune*" *diseases* like disseminated lupus erythematosus, rheumatoid arthritis, and scleroderma. The excess *immunoglobulins are polyclonal* and may represent specific antibody in some of these cases.

Neoplasms of immunoglobulin-producing cells, on the other hand, since they are in most instances clones derived from single abnormal cells, produce *monoclonal paraproteins*. These are indistinguishable from typical antibody molecules and have been shown in a few cases to react specifically with a very limited range of antigenic determinants. *Myelomas* are plasma cell tumors producing γG-, γA-, γD-, or γE-immunoglobulin and/or free L chains (Bence-Jones protein) (Figs. 8.6–8). In *Waldenström's macroglobulinemia*, γM-immunoglobulin is produced; and in *H chain disease*, Fc fragments. Infiltrates of neoplastic cells are characteristically found in spleen, nodes, marrow, etc. (Fig. 8.5). They may resemble morphologically any of the normal antibody-forming cell types (Section 6), but plasma cells are the most common form in myeloma and large lymphoid cells in macroglobulinemia and H-chain disease. Many of these show karyotypic abnormalities. A well-known animal model is Aleutian disease, induced by a slow virus infection in genetically suceptible strains of mink and characterized by massive plasma cell infiltrates in various organs, an extremely high level of plasma γG-globulin, and secondary changes attributable to the γG level in, e.g., the kidney (Fig. 8.4). Equally interesting are the plasma cell tumors induced in mice of the BALB/c strain by mineral oil or other irritants. These may be virus-induced.

Neoplasms of the central lymphoid organs or of lymphocytes in the peripheral pool are lymphomas. These do not in general produce paraproteins. Several animal models have been carefully investigated. *Thymus neoplasia*, whether induced by X ray, carcinogenic chemicals, or virus infection, is expressed as chronic lymphocytic leukemia. The circulating neoplastic cells may continue to express surface antigens normally restricted to cells in the thymus (the TL antigen). Certain murine leukemia viruses (Gross) may act only on thymus cells while others (Rauscher) may affect peripheral cells as well. The fowl leukoses involve virus-induced *neoplasia of the bursal lymphocytic system* and give rise to a condition resembling giant follicular lymphoma in man. In all these the neoplastic lymphocytes lack immunologic function and show abnormally reduced responsiveness to mitogens such as phytohemagglutinin. In *NZB mice*, however, which have a viral lymphoma affecting the thymus, there is an abnormality of the tolerance mechanism but the peripheral lymphocytes retain immunocompetence. In these animals there is extensive autoimmunization and a condition resembling human systemic lupus erythematosus. Finally, herpes-like viruses are responsible for Marek's disease (neurolymphomatosis) in chickens and *infectious mononucleosis* in man, a transient leukemia-like state in which autoimmunization is very common. No neoplasm is recognized at present which involves the effector cells of delayed hypersensitivity.

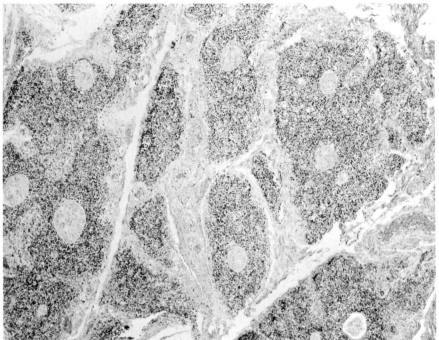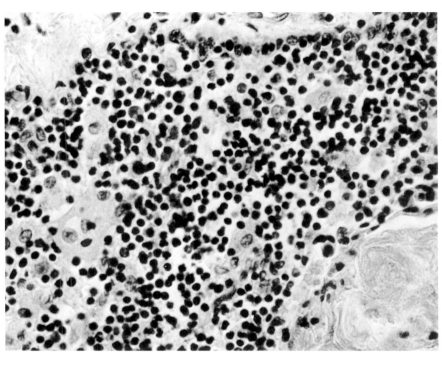

Fig. 8.1. Thymus in congenital agammaglobulinemia without lymphopenia. Low- and high-power view of thymus, showing well-developed lobules, poor corticomedullary differentiation, sparse population of lymphocytes, and prominent Hassall's corpuscles.

Hematoxylin-eosin; ×105, ×975. From Gitlin and Craig, *Pediatrics 32*: 517–30 (1963).

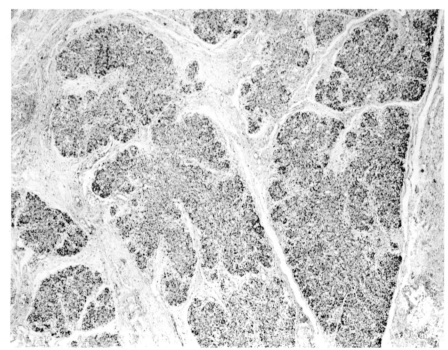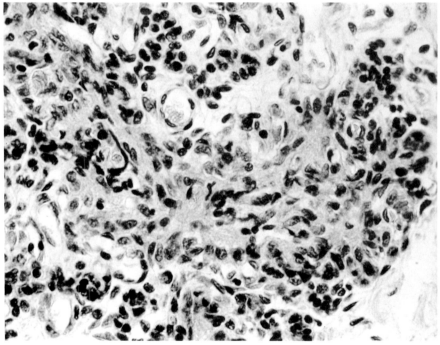

Fig. 8.2. Thymus in agammaglobulinemia with lymphopenia. Low- and high-power views of thymus from patient aged 5 months at time of death. The thymus shows fair lobular development but no corticomedullary differentiation and no Hassall's corpuscles. There are few small lymphocytes, and mononuclear reticulum cells predominate.

Hematoxylin-eosin; ×105, ×975. From Gitlin and Craig, *Pediatrics 32*: 517–30 (1963).

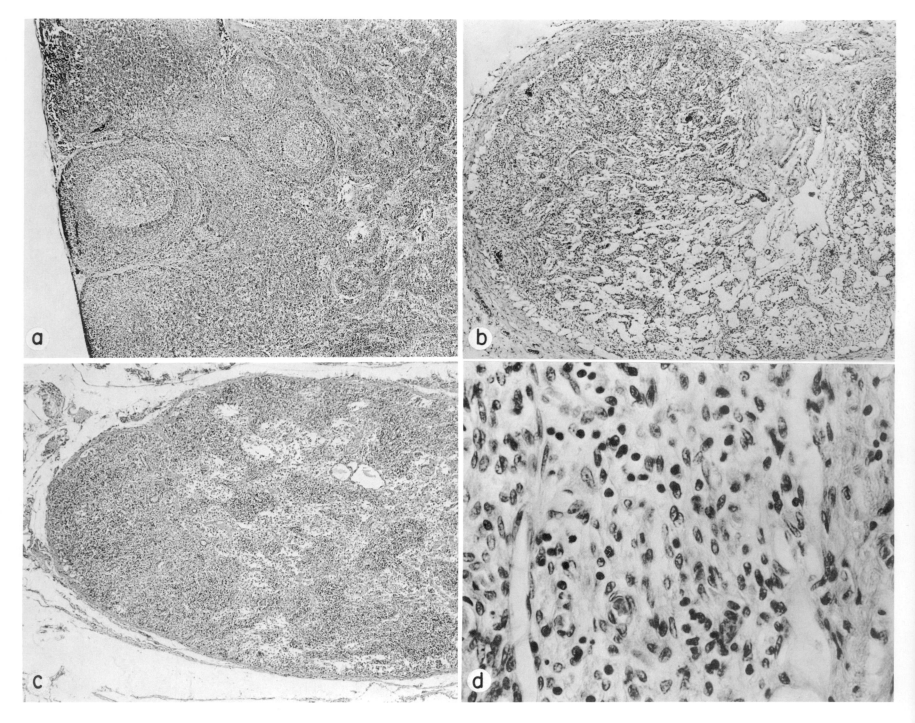

Fig. 8.3. Comparison of normal human lymph node (from 8-day infant stimulated with multiple antigens) (a) with nodes from children with agammaglobulinemia (c) and agammaglobulinemia with lymphopenia (b, d). Lymphocytes are reduced in number in the former and almost absent in the latter. Germinal centers are lacking in both.

Hematoxylin-eosin; (a–c) ×100, (d) ×970. From Gitlin and Craig, *Pediatrics 32*: 517–30 (1963).

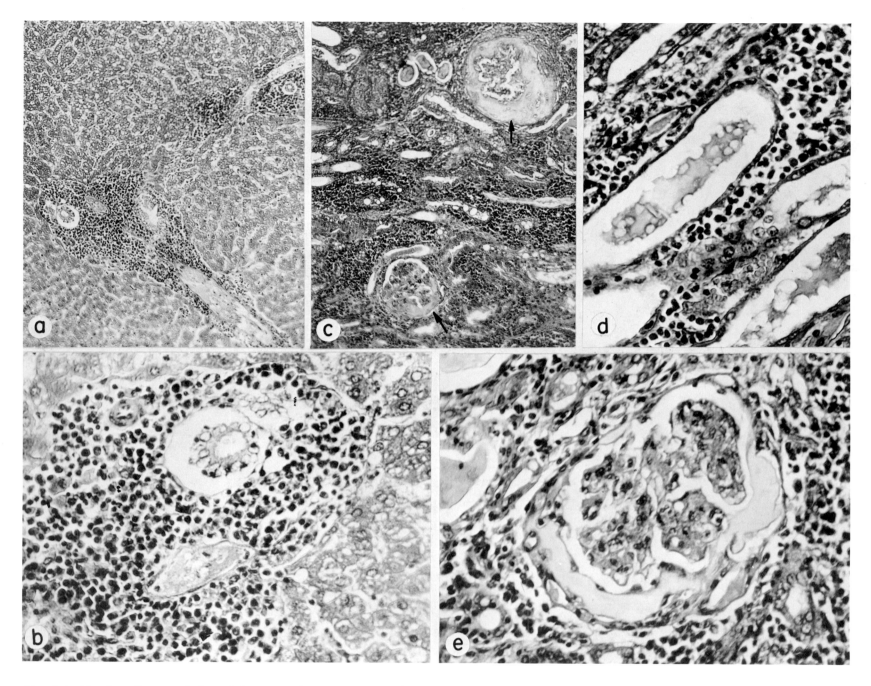

Fig. 8.4. Aleutian disease of the mink, a neoplasm of plasma cells producing immunoglobulin (paraprotein), induced by vertically transmitted infection with a slow virus in a genetically susceptible strain of mink. This is one of several experimental models for human neoplasms of antibody-forming cells. (a, b) Periportal infiltrates of plasma cells and large blast-like cells in the liver. (c–e) Renal lesions. (c) Massive cell infiltrates, like those seen in the liver, and inspissated protein occupying Bowman's space and compressing the glomerulus (arrows). (d) Higher-power view of cell infiltrate and protein in tubules. (e) A glomerulus, relatively unaffected by the disease. Bowman's space is dilated and filled with protein.

Hematoxylin-eosin; (a, c) ×150, (b, d, e) ×400. Courtesy of Dr. C. F. Helmboldt.

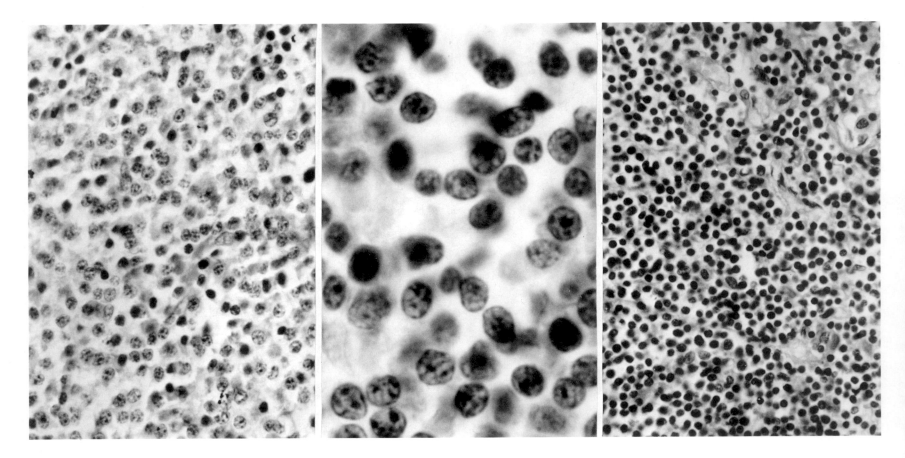

Fig. 8.5. Malignancies of immunologically active cells. (Left) Plasma cell myeloma; × 650. (Center) Waldenström's macroglobulemia; × 2,000. (Right) Lymphocytic lymphoma; × 500. Hematoxylin-eosin. Courtesy of Dr. B. Castleman.

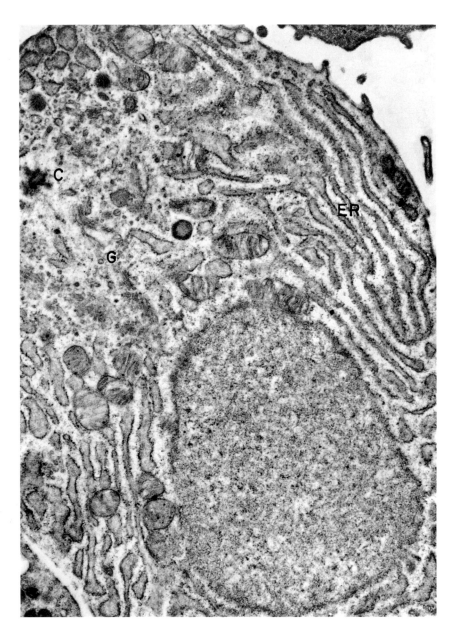

Fig. 8.6. Plasma cell from γG myeloma. Note flat endoplasmic reticulum (ER) and conspicuous centriole (C) and Golgi apparatus (G).

Electron micrograph; magnification not given. From Bessis, Breton-Gorius, and Binet, *Nouv. Rev. Franç. Hémat. 3*: 159–84 (1963).

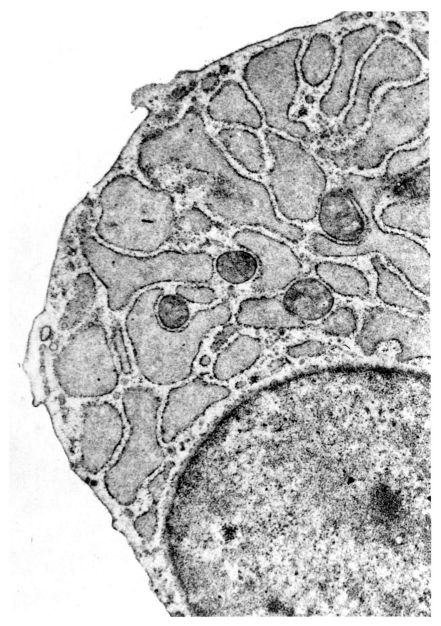

Fig. 8.7. Plasma cell from γA myeloma. Note swollen ergastoplasm, corresponding to violet staining in Giemsa preparations (flame cell or thesaurocyte).

Electron micrograph; magnification not given. From Bessis, Breton-Gorius, and Binet, *Nouv. Rev. Franç. Hémat. 3*: 159–84 (1963).

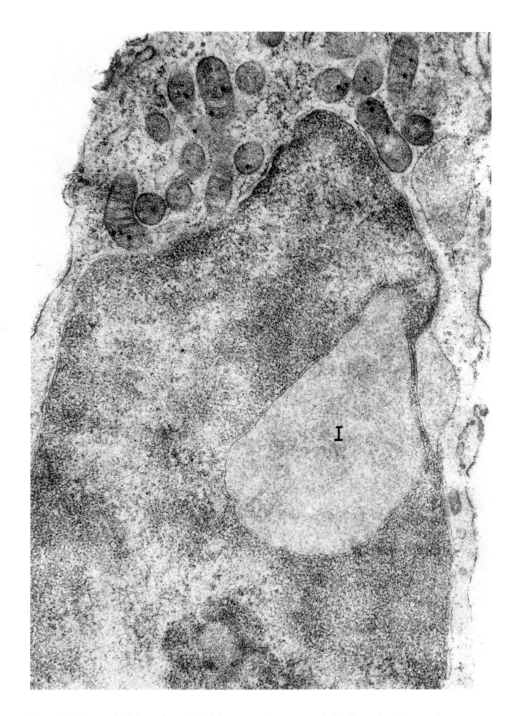

Fig. 8.8. Lymphoblast from Waldenström's macroglobulinemia. Note characteristic large nuclear inclusion (1), absence of endoplasmic reticulum, and numerous free ribosomes.

Electron micrograph; magnification not given. From Bessis, Breton-Gorius, and Binet, *Nouv. Rev. Franç. Hémat. 3*: 159–84 (1963).

9. Neutralization by Antibody

Antibody can neutralize *in vivo* the biologic activity of molecules present in solution in the blood or body fluids such as hormones, intrinsic factor, extracellular enzymes, and so on. Hetero-, iso-, and autoantibody are equally effective. The quantitative and qualitative aspects of neutralization are similar whether antibody is introduced by purposeful transfer or transplacentally into the individual possessing the antigen; or whether antigen is introduced into the individual who has formed antibody, as when insulin is injected into an insulin-resistant subject; or when antigen–antibody mixtures prepared *in vitro* are injected into a normal individual, as in the immunoassay of hormones; or when the host forms antibody against an autogenous antigen. There is of course no equivalent *in vitro* of neutralization, but a variety of laboratory techniques has been devised for demonstrating the ability of antibody to form a complex with any given antigen (Fig. 9.1). The only decisive proof that such complex formation plays a role in disease is passive transfer of serum, with or without a standard test dose of antigen, to the living host.

The usual *in vivo* effect of antibody against protein hormones is *anatomic and functional atrophy of the target organ* (thyroid, gonads, adrenal, etc.) and *compensatory change in the source organ* (e.g. pituitary). Experimental and naturally occurring cases involve pituitary hormones (somatotropin, TSH, gonadotropins, prolactin), thyroglobulin, parathormone, gastrin, erythropoietin, and nerve growth-promoting factor. A suppression of function by autoantibody is seen, for example, in hypopituitary dwarfs. Conventional heteroantibody against injected hormone preparations is responsible for resistance to hormone therapy, with insulin, chorionic or pituitary gonadotropins, etc. Heteroantisera against polypeptide hormones such as ACTH, vasopressin, oxytocin and glucagon are also highly effective in animal experiments but play an unknown role in human disease. Specific antibodies have been experimentally produced against a variety of still smaller biologically active molecules by using conjugates of these with carrier protein for immunization. The antibodies are effective in neutralization but are not recognized at present as causes of disease. Examples include thyroxine, estrone and other steroids, angiotensin, and bradykinin. In subjects treated with hydrochlorothiazide, the reverse situation has been described: formation *in vivo* of an immunogenic conjugate of the drug with insulin and antibody synthesis against the conjugate, with a consequent fall in insulin level and diabetes as a result of drug therapy.

Multiple situations involving a single biologically active substance may be recognized. With intrinsic factor, autoantibody may inhibit the binding of vitamin B_{12} and its absorption by the living subject, the secondary consequence being pernicious anemia. On the other hand, heteroantibody against hog intrinsic factor may be responsible for resistance of the subject with pernicious anemia to treatment. Autoantibody against thromboplastin, formed in systemic lupus erythematosus and related diseases, blocks the conversion of thromboplastin to thrombin and is in part responsible for the hemorrhagic tendency in these diseases. At the same time, iso-antibody against other proteins in the clotting sequence is responsible for resistance of patients with hemophilia to treatment with human plasma fractions. This case is unique in that the patient is immunized against a protein which he lacks for genetic reasons and for which he presumably has failed to develop tolerance. With such extracellular enzyme systems as pepsinogen and the various proteins in the complement sequence, heteroantibody has been shown experimentally to neutralize these *in vitro* and *in vivo*, but naturally occurring cases are not as yet known.

The list of possible examples of neutralization *in vivo* has by no means been fully explored. There is speculation that some cases of deficient plasma protein synthesis may be due to autoantibody formation or auto-allergy, but the mechanism may be more closely comparable to that of allotype suppression (Section 4) than neutralization.

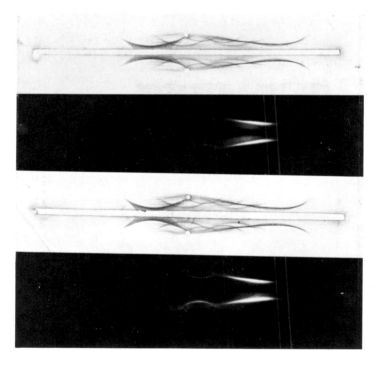

Fig. 9.1. Combination of insulin with antibody in serum of
patient with insulin-resistant diabetes: radioimmunoelectro-
phoretic patterns. Serum incubated with radioactive insulin,
heavily labeled with I^{125}, for 2 and 4 hours, then subjected
to immunoelectrophoresis against rabbit antiserum. Autoradiograph after 2-hour incubation (above) shows that insulin
is bound by antibody in the γG-globulin. However, after
4 hours (below), there is also binding by an α_2-macroglobulin.
This is interpreted as an artefact due to progressive denatura-
tion of protein in the test system and illustrates one of the
hazards of this technique of diagnosis. The specific binding
presumably occurs *in vivo* and is responsible for the patient's
resistance to treatment.

From Kantor and Berkman, *Yale J. Biol. Med. 40*: 46–56,
(1967).

10. Single Cell Lesions

The effect of antibody directed at an antigenic constituent of the cell surface membrane has been studied *in vitro* and *in vivo* with a variety of cell types. Striking effects are produced on cells in suspension, notably erythrocytes, leukocytes, sperm, or ascites tumor cells, and cells growing as a monolayer in tissue culture, among them such diverse cell types as amnion, liver, thyroid, glia, and various tumors (HeLa, mammary carcinoma). In the absence of complement, the principal effect of the antigen–antibody reaction is agglutination (Figs. 10.1, 2,8,14), frequently accompanied by changes in mechanical or osmotic fragility.

Agglutination as such is specific (Fig. 10.2). The antigen may be a cell constituent, an adherent antigenic substance (protein, polysaccharide), or a complex of exogenous allergen with a component of the cell surface membrane (Fig. 10.17). Hetero-, iso-, and autoantibodies all give agglutination, though some types of antibody (incomplete antibody) may fail to agglutinate. In such cases, agglutination may be enhanced by increasing the concentration of large, anisotropic molecules in the ambient medium, by trypsinizing the cells or treating them with other enzymes, or indeed by use of agglutinating antibody directed at the antibody attached to the cells (the Coombs antiglobulin technique). Formation of grossly visible aggregates (Fig. 10.1) requires formation of a lattice and depends, therefore, on the presence of a sufficient number of antigenic sites on the cell and on the bi- or multivalency of the antibody. The Fab fragment of agglutinating antibody, consisting of a single combining site, does not agglutinate. Antibody molecules bridging agglutinated cells or particles may actually be visualized by electron microscopy. The surface membrane of agglutinated cells may show focal projections or invaginations (Fig. 10.8). However, antibody does not penetrate the interior of the cell (Fig. 10.9), the various organelles remain unaffected, and there is no change in cell permeability, chemical constitution, or metabolic properties. Cells grow actively in the presence of agglutinating antibody, though clumping may decrease the growth rate.

When cells are coated (sensitized) with antibody but fail to aggregate, as with incomplete antibody or subthreshold concentrations of agglutinating antibody, the immunoglobulin coating enhances their susceptibility to phagocytic uptake (*opsonization*) (Figs. 10.14,15; see also Postscript) and to *immune adherence* (Fig. 10.5). In the latter, the coated cells stick to primate erythrocytes or to platelets of any of a number of mammalian species, a mechanism presumed to facilitate their uptake by adjacent phagocytes. These mechanisms both involve the participation of part of the complement sequence. The coated cells are also sensitized to the lytic action of complement (discussed below), and may be identified by laboratory artifices such as the Coombs method (agglutination by antiglobulin), mixed agglutination (Fig. 10.3), or the immunofluorescence technique (see other sections). In a mechanism related to opsonization and immune adherence, a type of γ_2G-antibody (*cytophilic antibody*) possesses the special property of adhering to as yet unknown receptors on the macrophage surface and endowing it with an enhanced capacity to take up specific antigen (Fig. 10.4). In opsonization, different surface receptors (of both polymorphs and macrophages) are involved in uptake of immunoglobulin-coated antigenic cells or particles; and in immune adherence still another receptor, present in platelets and primate erythrocytes, plays a role. The fixation of γE-antibody and foreign γG on certain cell types (mast cells, basophils, platelets) involves still another set of cell receptors. Reaction of antigen with these sensitized cells leads to release of vasoactive mediators and is a major mechanism of anaphylaxis (Section 11). Finally, soluble antigen–antibody complexes tend to produce agglutination of platelets and may also result in platelet damage and release of anaphylactic mediators.

In the presence of a complete array of complement components, cells sensitized by complement-fixing antibody (γM, some γG) undergo *immune lysis*. Small holes are formed in the cell membrane (Fig. 10.11), and there is rapid equilibration of ions and small molecules such as K^+, Na^+, $PO_4^=$, amino acids, and ribonucleotides between the cytoplasm and the medium, followed by osmotic entry of water into membrane-bounded compartments of the cell (Figs. 10.8–10). The consequent swelling of the cell and stretching of its surface membrane enlarges the holes sufficiently to permit escape of macromolecules, among them proteins such as hemoglobin and even entire ribosomes. These changes are readily visible in light microscopic or stained preparations as cytoplasmic swelling, vacuolation, and loss of basophilia, usually accompanied by nuclear changes such as pycnosis with clumping and margination of chromatin (Figs. 10.6,7,16,17). The loss of soluble enzymes and coenzymes as well as of their substrates results in progressive death of the cell. An exactly comparable sequence of changes occurs in erythrocytes, nucleated mammalian cells, and bacteria (Gram-negative organisms and protoplasts of Gram-positive) undergoing immune lysis. In erythrocytes, a single hole is sufficient to initiate lysis, and this requires the action of a single molecule of γM-antibody or two or more of γG. In nucleated cells it appears that multiple antigenic sites must be affected to give the production of a single hole and lysis. The size and pattern of the holes formed vary slightly, depending on the type of complement tested and the distribution of antigenic sites.

Immune lysis cannot be reproduced *in vitro* in systems other than those involving cells in suspension or in monolayer culture. Cells growing in a well-fused mass may be completely resistant to the action of antibody. Thus human thyroid epithelium, freshly trypsinized and placed in culture in the presence of specific antibody and complement, undergoes a cytotoxic effect comparable to lysis. Antibody and complement added to cultures more than 36 hours old, however, are without effect. The difference must be attributed to the development of barriers in the organized tissue which inhibit the access of the antibody molecules.

There exist special types of lysis such as the *nuclear lysis* produced in slightly injured cells by antibody against DNA, the so-called LE factor. This lysis is usually accompanied by the formation of rosettes of phagocytic cells adherent to the damaged nucleus or actual ingestion of the nucleus by a phagocytic cell with formation of an LE cell (Figs. 10.12–15). Antibody against microsomal (i.e. membrane) constituents of the cell are almost always cytotoxic. However, one instance is known at present in which *autoantibody*, *against a thyroid microsomal antigen* (long-acting thyroid stimulator), *augments function* by an as yet unknown mechanism. *Mast cell and platelet degranulation* and discharge of anaphylactic mediators (Figs. 11.3–5) represent a special type of immune lysis not involving complement (Section 11). In this case the cell is not destroyed.

Other changes may be initiated in special types of cells by the antigen–antibody reaction. Polymorphonuclear leukocytes synthesize and release *endogenous pyrogen*, a heat-labile protein, capable of acting directly on the thermoregulatory center in the brain to cause a monophasic fever and antagonized by aspirin, amidopyrine, etc. Endotoxin (Section 15), which is lipopolysaccharide and therefore heat-stable, also damages polys (polymorphonuclear leukocytes) and causes them to release endogenous pyrogen. It is not clear whether this action is a direct toxic event or results from interaction of endotoxin with natural antibody in the serum, i.e. is a special case of the antigen–antibody reaction. In this context endotoxin is called *exogenous pyrogen*. It may also act directly on the thermoregulatory center. In the intact organism, endotoxin produces leukopenia and a biphasic fever. If administered repeatedly, it gives "tolerance" (not to be confused with specific immunologic tolerance) due to formation of specific antibody (γM) and activation of the RE system. This tolerance may be overcome by increasing the dose of endotoxin or by RE blockade. Endogenous pyrogen is also released in situations involving cellular hypersensitivity (Sections 17, 18), in situations which may or may not involve an immunologic reaction (bacterial and viral infection, neoplasia) and in nonimmunologic situations (vascular occlusion metabolic abnormalities such as gout, porphyria, thyroid storm).

The findings in intact animals and human subjects duplicate quite well what is found *in vitro*. Only accessible cells—i.e. red cells, white cells, platelets, sperm, ascites tumors, and lymphomas under suitable conditions, and cells disposed in a monolayer, notably vascular endothelium and possibly the cells of serous surfaces—are directly affected by circulating antibody. The patterns of disease are well illustrated in various conditions affecting the red cell. Transfusion reactions occur when cells are accidentally transferred to an individual possessing antibody against an antigen of those cells or when substantial amounts of antibody are given to a recipient whose cells possess the corresponding antigen. Transplacental passage of antibody against fetal red cells causes hemolytic disease of the newborn and erythroblastosis. Autoantibody against antigens of one's own erythrocytes causes several syndromes which include acquired hemolytic anemia, paroxysmal cold hemoglobinuria, and possibly others such as blackwater fever. Finally, antibody directed at a complex of drug (quinidine, fuadin, etc.) with red cells produces an acute "allergic" hemolytic reaction whenever the corresponding drug is administered. The details vary a good deal, depending on the molecular class of the antibody and the relative total amounts of antibody and cells. Thus under different conditions red cell destruction may occur primarily by means of intravascular complement-mediated lysis, by phagocytic uptake and destruction in reticuloendothelial cells of the liver, or more slowly by mechanical as well as phagocytic breakdown in the spleen.

Similar patterns may be seen with the other cell types mentioned. In each case the character of the disease is, of course, determined by the identity of the cell affected. Destruction of red cells, as noted, results in anemia, hemoglobinuria, and so on. White cell destruction may give rise to febrile transfusion reactions or febrile reactions to drugs (sulfonamides, quinidine, thiouracil, PAS, streptomycin), neonatal neutropenia produced by maternal antibody against paternal white cell antigens, chronic leukopenia produced by autoantibody, and allergic agranulocytosis with certain drugs (amidopyrine, sulfapyridine). Fever also occurs as a result of immunologic leukocyte damage in hemolytic transfusion reactions, paroxysmal cold hemoglobinuria, and serum disease. Platelet destruction is readily produced with hetero- or isoantisera and is seen especially in man in neonatal thrombocytopenia and allergic thrombocytopenic purpura due to drugs (Sedormid, quinidine). It is not clear at present whether idiopathic thrombocytopenic purpura is indeed mediated by an autoantibody, though this has been suggested. The possibility that certain types of marrow aplasia involve the action of antibody directed at hemopoietic cells or at complexes of those with specific drugs has not been validated in cases of human disease, though such lesions are produced experimentally with heteroantisera. Antibodies giving sperm agglutination have been incriminated in human infertility. Finally, tumor immunity involving ascites tumors is antibody-mediated. Vascular purpura may be easily produced experimentally with heteroantiserum against endothelium, and both heterograft rejection and some instances of "white graft" rejection affecting skin homografts are clearly due to antibody acting on endothelium. A similar mechanism has not, however, been clearly demonstrated in human vascular disease. Several immunological conditions affecting serous surfaces, notably the post-myocardial infarction, post-commissurotomy, and post-pericardiotomy syndromes, may well be mediated by humoral antibody against tissue antigens. Here too the mechanism remains to be demonstrated. Satisfactory proof of mechanism would require production of disease in normal recipients by passive transfer of antibody (and challenge with drug, if a drug is involved).

In general, antibody against cells in formed tissues has no cytoxic effect in the intact animal, probably because of the barrier noted in tissue-culture systems. Thus passive transfer of high-titered heteroantibody against thyroid, myelin, pancreas, adrenal, and so on does the recipient no visible harm. In human subjects with "autoimmune" disease affecting the thyroid, for example, passive transfer of antibody or transplacental passage of γG-antibody fails to produce corresponding disease in the recipient. As will be noted later (Sections 21,22), parenchymal lesions in these organs depend in most instances on the cellular (delayed) type of sensitization. Except for the case of the long-acting thyroid stimulator (LATS), which produces an effect on cells *in vivo*, all instances in which antibodies to tissue constituents produce lesions involve extracellular antigens. Antibody against basement membrane constituents may produce vascular or pulmonary lesions, but its best known effect is the production of an Arthus-like lesion in the renal glomerulus, so-called nephrotoxic nephritis, illustrated in detail in Section 14. Another Arthus-like lesion is produced with local introduction of antibody against components of the connective tissue ground substance. Antibody against intercellular cement substance of the epidermis appears to be responsible for the bullous lesions of different types of pemphigus (Fig. 22.4); the mechanism here is unknown but may involve some sort of lysis of the cement substance itself. A similar antibody against the epidermal basement membrane produces the lesions of bullous pemphigoid or dermatitis herpetiformis. Finally, an eosinophilic infiltrate appears in the thyroid treated with high-titered heteroantibody against thyroglobulin, presumably as a reaction to local formation of immune complexes. The production of membranous glomerulonephritis (wire-loop lesions) in systemic lupus erythematosus and in the NZB mouse, which develops a disease resembling lupus (illustrated in Section 13), is due to glomerular deposition of circulating immune complexes formed between nuclear constituents and antoantibody and not to autoantibody against renal antigens as such.

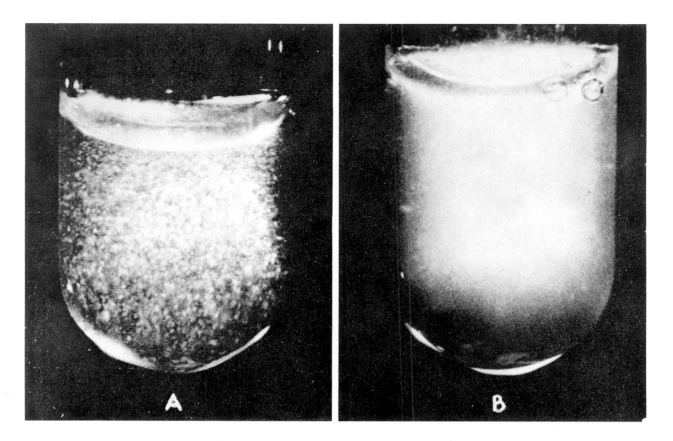

Fig. 10.1. Leukocyte agglutination. White cells of patient with myeloid leukemia agglutinated by rabbit antibody against human leukocytes (A). Control serum produces no agglutination (B).
From Steinberg and Martin, *J. Immunol. 51*: 421–26 (1945).

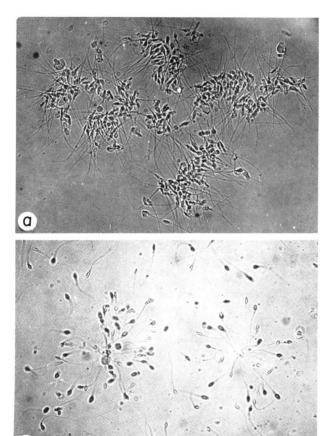

Fig. 10.2. Agglutination of human sperm by autoantibodies present in the ejaculate. (a) Head-to-head agglutination. (b) Tail-to-tail agglutination. (c) Gross tube agglutination of sperm by serum antibody. A serial dilution titration is illustrated. (a, b) phase photomicrographs; magnifications not given. From Rümke, in *First International Symposium on Immunopathology*, P. Grabar and P. Miescher, eds., Schwabe, Basel, 1959, pp 145–53.

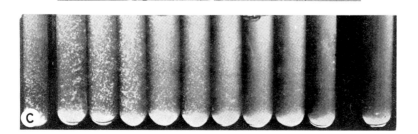

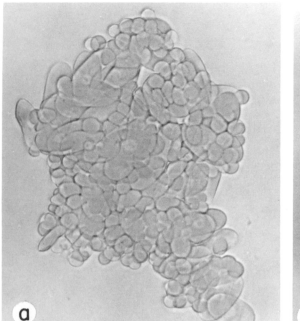
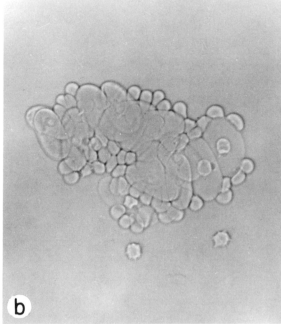
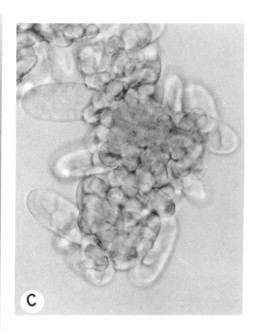

Fig. 10.3. Mixed agglutination of alligator erythrocytes, sensitized by subagglutinating dose of rabbit antialligator erythrocyte serum, and rabbit red cells of blood group G, sensitized by incomplete rabbit anti-G isoantiserum, when these are allowed to react with serum of a patient with rheumatoid arthritis. The serum contains antibody specifically reactive with rabbit immunoglobulin. Distinct patterns result when the three reactants are mixed at once (a); when alligator cells are first allowed to react with the rheumatoid serum, washed, and then mixed with sensitized rabbit cells (b); when the rabbit cells react first with rheumatoid serum and are subsequently exposed to alligator erythrocytes (c).

Fresh preparations; × 400. From Milgrom, Witebsky, Goldstein, and Loza, *J. Am. Med. Ass. 181*: 476–84 (1962).

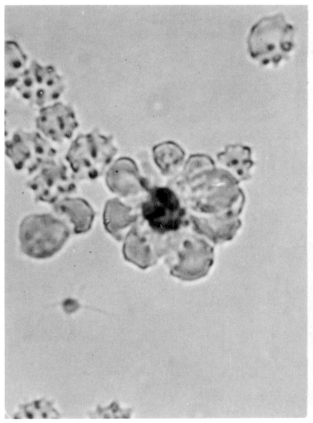
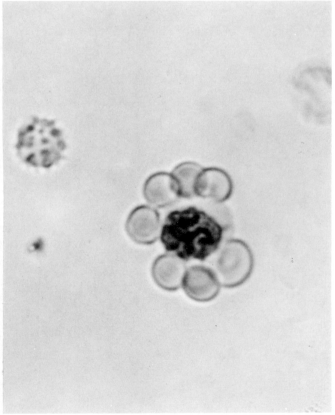

Fig. 10.4. Uptake of antigen by cells coated with cytophilic antibody. Human red cells sensitized with anti-D antibody, incubated for 30 minutes at 37°C with leukocytes of D-sensitive subject, show formation of rosettes, in which individual erythrocytes are firmly adherent to a central cell, here a monocyte. Specimens were diluted with saline (causing slight crenation of the erythrocytes) and stained with neutral red. Note absence of agglutination of the red cells and complete absence of any involvement of platelets. Mediator in this case is non-complement-fixing γG antibody. Binding is entirely specific for monocytes and macrophages and does not occur with other cell types. It leads to cell injury, indicated by spherocytosis of the red cells, as shown here, but rarely to phagocytosis.

From Jandl and Tomlinson, *J. Clin. Invest. 37*: 1202–28 (1958); (see also LoBuglio and Jandl, *ibid., 46*: 1087, 1967, abstr.).

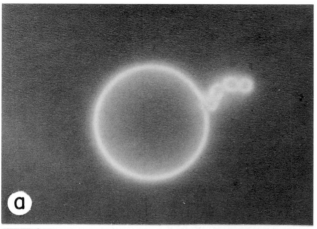

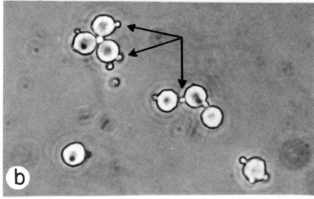

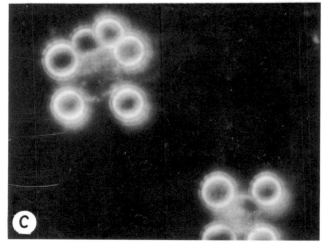

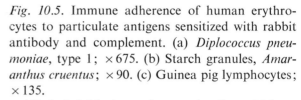

Fig. 10.5. Immune adherence of human erythrocytes to particulate antigens sensitized with rabbit antibody and complement. (a) *Diplococcus pneumoniae*, type 1; ×675. (b) Starch granules, *Amaranthus cruentus*; ×90. (c) Guinea pig lymphocytes; ×135.

All dark-field photomicrographs. From Nelson, *Science 118*: 733–37 (1953), and *Transfusion 3*: 250–59 (1963).

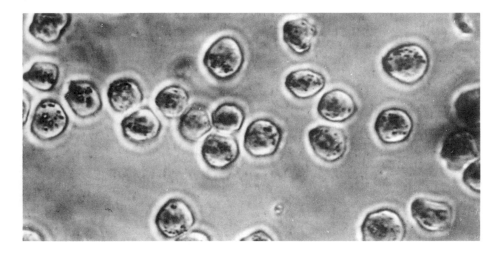

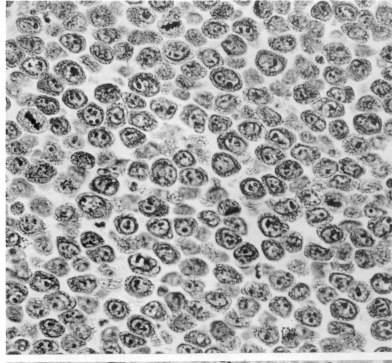

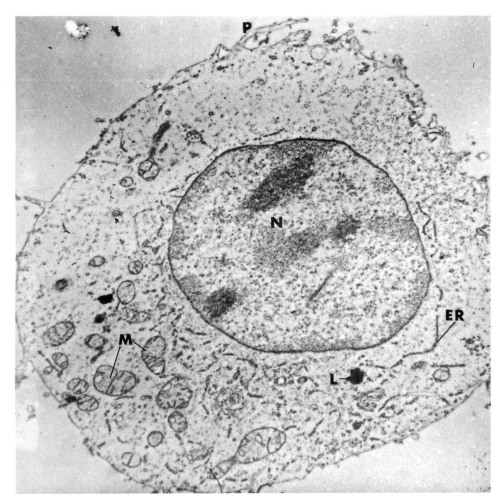

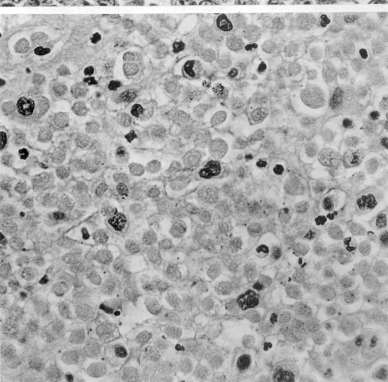

Fig. 10.6. Effect of antibody on Krebs ascites tumor cells. (Above) Normal cells in phase photomicrograph, showing uniform size, sharp cytoplasmic borders, moderate cytoplasmic granulation, and indistinct nuclear outlines; × 640. (Below) Normal cell in electron micrograph, showing variability in shape of mitochondria (M) and arrangement of mitochondrial cristae, poorly developed endoplasmic reticulum (ER), small, free osmiophilic granules in cytoplasm, lipid droplets (L), and projections of surface membrane (pseudopods) (P); × 10,500.

From Goldberg and Green, *J. Exp. Med. 109*: 505–10 (1959).

Fig. 10.7. Ehrlich ascites tumor cells 7 days after transplantation (above) and 36 hours after ip injection of 4.5 mg rabbit antibody globulin plus 3 ml guinea pig complement (below). Normal cells show nuclei rich in chromatin and many mitoses. Lysed cells show nuclear shrinkage, ballooning of cytoplasm, and loss of stainable material from both nucleus and cytoplasm. A few unlysed cells remain.

Feulgen-fast green; × 600, × 650. From Flax and Wissler, *Ann. N.Y. Acad. Sci. 69*: 773–94 (1957).

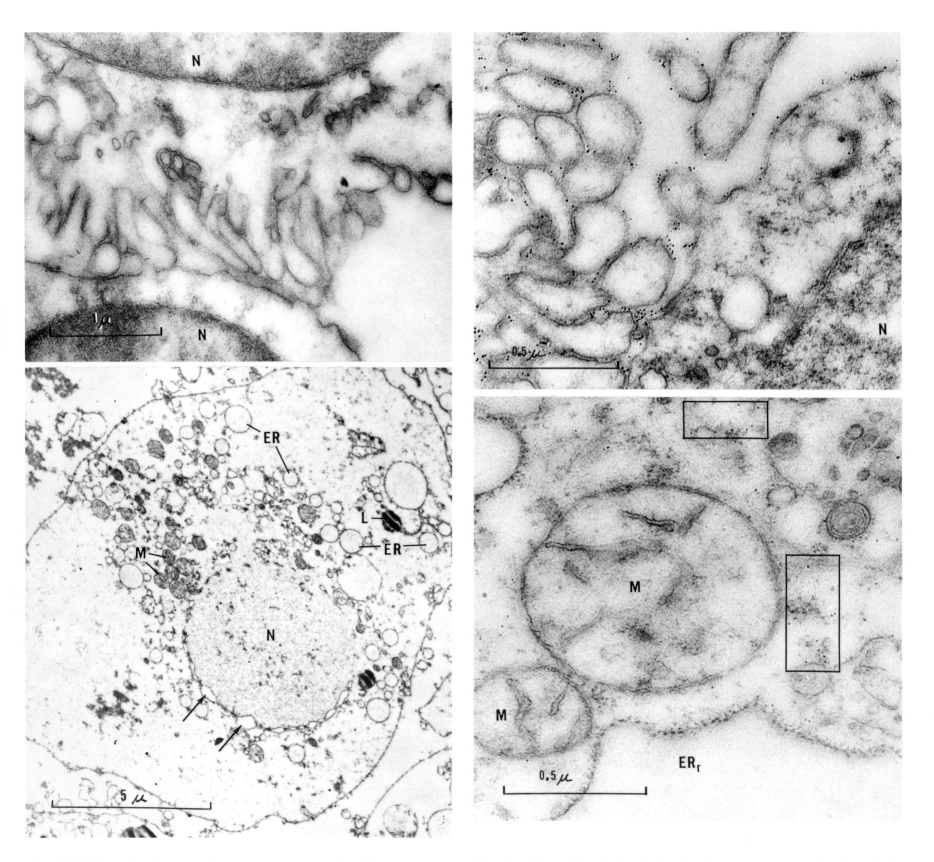

Fig. 10.8. Effect of antibody on Krebs ascites tumor cells. (Above) Agglutination of two cells in absence of complement. Surface membranes show focal zones of invagination and evagination and interdigitation of the surface projections from each cell; ×30,000. (Below) Cell treated with antibody and complement. Expanded cavities in endoplasmic reticulum and perinuclear space (arrows) and widened nuclear pores. Mitochondria are swollen to varying degrees; ×8,500.

Electron micrographs; abbreviations as in Fig. 10.6. From Easton, Goldberg, and Green, *J. Exp. Med. 115*: 275–88 (1962), and *J. Biophys. Biochem. Cytol. 7*: 645–50 (1960).

Fig. 10.9. Use of ferritin-labeled antibody to demonstrate site of antibody action on Krebs ascites tumor cells. (Above) In absence of complement, antibody is distributed on both folded and unfolded segments of surface membrane and inside occasional pinocytotic vesicles; ×68,000. (Below) In cell undergoing lysis by excess labeled antibody and complement (note swelling of mitochondria) additional label is seen scattered throughout cytoplasmic matrix; ×75,000.

Electron micrographs. From Easton, Goldberg, and Green, *J. Exp. Med. 115*: 275–88 (1962).

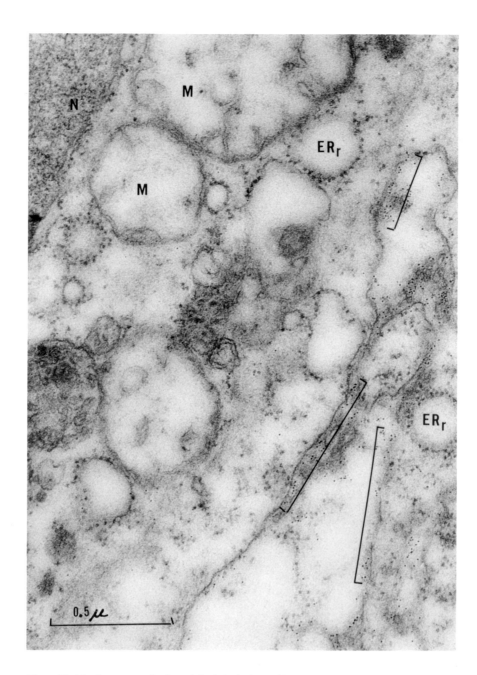

Fig. 10.10. Immune lysis with labeled antibody and complement. Mito-chondria and endoplasmic reticulum are swollen. Antibody is largely limited to cell surface membrane (brackets).

Electron micrograph; ×63,000. From Easton, Goldberg, and Green, *J. Exp. Med. 115*: 275–88 (1962).

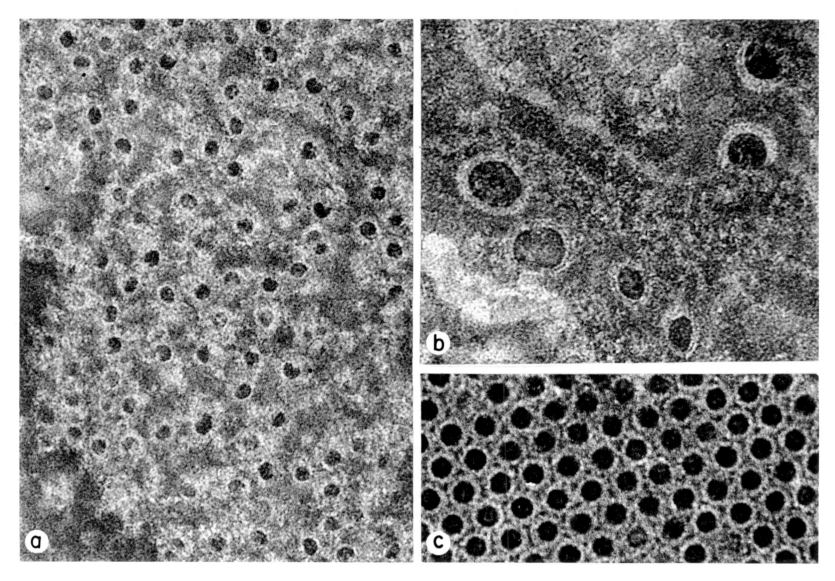

Fig. 10.11. Comparison of immune lysis with lysis produced by physical or chemical agents. (a) Human erythrocytes lysed by 18S antibody (anti-I) and human complement; ×374,000. (b) Cells lysed by streptolysin 0; ×400,000. (c) Liver cell membranes treated with saponin. The cell membrane in each case shows holes characteristic in size, shape, variabilty, and distribution; ×640,000.

Electron micrographs. (a) From Rosse, Dourmashkin, and Humphrey, *J. Exp. Med. 123*: 969–84 (1966). (b) Humphrey and Dourmashkin, unpublished. (c) Dourmashkin, Dougherty, and Harris, *J. Roy. Micr. Soc. 81*, pts. 3, 4: 215–18 (1963). See also *Nature 196*: 952–55 (1962).

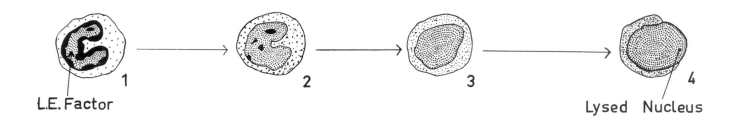

L.E. Factor

1 → 2 → 3 → 4

Lysed Nucleus

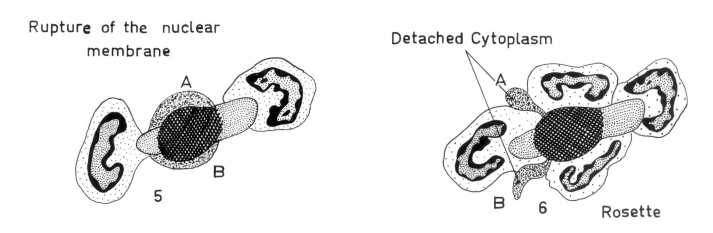

Rupture of the nuclear membrane

Detached Cytoplasm

A

A

B

5

B 6

Rosette

NUCLEAR LYSIS AND FORMATION OF ROSETTES

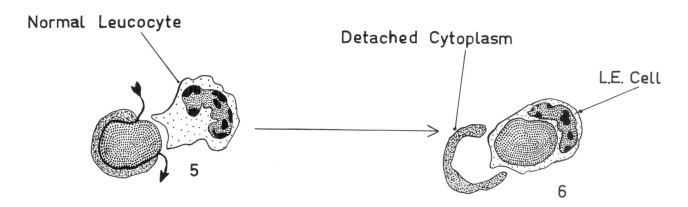

Normal Leucocyte

Detached Cytoplasm

L.E. Cell

5 →

6

NUCLEAR LYSIS AND L.E. CELL FORMATION

Figs. 10.12 and 10.13. Sequence of events in lysis and opsonization of leukocyte nucleus by L. E. factor (antinuclear antibody), with subsequent formation of a rosette of attached phagocytes, or actual ingestion of the lysed nucleus by a phagocytic cell with formation of an L. E. cell.

From Robineaux, in *Henry Ford Hospital Symposium on Mechanisms of Hypersensitivity*, J. H. Shaffer et al., eds., Little, Brown, Boston, 1959, pp. 371–95.

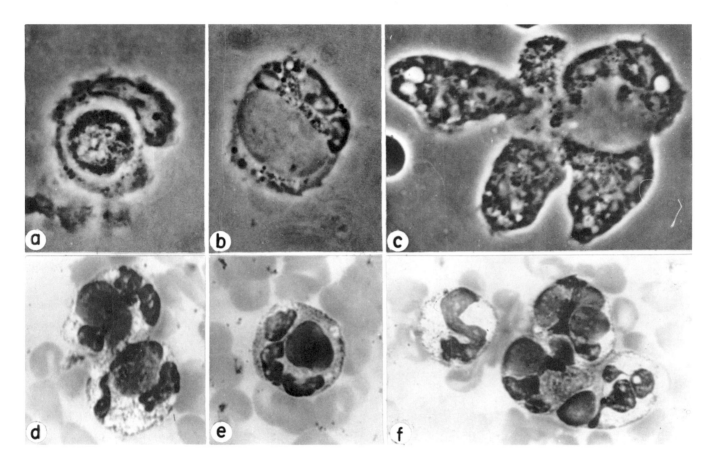

Fig. 10.14. Opsonization of the nucleus by antinuclear antibody with varying degrees of nuclear homogenization and phagocytosis by polymorphonuclear leukocytes (the LE phenomenon). All figures except (c) are from preparations of human leukocytes incubated with serum of patients with lupus erythematosus; (c) is from a similar preparation in which purified antibody against DNA, obtained from a lupus patient's serum (Seligmann), was employed. (a) Phagocytosis of normal-appearing nucleus, the pseudo-LE cell. (b, e) Typical LE cells, with phagocytosis of markedly altered nuclear material. (c) Rosette, with adherence of several polymorphs to a homogenized nucleus. (d) Phagocytosis of partially altered nuclei. (f) Aggregate of LE cells.

(a–c) Phase contrast; (d–f) Giemsa stain. See Robineaux, in *Henry Ford Hospital Symposium on Mechanisms of Hypersensitivity*, J. H. Shaffer et al., eds., Little, Brown, Boston, 1959, pp. 371–95.

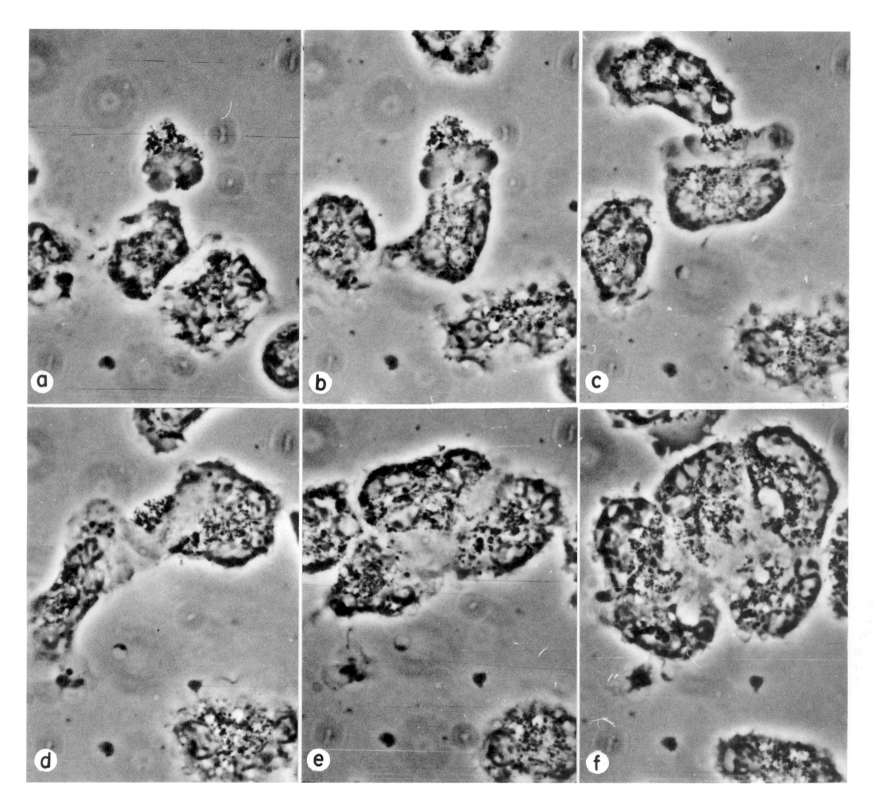

Fig. 10.15. Opsonization of the nucleus by antinuclear antibody with successive stages in the formation of a rosette. Washed normal human blood leukocytes, mixed with serum of a lupus erythematosus patient containing antinuclear factor, and incubated at 37°C for 2 hours. (a) Damaged leukocyte with homogenized nucleus. (b–d) Successive adherence of one, two, and three normal polymorpho-nuclear leukocytes to the altered nuclear mass. A small tag of the damaged cell's cytoplasm remains attached to the nucleus. (e, f) Formation of rosette with four and five adherent polys.

Phase contrast; time-lapse cinematography. From Robineaux, *Henry Ford Hospital Symposium on Mechanisms of Hypersensitivity,* J. H. Shaffer et al., eds., Little, Brown, Boston, 1959, pp. 371–95.

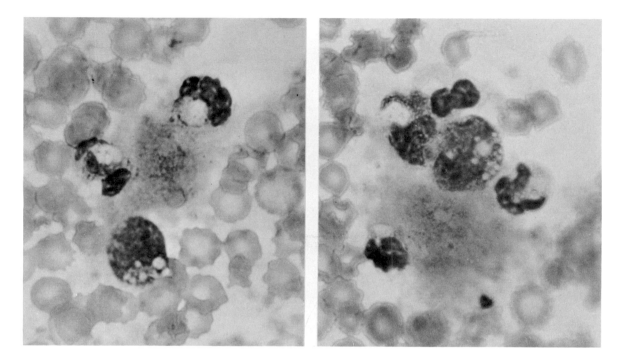

Fig. 10.16. The "lympholysis" phenomenon of Favour, produced by tuberculoprotein, specific anti-body, and complement acting on blood leukocytes and lymphocytes. Fresh blood of rabbit, sensitized by repeated iv injection of heat-killed tubercle bacilli, incubated with old tuberculin 1:20 for 1 hour. Both fields show amorphous, basophilic masses of fused platelets with adherent polymorphs and lymphocytes showing varying degrees of vacuolation and nuclear alteration. In this experiment the total counts of polys and lymphocytes were reduced by 40 per cent and 11 per cent respectively after 6-hour incubation.

Wright's stain; ×1,000. From Waksman and Bocking, *Am. Rev. Tuberc. 69*: 1002–15 (1954).

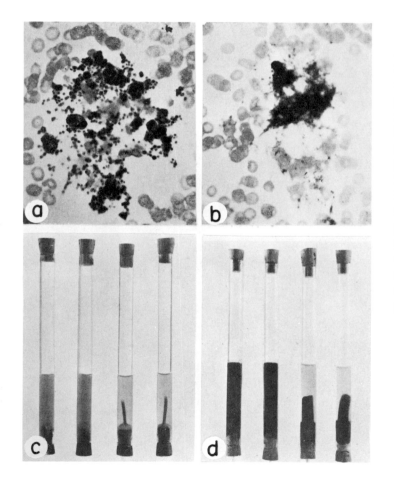

Fig. 10.17. (a, b) Photomicrographs of Leishman-stained blood films showing lysis of platelets by sedormid during coagulation of blood from patient who has recovered from Sedormid purpura. (a) Blood diluted with saline; sample aspirated at 5 minutes. Large clump of platelets, essentially unlysed. (b) Same blood sample, diluted with saturated solution of Sedormid in saline; sample aspirated at 2½ minutes. Large clump of platelets undergoing lysis. Platelets in center are fused and few of these in periphery remain recognizable. By 2½ minutes later, almost no recognizable platelets remained. (c, d) Effect on clot retraction of removal of platelets. Blood of same patient illustrated above. (c) Plasma clotted with thrombin after centrifugal removal of platelets (first two tubes) compared with normal plasma clotted with plasma. (d) Blood plus saturated solution of Sedormid in saline (first two tubes) compared with blood plus saline. In each case, platelet removal or destruction results in failure of clot retraction.

From Ackroyd, *Clin. Sci. 8*: 235–67 (1949).

11. Anaphylaxis and Related Phenomena

Anaphylaxis, classically, is the reaction induced by a systemic dose of antigen in a sensitized animal possessing humoral antibody. Gross manifestations in the guinea pig include itching, sneezing, coughing, respiratory embarrassment, involuntary urination and defecation, convulsions, prostration, and death in 2–5 minutes. Autopsy shows severe bronchoconstriction and inflated lungs (Fig. 11.7). In the rabbit, death occurs in minutes, but there is little respiratory difficulty, and autopsy shows pulmonary circulatory obstruction and right heart failure. Dogs show profound prostration with vomiting and bloody diarrhea, death following in 1–2 hours. At postmortem, hepatic vein obstruction and liver engorgement are found. The picture of anaphylaxis in man is a combination of several of the above elements.

The *pathophysiologic findings* associated with anaphylaxis fall into two major groups. On the one hand there is degranulation of the mast cells near blood vessels and circulating basophils (Figs. 11.3,4). There may be a comparable "lysis" of platelets and in some instances degranulation of polymorphs and even reticuloendothelial cells in the liver. In each case the *cell releases* one or more *pharmacologically active materials* without itself being killed. These include histamine, heparin, 5-hydroxytryptamine, slow-reacting substance (SRS–A), kinins, and lysosomal enzymes. These in turn produce a striking increase of vascular permeability affecting venules and small veins (frontispiece; Figs. 11.2,5,6), smooth muscle contraction, glandular hypersecretion, incoagulability of the blood, changes in heart rate, etc.; also secondary physiologic changes including the bronchial obstruction seen in guinea pigs and the localized vascular obstruction in rabbits and dogs, as well as shock, hypothermia, anoxia, and so forth. On the other hand one sees *noncellular emboli*, consisting of antigen–antibody aggregates and possibly other proteins (Figs. 11.8,9), a fall in complement, and formation of *poly–platelet aggregates*, with resulting leukopenia, thrombocytopenia, and embolization of small vessels. These are followed by vascular necrosis, hemorrhage, and focal necrosis of, e.g., the liver and myocardium. This group of changes is closely related to the Arthus mechanism (Section 12).

The relative importance of the two groups of findings differs in different species of animals, with different types of antibody, and with different durations. *Acute anaphylaxis* is dominated by the release of mediators. Histamine and heparin are formed and stored in mast cells (and basophils and platelets), for example, and released by the mechanism triggered by the antigen–antibody reaction. 5-Hydroxytryptamine is made in enterochromaffin cells, taken up by platelets from the plasma, stored, and released; SRS–A is newly formed after the antigen–antibody reaction, apparently in polys. Kinins are formed from serum proteins by an enzyme (kallikrein) released at the time of the trigger reaction. Lysosomal enzymes may be released from polys and liver macrophages. Finally, different "anaphylatoxins" are formed by the splitting of certain complement components (C′3 and C′5) when complement is activated by the antigen–antibody reaction. The relative importance of these different agents varies in different situations. *Protracted anaphylaxis* is dominated by embolic phenomena, hemorrhage, and necrosis.

The major determinant of the type of anaphylaxis observed is the nature of the participating antibody. *Cytotropic anaphylaxis* involves antibodies fixed in the tissues from the circulation, a process requiring some time (hours). Homocytotropic antibody can sensitize the individual's own tissues. One or two types are recognized in each species studied (man, dog, rabbit, rat, mouse, guinea pig), one being comparable to γE-globulin (atopic reagin) in man. Heterocytotropic antibody is active when transferred to other species. Only slow-migrating γG-globulin has this property. *Aggregate anaphylaxis* is produced by formation of soluble antigen–antibody aggregates, e.g. in rabbits or guinea pigs with high titers of circulating γG-antibody, and can be mimicked by injection of antibody against the individual's own γG-globulin or indeed injection of preformed, aggregated

γG-globulin alone. Here no tissue fixation is involved, and no latent period for "sensitization" with passive antibody is required. *Cytotoxic anaphylaxis* is produced with complement-fixing antibody (γM or γG) directed at specific cells, e.g. endothelium, and is identical with immune lysis as defined in Section 10. In species such as the guinea pig, which easily form homocytotropic antibody, anaphylaxis is predominantly a tissue reaction. In species which form large amounts of γG (rabbit), the usual reaction is aggregate anaphylaxis in the blood stream. Many species (man, rat, mouse) commonly exhibit both mechanisms.

Anaphylaxis may be investigated at the level of the intact individual (Fig. 11.1). However, much of our knowledge of both its immunologic and its physiologic mechanisms is derived from the study of cutaneous anaphylaxis and passive cutaneous anaphylaxis (PCA), with observation of edema or blueing, the local leakage of intravenously injected dye (frontispiece; Fig. 11.2). Isolated tissues (perfused or chopped lung, uterus, ileum, mesentery) have been studied grossly for contraction, histologically for degranulation of mast cells, or physiologically for release of mediators. Cell suspensions (peritoneal mast cells, blood leukocytes, platelets) similarly have been examined for degranulation or release. In studies of the immunologic reactants, both antigen and antibody are passively administered to normal recipients. Either reactant may be given systemically and the other locally, both may be systemic, or both local; and antibody may be injected before antigen (direct passive sensitization) or after (reversed passive sensitization). The same maneuvers can be performed with isolated tissues or cell suspensions.

Fixation of cytotropic antibodies in tissue is a process taking several hours and is affected by such factors as temperature, ionic strength of the medium (affecting charge of the antibody molecule), pCO_2 (affecting intracellular pH), and the presence and concentration of competing "normal" immunoglobulin. Nanogram amounts of antibody per gram of tissue suffice to sensitize. Preformed aggregates, on the other hand, are effective releasers only in 100- to 1,000-fold greater concentrations. The role of the *Fc* portion of the antibody molecule, which does not contain specific antibody-binding sites, in fixation and in the action of preformed aggregates, and the role of molecular distortion in the Fc portion of the molecule in the triggering process, are under active investigation.

The release phenomenon in cytotropic systems involves activation of a chymotrypsin-like enzyme and requires Ca^{++}, free SH groups, and thermolabile components which may overlap in part the system of complement components. The mast cell extrudes its granules without losing the integrity of the plasma membrane a process comparable to exoplasmosis or to the discharge of zymogen granules from pancreatic cells (Figs. 11. 3, 4). In aggregate anaphylaxis, platelets actually phagocytize specific precipitates and release mediators by a process analogous to explasmosis, and a similar mechanism accounts for release of lysosomal enzymes from polys and macrophages. Soluble complexes produce a cytotoxic (complement-mediated) release from platelets, accompanied by leakage of intracellular contents such as K^-.

Eosinophilic cell infiltrates are characteristic of certain responses thought to involve antigen–antibody reactions (Figs. 2.18,19; 11.10–12). Available evidence suggests that antibody of the γE type is involved. However, the conditions under which such responses are seen are as yet inadequately defined.

Anaphylactoid phenomena are produced in normal individuals by injection of any of a variety of materials capable of releasing mediators such as histamine without the intervention of an antigen–antibody reaction. The resulting clinical, physiological, and pathological picture may be virtually indistinguishable from that of true anaphylaxis. Effective releasers include proteolytic enzymes, surface-active materials, peptones, a variety of simple and complex organic bases which act to displace histamine from its complex with heparin, certain large molecules such as dextran, and anaphylatoxin. Releasers are present in bee and wasp venoms and in certain foods (lobster, strawberries).

Atopic allergy is the group of naturally occurring human allergies to pollens, foods, insect stings, etc., which includes asthma, hay fever, urticaria (hives), and atopic eczema. Contrary to statements in many texts, animals get typical atopy, e.g., dogs suffer from hay fever during ragweed season (Fig. 11.1). Most atopy is anaphylactic. The same clinical elements are present (itching and whealing, sneezing, respiratory embarrassment), the same pathophysiologic elements (edema, smooth muscle contraction, hypersecretion, leukopenia), and the same pharmacologic findings (release of histamine, SRS-A, etc. as part of the process and partial protection by anti-histaminic drugs). Histamine is released from sensitized tissues triggered by allergen *in vitro*. The atopic subject is exposed only to low dosage of antigen reaching sensitized tissues by inefficient routes, i.e. across mucous membranes. This accounts for the lesser degree of symptomatology, as compared with anaphylaxis, and for the frequent localization of disease to one organ. However, a sufficiently large systemic dose of antigen, administered parenterally by some mischance, causes typical anaphylactic shock, often with death in 2–5 minutes. Conversely, anaphylactically sensitized guinea pigs exposed to an aerosol of antigen develop typical asthma.

The antibody responsible for atopic allergy, *atopic reagin*, is a homocytotropic γE-globulin. It is heat-labile (56°C, 4 hours), fixes in tissues such as skin for long periods of time (8–10 weeks or more), and sensitizes the site at which it is fixed in amounts as low as 1–2 ng for a passive wheal and flare (the Prausnitz-Küstner or P-K reaction) (Fig. 11.1). It can sensitize the tissues (lung, ileum, skin) of other primates (frontispiece) but does not give precipitation, complement-fixation, or passive anaphylaxis in the guinea pig. It is most easily identified by its ability to mediate histamine release from normal human white cells sensitized *in vitro*. Members of families showing unusual susceptibility to atopic allergy apparently have an increased ability to produce antibody of reagin type in response to antigenic stimuli (pollen, foods, insect bites) to which most of the population do not respond. However, nonatopic individuals produce reagin and develop anaphylactic responses to antigens of helminth parasites and to certain antigens in injected horse serum. Thus the formation of reagin is itself a normal defensive mechanism. In atopics treated with repeated small doses of antigen (hyposensitization), there appears a thermostable *blocking antibody*, which does not give a P-K reaction and blocks the P-K when added to serum containing reagin. This antibody has now been definitely identified as γA-immunoglobulin.

The fact that atopic allergy is frequently expressed in a single organ, the *shock organ*—the lung in asthma, the skin in food allergies, the upper respiratory mucosa in hay fever due to pollens—is accounted for in part by the route of exposure to allergen and in part by the enhanced localization of antibody occurring at a site of existing inflammation. However, the shock organ also shows an abnormal sensitivity to histamine and other mediators, which has been attributed to "induced histamine" synthesis within the organ itself. It follows that any agency causing histamine release for physiologic purposes, such as trauma, heat, exercise, or psychogenic stimuli, will tend to cause symptoms in the shock organ and exacerbate effects produced by the immunologic reaction.

Nonimmunologic disease, which resembles atopic allergy, occurs in a number of situations (Fig. 11.1). Any abnormality in the pathway of histamine release or the sensitivity of target cells to histamine and other mediators may result in wheal and flare or bronchoconstrictive reactions. Examples are dermographism (trauma), physical allergy (heat, cold), urticaria occurring with heat, exercise, or emotion in young girls, and atopic phenomena occurring on psychiatric grounds. In any individual case, the mechanism may prove quite simple. Hereditary angioneurotic edema, for example, is directly attributable to a deficiency of complement C'la esterase inhibitor, which leads to hyperactivity of the complement system after any of the usual trigger reactions. Conversely, a given situation may be more complicated than it seems. Certain cases of physical allergy have an immunologic basis, the physical agency producing altered tissue antigens to which the patient is sensitized.

Few cases of atopy present a simple anaphylactic situation. Asthma, in particular, is frequently complicated by infection, bacterial allergy, bronchiectasis, and by the abnormal pharmacologic response to all sorts of stimuli.

There is a separate group of pulmonary diseases associated with circulating precipitating antibody against inhalant allergens, derived especially from thermophilic actinomycetes in moldy hay (farmer's lung) or other plant or animal products (maple bark stripper's disease, pigeon fancier's lung, mushroom picker's disease, bagassosis, etc.). These are characterized by interstitial inflammatory lesions, fibrosis, and granuloma formation and may involve Arthus and delayed reaction mechanisms rather than anaphylaxis.

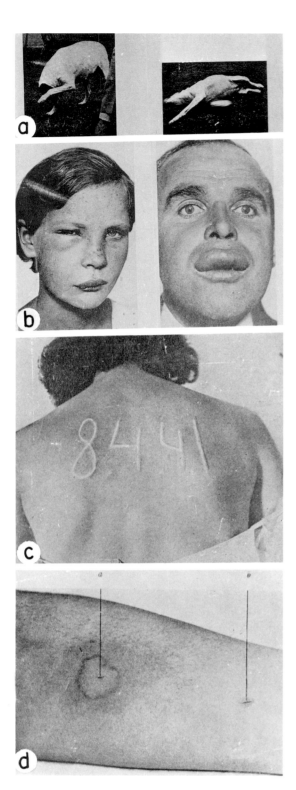

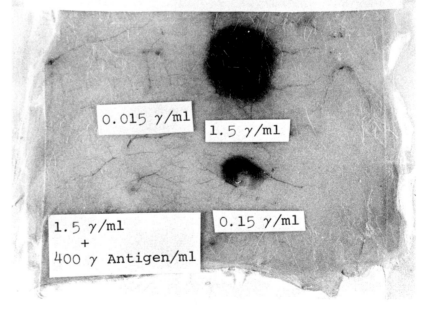

Fig. 11.1. Anaphylactic and anaphylactoid manifestations. (a) Naturally occurring hay fever in dog sensitive to ragweed pollen. Characteristic movements observed during pollination season. The same responses could be elicited by ophthalmic and nasal tests with ragweed pollen out of season. (b) Angioneurotic edema of periorbital and perioral tissues and of upper lip in specifically sensitive subjects after ingestion of sardines and acetylsalicylic acid (aspirin) respectively. (c) Dermographism: wheal and flare reaction elicited by mild trauma. (d) Cutaneous anaphylaxis: wheal and flare reaction elicited by scratch test with ragweed pollen in sensitive subject (*a*) and control test with diluent alone (*b*).

(a) From Wittich, *J. Allergy 12*: 247–51 (1941), C. V. Mosby, St. Louis. (b–d) From E. Urbach and P. M. Gottlieb, *Allergy*, Grune and Stratton, New York, 1946.

Fig. 11.2. Quantitative study of passive cutaneous anaphylaxis (PCA) in guinea pig, sensitized with rabbit γG-globulin antibody against DNP-BGG injected intradermally in various doses, and challenged 4 hours later with a large dose of DNP-BSA injected iv with Evans blue dye. DNP-specific reaction (at 20 minutes) is seen at site sensitized with 0.015 μg of antibody, but not 0.0015 μg. Addition of excess antigen (40 μg) effectively neutralizes largest dose tested (0.15 μg). Note that identity of carrier protein does not affect nature of reaction, which is hapten-specific.

Courtesy of Dr. Z. Ovary.

PCA in Guinea Pig. Latent Period 4 h.
Antibody: Rabbit IgG anti-$DNP_{55}BGG$.

Antigen : $DNP_{37}BSA$ (500 γ protein iv).
Intradermal injections: 0.1 ml/sites.

0.015 γ/ml

1.5 γ/ml

1.5 γ/ml
+
400 γ Antigen/ml

0.15 γ/ml

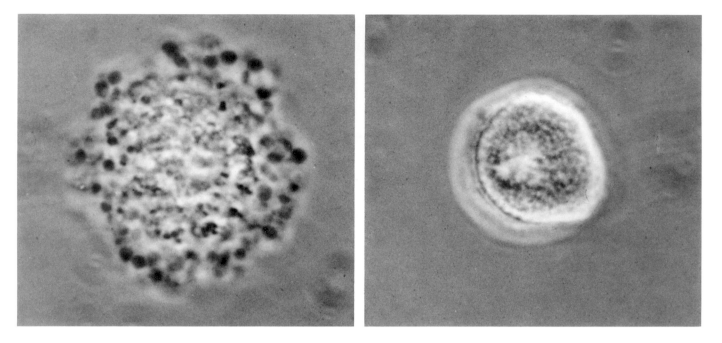

Fig. 11.3. Anaphylactic mast cell degranulation. Sensitized rat peritoneal mast cells incubated 3 minutes at 37°C in presence and absence of specific antigen, left and right respectively. Phase contrast; × 2,300. Courtesy of Dr. J. H. Humphrey.

FIGURES 11.4 and 11.5

Mast cell degranulation in rat skin during passive cutaneousa naphylaxis. Electron micrographs; magnifications not given. Courtesy of Dr. D. Lagunoff.

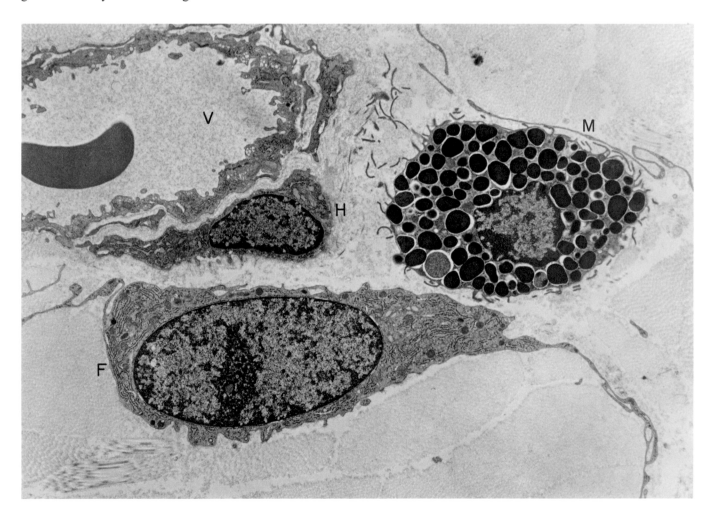

Fig. 11.4. Normal mast cell (M) located close to venule (V) in deep dermal connective tissue. An adventitial histiocyte (H) is situated at the surface of the vessel and a fibroblast (F) is seen adjacent to this group of tissue elements, with processes extending between bundles of collagen fibers.

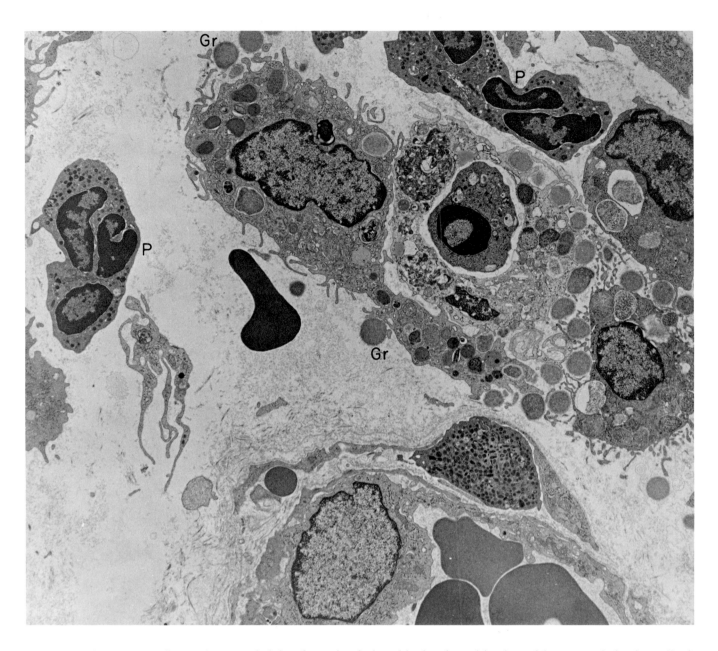

Fig. 11.5. Two mast cells are shown at height of reaction induced by local sensitization with rat anaphylactic antibody (formed after immunization with human serum albumin and pertussis as adjuvant) and later systemic challenge with homologous antigen. Lysis of the cytoplasmic granules is shown by their change in electron density, and many granules (Gr) are seen escaping from the cell surface (degranulation). The connective tissue elements are widely separated by fluid (edema) and there are a few polymorphonuclear leukocytes (P) in the perivascular zone of inflammation.

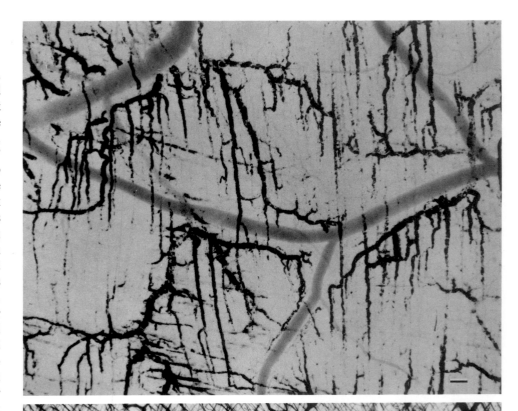

Fig. 11.6. Vessel permeability in anaphylactoid states. Thin sheets of striated muscle (rat cremaster), prepared in different ways and shown at the same enlargement (×45) to demonstrate the selective nature of leakage induced by the action of serotonin (or histamine). (Above) Typical example of "vascular labeling," whereby leaking blood vessels are marked *in vivo* with carbon black. Serotonin was injected over the cremaster muscle, and a suspension of carbon black injected iv. As a result of the serotonin injection, gaps developed between endothelial cells in the venules; plasma, loaded with carbon black, escaped through these gaps; the basement membrane, however, remained intact, and acting as a filter retained the carbon particles in amounts large enough to form visible deposits. One hour later the animal was killed, the cremaster was fixed in formalin, cleared in glycerin, and examined by transillumination. No carbon is visible in the blood stream because it has been removed by the reticuloendothelial system, but some is quite obviously trapped within the wall of the leaking vessel. *The vessels which appear in heavy black are those that have been induced to leak by the local injection of serotonin.* Scale = 100 μ. (Below) Cremaster of normal rat in which the entire vascular system has been injected with a mixture of carbon and gelatin. Note large number of very fine vessels (capillaries, in the strictest sense) superimposed in different planes. By comparing this photograph with the one above, it becomes apparent that the great majority of these fine vessels are not blackened by the method of vascular labeling: i.e. are not induced to leak by serotonin (histamine would give the same effect). From Majno and Palade, *J. Biophys. Biochem. Cytol. 11*: 607–26 (1961).

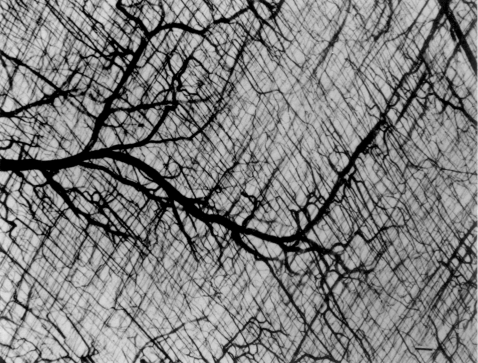

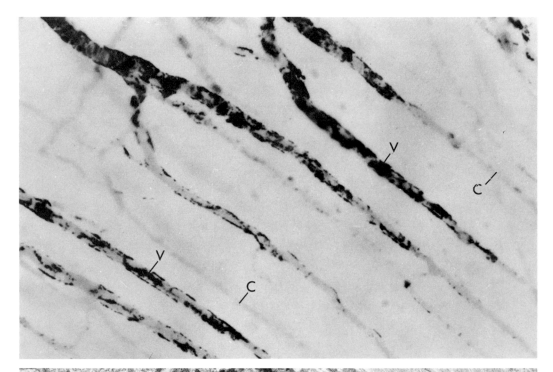

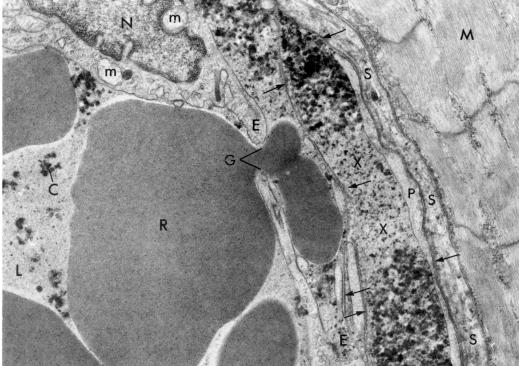

Fig. 11.7. Detail from preparations similar to that of Fig. 11.6 (upper). Vascular leakage was induced with histamine, and the leaking vessels were marked *in vivo* with carbon black. (Above) High-power view (×300). Note abundant deposits of carbon in the venules (V), whereas in the capillaries (C) carbon deposits are minimal or absent. (Below) Electron micrograph, demonstrating typical endothelial gap in the wall of a venule 3 minutes after local injection of histamine (and iv injection of colloidal carbon black). L, lumen of venule; SSS, extravascular space; M, fiber of striated muscle; R, red blood cell which is partially engaged in a gap (G) between the endothelial cells E, E. Note the multiple layers of cells and of basement membrane (arrows), a structural characteristic of the venules. The wall of this leaking vessel is partially dissociated —in the manner of a dissecting aneurysm—by deposits of retained materials (X, X): carbon particles, and very small osmiophilic bodies presumably chylomicra and lipoprotein aggregates. N, nucleus of endothelial cell; m, m, dilated mitochondria (this dilation is not constant and probably artefactual); C, carbon particles still present in the circulating plasma.

×17,800. Courtesy of Drs. G. I. Schoefl and G. Majno.

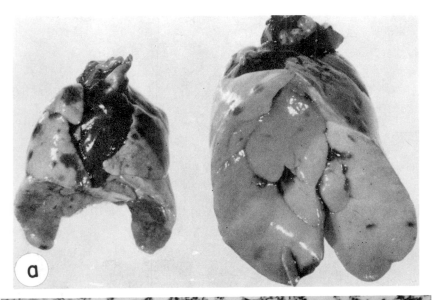

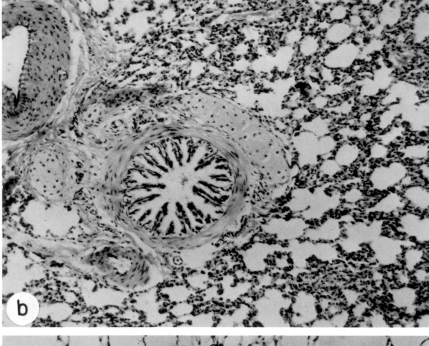

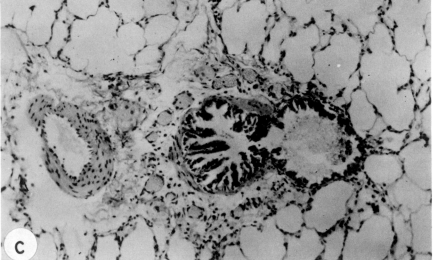

Fig. 11.8. Systemic anaphylaxis. (a) Gross appearance of lungs from a normal guinea pig, sacrificed by a blow on the head and from one dying in anaphylactic shock within several minutes after iv injection of soluble antigen–antibody complexes in antigen excess. Note increase in lung size due to bronchiolar constriction and extensive emphysema. The heart is hidden from view by the overinflated lungs. Small pulmonary hemorrhages are characteristic feature of shock induced in this manner. (b, c) Sections of the lung from a normal guinea pig and from one dying in anaphylactic shock. The only abnormalities in the latter are vascular stasis and marked emphysema. Hematoxylin-eosin; ×115.

(a) From Germuth and McKinnon, *Bull. Johns Hopk. Hosp. 101*: 13–43 (1957). (b, c) Courtesy of Dr. F. J. Dixon.

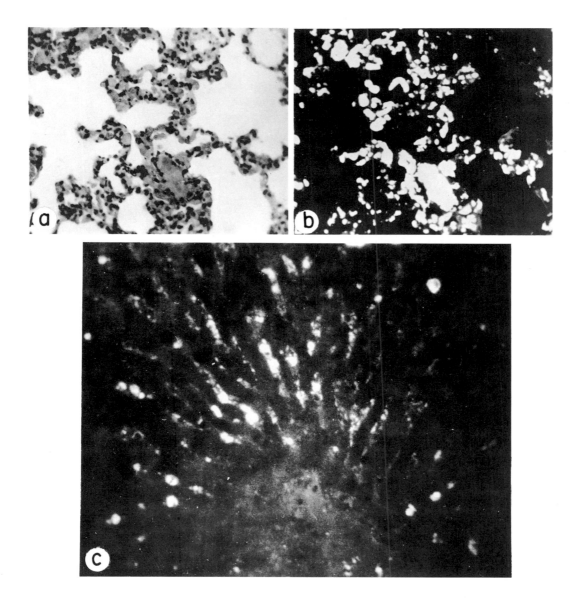

Fig. 11.9. Antigen–antibody complexes in anaphylaxis. (a) Rabbit sensitized to BSA and challenged with fluorescein-labeled BSA. Lung showing amorphous, eosinophilic intra-capillary "thrombi." (b) Same microscopic field under ultraviolet illumination, showing presence of fluorescent antigen in "thrombi." (c) Rat sensitized with HSA, shocked with iv antigen, and sacrificed at 6 hours. Liver section, stained with fluorescent anti-HSA, shows intravascular aggregates containing antigen in sinusoids about portal triad. Rat γ-globulin is also found in these deposits by suitable stains.

(a) Hematoxylin-eosin and (b) direct fluorescence method; both ×150. (c) Indirect fluor-escence technique; ×200. (a, b) From McKinnon, Andrews, Heptinstall, and Germuth, *Bull. Johns Hopk. Hosp. 101*: 258–80 (1957). (c) From Fennell and Santamaria, *Am. J. Path. 41*: 521–34 (1962).

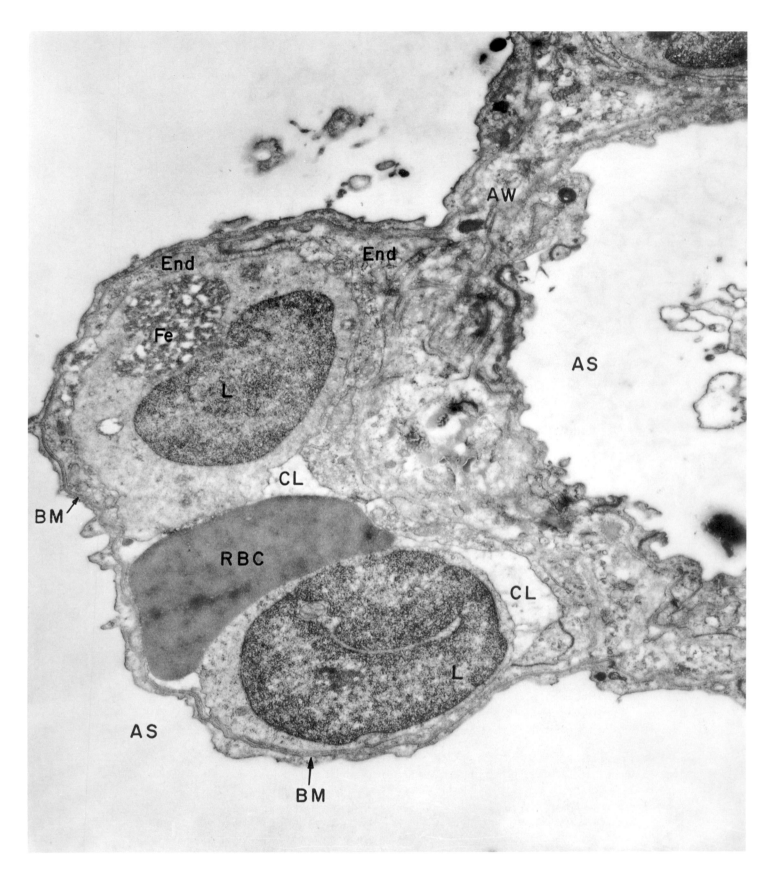

Fig. 11.10. Pulmonary anaphylaxis, rabbit. A single capillary from the lung of a rabbit immunized with horse ferritin and injected iv with 48 mg of ferritin at the time circulating antibody reached 500 μg/ml. Several minutes after onset of anaphylaxis, one sees within the capillary lumen (CL) an antigen–antibody precipitate (Fe) encircled by cytoplasm of a wandering blood cell (L). Antigen was not found in endothelium (End), in basement membrane (BM), in alveolar epithelium, or alveolar spaces (AS) but always as a precipitate within the vascular lumen. RBC, red cells; AW, alveolar wall.

Electron micrograph; ×19,800. Courtesy of Dr. F. J. Dixon.

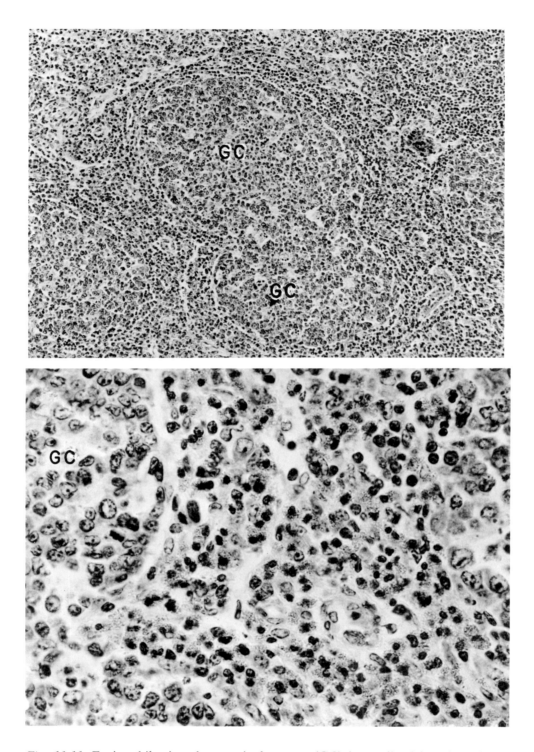

Fig. 11.11. Eosinophils ring the germinal centers (GC) in popliteal lymph node of guinea pig 1 day after the last of seven weekly footpad injections of hemocyanin. In black and white photomicrographs, they are conspicuous by their dark, compact nuclei and cytoplasmic granules. Presumably they are present as a response to complex of antigen with one molecular form of antibody (γE?).

Dominici stain; ×150, ×600. From Litt, *Am. J. Path. 42*: 529–49 (1963).

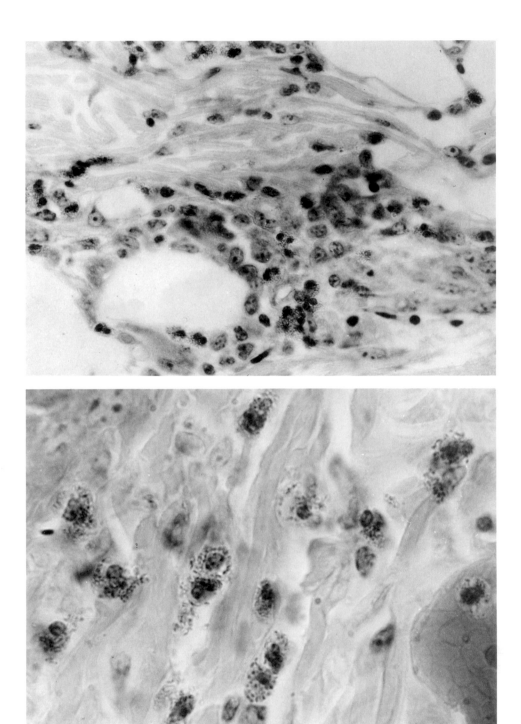

Fig. 11.12. Eosinophils at site of retest reaction in guinea pig with mild delayed sensitization, induced by footpad inoculation of 0.28 μg diphtheria toxoid in saline. Skin site is shown after elicitation of a delayed skin reaction with 2.8 μg toxoid at 7 days and retest with the same dose at the same site at 12 days. (Above) Infiltration of eosinophils in nest of residual histiocytes in the deep dermis, 24 hours after retest; ×600. (Below) Eosinophils in superficial dermis; ×1,200. Dominici stain. From Arnason and Waksman, *Lab. Invest. 12*: 737–47 (1963).

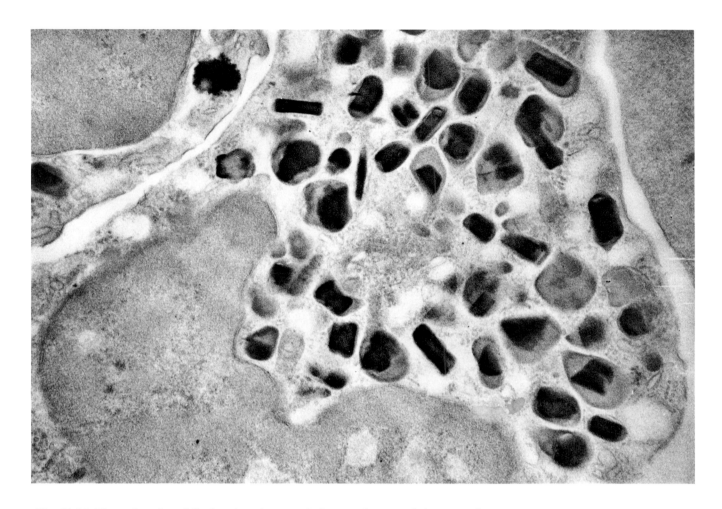

Fig. 11.13. Normal eosinophil, showing characteristic granules containing crystals.
Electron micrograph; ×15,000. From Bessis, in *Electron Microscopic Anatomy*, S. M. Kurtz, ed., Academic Press, New York, 1964.

12. Local Phenomena of Arthus Type

The reaction to skin test with antigen in a suitably sensitized individual consists of local *edema, erythema*, and *hemorrhage*, appearing over a half hour or more, reaching a *maximum at 2–5 hours* (later if the reaction is very severe), and presenting gross necrosis secondarily (in reactions of maximal intensity) (Fig. 12.1). This is the local Arthus reaction. The same lesion can be elicited by injection of antigen into any vascular organ: brain, stomach, kidney, liver, lung, testis, joint, eye, etc. (Figs. 12.3,15). In the absence of vessels, as in the cornea, only a deposit of immune precipitate is formed, and damage is limited to cellular elements within the zone of precipitation (Figs. 12.12–14).

Arthus reactions may be produced passively with humoral antibody (Fig. 12.3). Precipitating complement-fixing (γM or γG) antibody must be present in the circulation in large amounts, as much as a thousand times more than is required for a strong local anaphylactic response. The antibody is not fixed in tissues; indeed cytotropic antibody, such as guinea pig γ_1-globulin in the guinea pig, will not mediate an Arthus reaction. As with anaphylaxis, passive sensitization may be local or systemic, and one may study direct or reversed passive lesions as well as lesions produced with preformed immune complexes (Figs. 12.6,8).

Histologically, the Arthus reaction is characterized by *vascular fibrinoid necrosis, edema*, massive *diapedesis of neutrophils* and some eosinophils, and *hemorrhage* (Figs. 12.2,3). There may also be thrombi of polys and platelets. Microscopic observations *in vivo* (ear chamber or exposed mesentery) show the same details: leukocyte and platelet clumping and sticking to vessel walls, thrombosis, diapedesis, and vascular necrosis, sometimes reaching a peak as late as 8–10 hours after administration of antigen.

Fluorescence microscopy shows the intraluminal formation and subendothelial deposition of antigen–antibody aggregates and the fixation of complement (Figs. 12.5,10). Activation of the complement leads to generation of chemotactic factors which in turn induce the local entry of granulocytes, apparently with the assistance of the clotting mechanism (Figs. 12.5,10). These phagocytize the immune complexes (Fig. 12.5) and there is intra- and extracellular discharge of their lysosomal contents, well visualized in electron micrographs (Figs. 12.9,11). The released acid hydrolases (cathepsins D and E) and "cationic protein" cause vascular necrosis and rupture of the basement membrane, with a secondary outpouring of protein and cells and hemorrhage. Thrombosis, when it occurs, may result in additional, ischemic damage. Arthus lesions produced passively by preformed complexes differ only insofar as the injected immune aggregates are outside the vessel at the initiation of the process (Fig. 12.6). In vessels altered by vasoactive amines such as histamine, there is preferential localization of complexes present in the circulation, with formation of typical local lesions (Fig. 12.8). This mechanism may play an important role in the pathogenesis of serum arteritis (Section 13).

The Arthus reaction can be mimicked by intradermal injection of poly granules or, indeed, of hydrolases derived from them. On the other hand, both active and passive Arthus lesions are suppressed by reduction in the available circulating granulocytes, as with irradiation, nitrogen mustard treatment, or injection of antipolymorph antiserum (Fig. 12.4), by reducing the number of platelets, by blocking the clotting mechanism with heparin, by use of antibody with the wrong properties (nonprecipitating, noncomplement-fixing), or by carrying out the correct procedures in complement-deficient animals. On the other hand, histamine injection does not duplicate the Arthus reaction, the reaction may occur in the absence of histamine release, and antihistaminic drugs have little or no effect on lesion formation. Release of other agents such as bradykinin, which affect vascular permeability, may, however, play a role. Since SH-dependent proteases (cathepsins) are major elements of the mechanism, increasing as the lesion grows, healed lesions may be reactivated (Fig. 12.7) by local injection of reduced glutathione or cysteine.

Late during the evolution of an Arthus reaction, there is a progressive *increase in* the number of *mononuclear cells*, and many of these undergo *transformation into plasma cells*. This change is comparable to the "progressive immunization reaction" seen at sites of antigen injection in normal animals (Section 5) but is relatively more intense in the Arthus site.

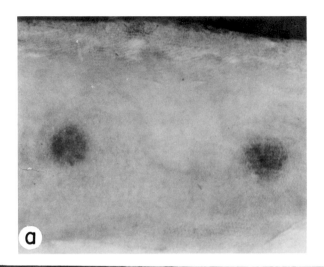

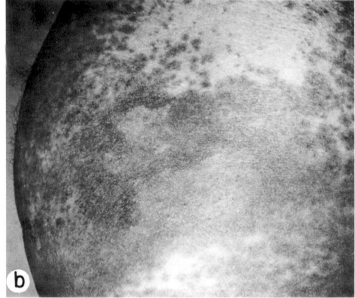

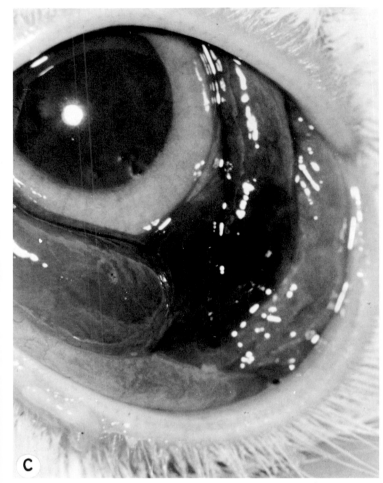

Fig. 12.1. Arthus reaction: gross manifestations. (a) Reversed passive Arthus reaction in rabbit given excess BSA iv and antibody (0.29 mg anti-BSA N) intradermally 6 hours earlier. Maximal response, showing pale erythema and edema, with central zone of hemorrhage. (b) Severe edematous and hemorrhagic lesion in buttock of previously sensitized human subject given local injection of penicillin. Character of reaction suggests that it depends on Arthus mechanism. (c) Arthus reaction in subconjunctival tissue of rabbit, passively immunized with iv antibody (12.1 mg N) and injected subconjunctivally at the same time with specific antigen (ovalbumin, 0.32 mg N). Severe edema (chemosis) and hemorrhage. Internal eye is normal.

(a) From Cochrane and Weigle, *J. Exp. Med. 108*: 591–604 (1958). (b) Courtesy of Dr. I. Braverman. (c) From Waksman and Bullington, *J. Immunol. 76*: 441–53 (1956).

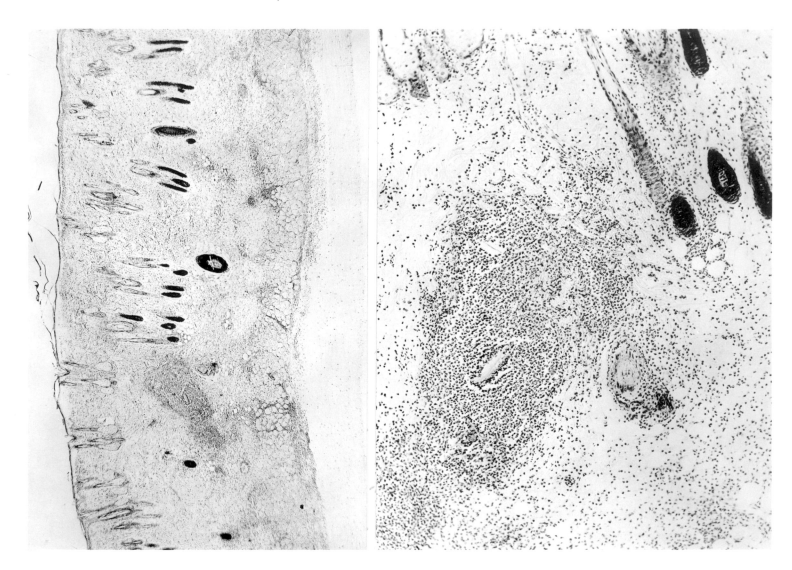

Fig. 12.2. Arthus reaction: microscopic character. Active 4-hour reaction, elicited with 30 μg BSA in flank skin of rat sensitized 2 weeks earlier with 500 μg BSA plus complete Freund adjuvant. Massive infiltration of vessel walls with polymorphs, and diffuse edema and poly infiltration. Hematoxylin-eosin; ×32 and ×120. From Janković, Waksman, and Arnason, *J. Exp. Med. 116*: 159–76 (1962).

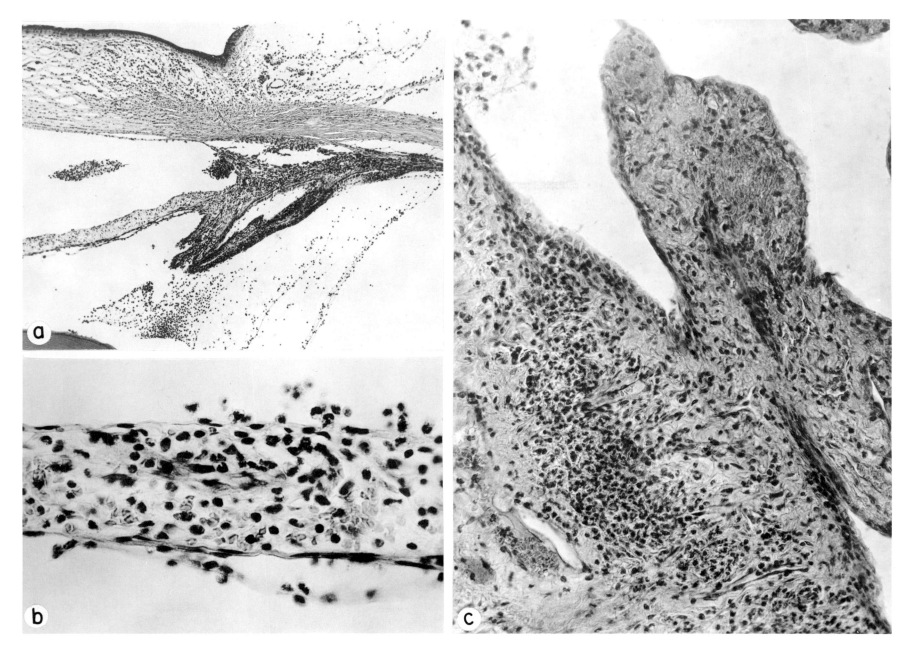

Fig. 12.3. Arthus reaction: microscopic character. (a, b) Passive Arthus reaction in guinea pig eye, elicited by rabbit antibody (1 mg) iv and ovalbumin (30 μg) in the vitreous. Iridocyclitis, showing exudation of polymorphonuclear leukocytes and petechial hemorrhages; ×35, ×440. (c) Similar lesion in rabbit eye, elicited by rabbit antibody (12.1 mg N) iv and ovalbumin (0.32 mg N) in the anterior chamber and photographed at 24 hours. Massive exudation of polys, iris edema, and hemorrhage in iris and ciliary body; ×200.

Hematoxylin-eosin. (a, b) Courtesy of Dr. A. Silverstein (AFIP negs. 59-3626, 3628). (c) From Waksman and Bullington, *J. Immunol. 76*: 441–53 (1956).

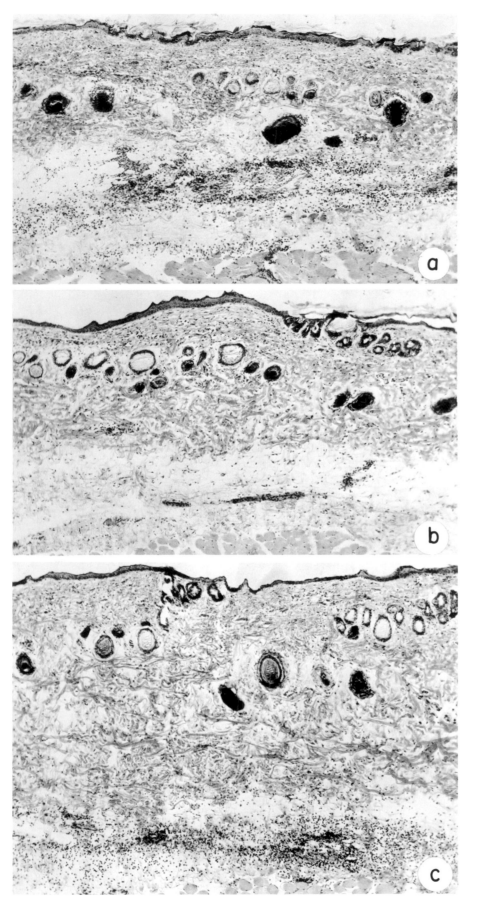

Fig. 12.4. Abolition of Arthus reaction by experimental production of leukopenia. Reversed passive Arthus lesions produced in guinea pigs by iv injection of 2 mg BSA, followed immediately by intradermal injection of specific rabbit antibody (0.1 mg N), and read at 2 hours. (a–c) Reactions in animals treated with rabbit antilymphocyte serum, antipolymorphonuclear serum, and normal serum respectively. In each case two doses of serum were given 18 hours and $\frac{1}{2}$ hour before the test. Reaction is suppressed specifically by antipolymorphonuclear serum.

Hematoxylin-eosin; ×55. From Waksman, Arbouys, and Arnason, *J. Exp. Med. 114*: 997–1022 (1961).

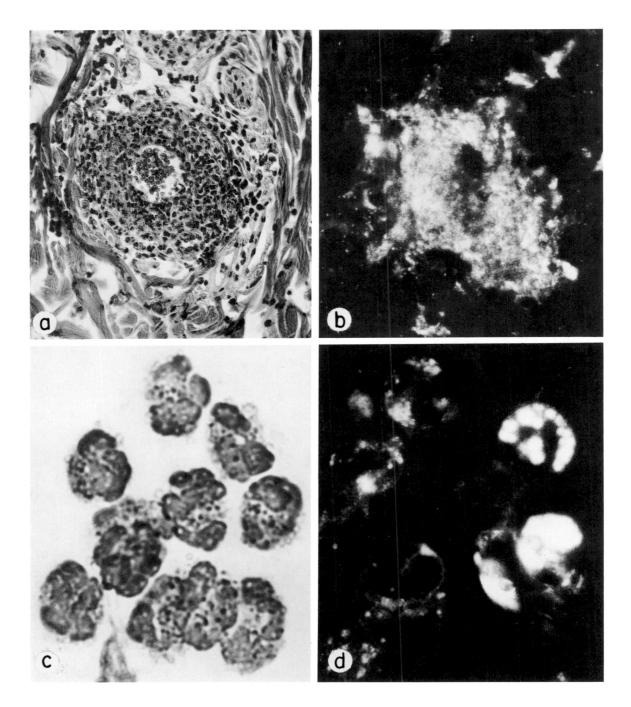

Fig. 12.5. Arthus reaction: immunochemical mechanism. (a) Classical Arthus reaction in rabbit skin at 8 hours, showing necrosis of vessel wall and massive infiltration of inflammatory cells. (b) Similar lesion stained for antigen (BSA), showing presence of immune complexes throughout area of inflammation. Essentially the same distribution is seen in reversed passive Arthus lesions. (c) Print of biopsied 7-hour lesion, showing predominantly polymorphonuclear character of cell exudate. (d) Similar print stained by fluorescence technique, showing uptake of BSA by these cells. Some contain a great deal of antigen, others very little. Stain for rabbit globulin shows its presence in the cells, presumably in immune complex with antigen; other serum proteins are not found. A similar pattern of staining is seen in mononuclear cells present in the Arthus lesions.

(a) Hematoxylin-eosin; ×280; (b) Fluorescence; ×240. (c) Wright's stain; ×2,700. (d) Fluorescence; ×2,700. From Cochrane and Weigle, *J. Exp. Med. 108*: 591–604 (1958) and Cochrane, Weigle, and Dixon, *J. Exp. Med. 110*: 481–94 (1959).

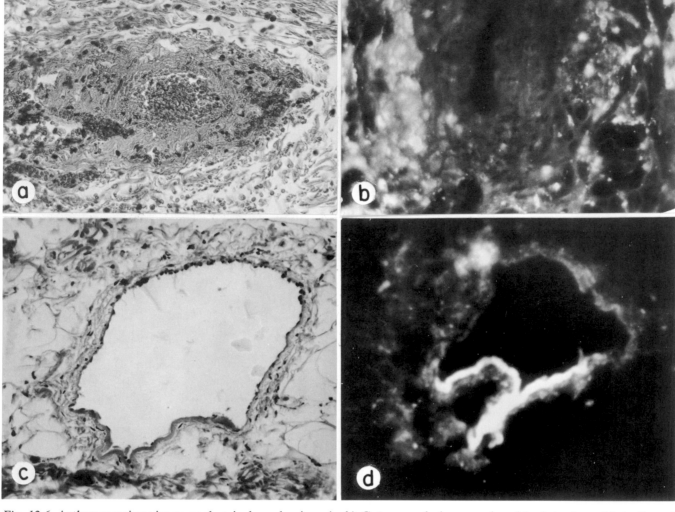

Fig. 12.6. Arthus reaction: immunochemical mechanism. (a, b) Cutaneous lesions produced by intradermal injection of soluble complexes, in conventional cell stain and stained by fluorescence for antigen (BSA). There is necrosis of vessel wall and hemorrhage but minimal cellular exudate. Correspondingly, antigen is abundant in connective tissue around vessel, but none is seen in vessel wall. (c, d) Active Arthus lesion (7 hours) in leukopenic rabbit, showing band of deposited material in lower portion of vessel wall but absence of any vascular reaction in the absence of polys. Material identified as antigen by fluorescence corresponds to line of deposit. Stain for rabbit globulin gives the same sharply localized line. Bright spot above is artefact.

(a, c) Hematoxylin-eosin; ×238, ×155. (b, d) Fluorescence technique; ×435, ×155. From Cochrane and Weigle, *J. Exp. Med. 108*: 591–604 (1958), and Cochrane, Weigle, and Dixon, *J. Exp. Med. 110*: 481–94 (1959).

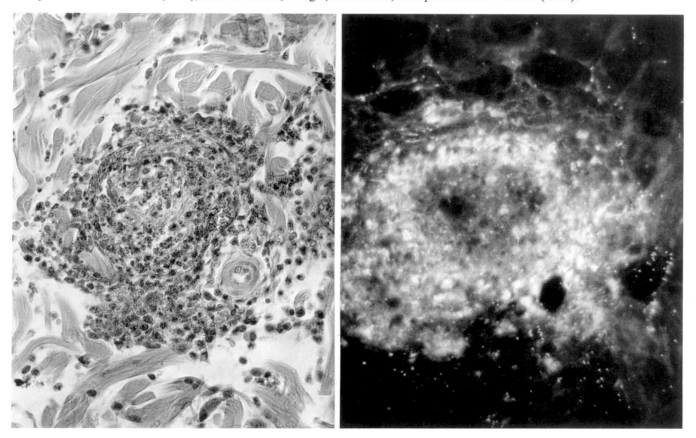

Fig. 12.7. Reactivation of Arthus lesion by injection of antigen (BSA, 75 μg N) into 72-hour site. Lesion photographed at 6 hours. Antigen (BSA) is localized, presumably as a complex with persisting antibody, throughout site of previous lesion in vessel wall, and zone of poly infiltration corresponds to this localization.

Hematoxylin-eosin; ×290; fluorescence technique; ×290. From Cochrane, Weigle, and Dixon, *Proc. Soc. Exp. Biol. Med. 101*: 695–99 (1959).

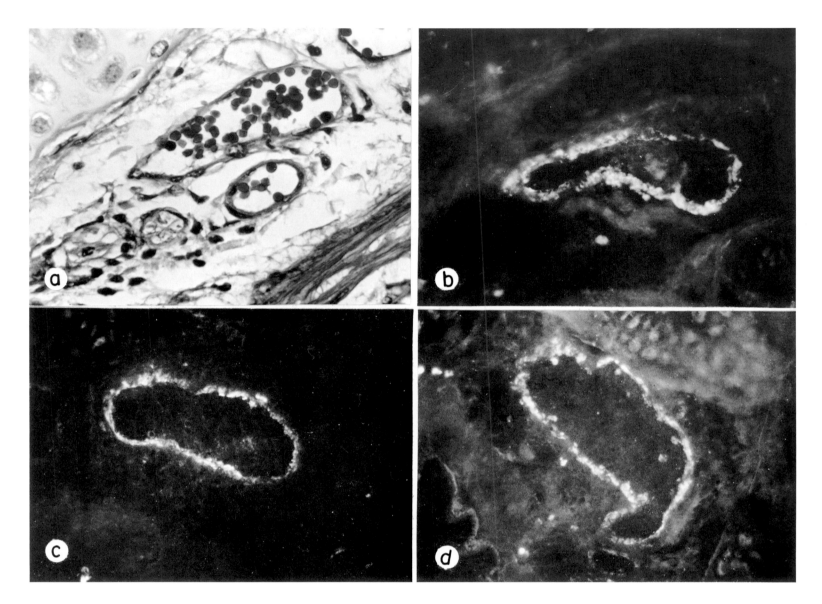

Fig. 12.8. Arthus reaction: immunochemical mechanism. Localization of circulating antigen–antibody complexes (BSA–anti-BSA) in walls of small pulmonary vessels in guinea pig subjected to histamine shock. (a) Vessel, a few minutes after initiation of process, shows dilatation but little sign of vessel-wall damage. (b–d) Similar vessels stained by fluorescence technique for antigen (BSA), antibody (rabbit γ-globulin), and host complement (guinea-pig C'3C). All show similar localization of immune complexes and complement fixation in vessel wall.

(a) Hematoxylin-eosin; ×340, (b–d) ×250. From Cochrane, *J. Exp. Med. 118*: 489–502 (1963).

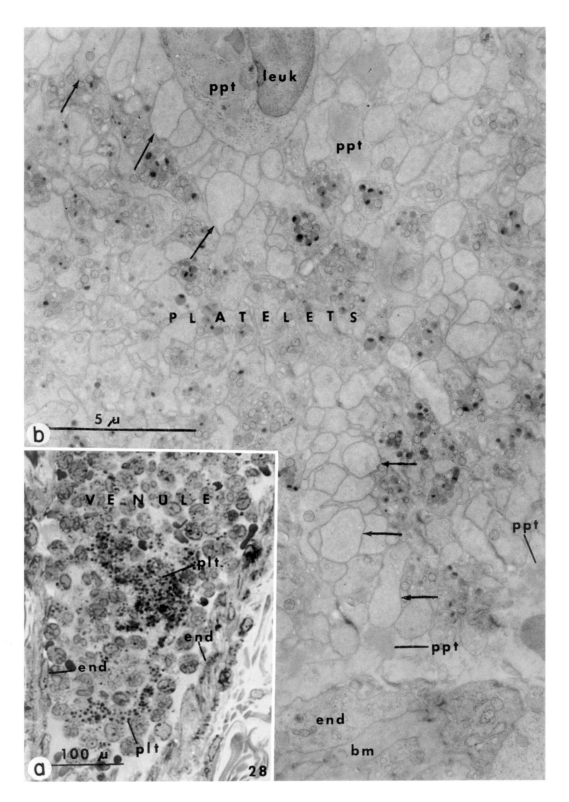

Fig. 12.9. Role of granulocytes and platelets in Arthus reaction. Two-hour reaction elicited by intradermal injection of 2.5 mg BSA in actively sensitized rabbit with high titer of circulating precipitating antibody (0.4–0.8 mg N/ml). (a) Light microscopic picture of large venule occluded by leukocytes and clumps of platelets (plt) (end, endothelium); ×200. (b) Low-power electron micrograph of same vessel. Precipitated material (ppt) is seen in leukocyte (leuk) and between leukocyte and platelets. Individual platelets are swollen (arrows) (bm, basement membrane); ×8,400.

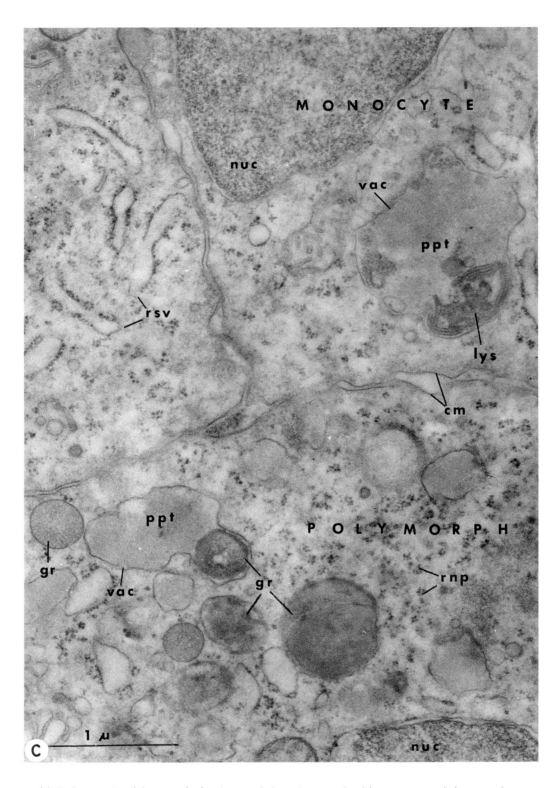

(c) Polymorph with vacuole (vac) containing phagocytized immune precipitate and granules (gr), one of which is discharging its contents into the vacuole. The monocyte shows similar vacuole and discharge of lysosome-like structure into it (nuc, nucleus; cm, cell membrane; rnp, ribosomes; rsv, endoplasmic reticulum); × 36,450.

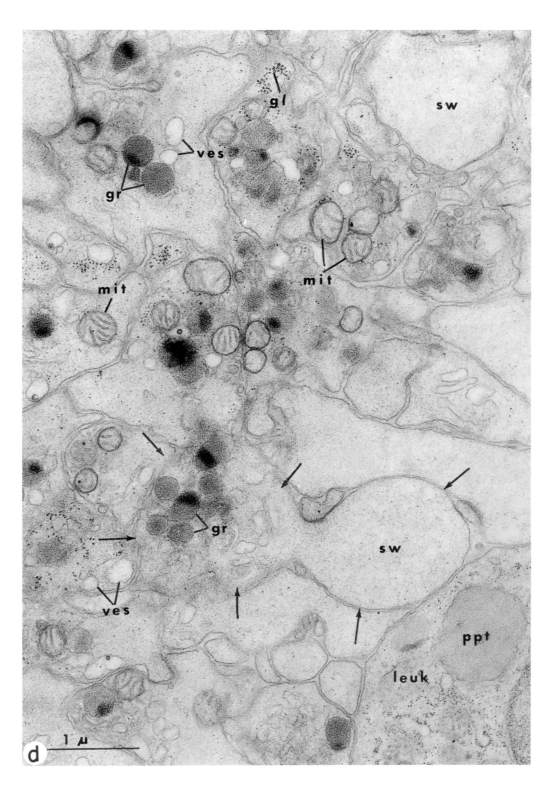

(d) Higher magnification and deeper cut of same area shown in (a). A single platelet is outlined by arrows. Its cytoplasm is swollen (sw). The granules show varying degrees of lysis. Some are dense and have well-marked limiting membrane; others are barely discernible. Leukocyte containing precipitate is seen at lower right (mit, mitochondria; ves, vesicles; gl, glycogen); ×26,900.

From Uriuhara and Movat, *Lab. Invest. 13*: 1057–79 (1964).

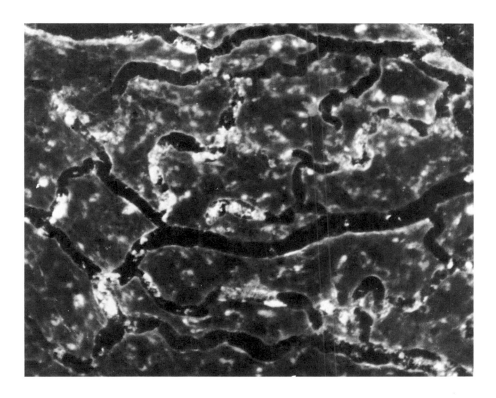

Fig. 12.10. Precipitated antigen (horse serum proteins) in lumen and walls of small vessels, as well as in smaller amounts in interstitial connective tissue of mesentery, 15 minutes after its surface application in actively sensitized rabbit.
Fluorescence technique; ×250. From Movat, *Verhandl. Deut. Ges. Path. 46*: 48–74 (1962).

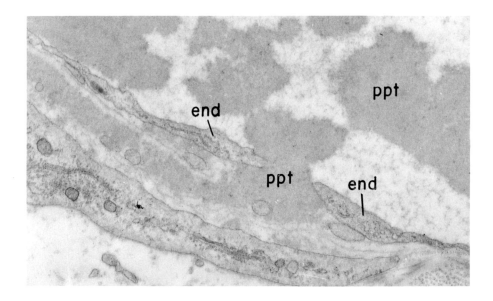

Fig. 12.11. Electron micrograph of similar lesion, showing gap in endothelium (end) and penetration of immune precipitate (ppt) into subendothelial zone. ×17,600. From Movat, *Verhandl. Duet. Ges. Path. 46*: 48–74 (1962).

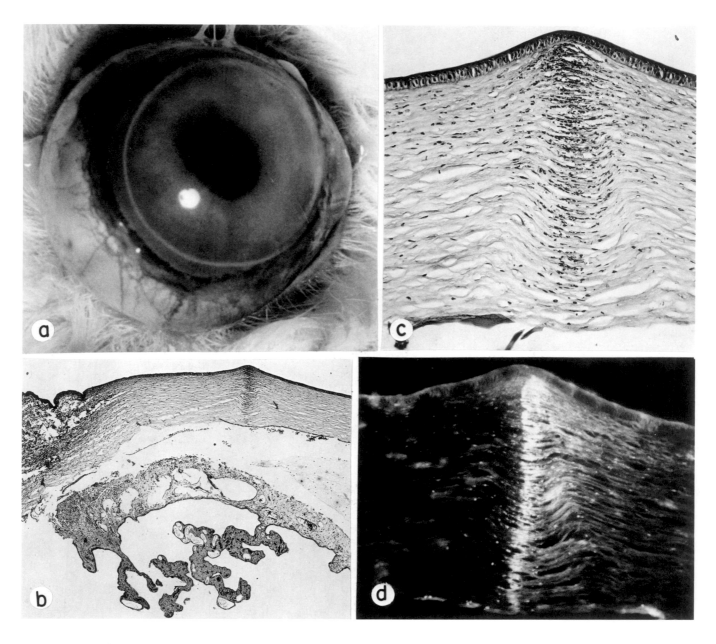

Fig. 12.12. Antigen–antibody reaction in avascular cornea. Lesion produced in eye of BSA-sensitized rabbit, injected intracorneally with 1 mg fluorescein-labeled BSA 24 hours earlier. (a) Opaque ring in cornea with clear area between ring and limbus. Note engorgement of limbal and bulbar vessels with petechial hemorrhages. (b) Section of cornea and adjacent limbus. Eosinophilic line of precipitate infiltrated by polymorphonuclear leukocytes corresponds to opaque ring seen grossly. There is acute inflammation at limbus. (c) Higher magnification, showing palisading of leukocytes, especially on side toward limbus (right). (d) Fluorescence photomicrograph of similar lesion, showing precipitation of fluorescent antigen diffusing from center of cornea (right).

(a) ×4.3. (b, c) Hematoxylin-eosin; ×29, ×145. (d) Fluorescence; ×115. From Germuth, Maumenee, Senterfit, and Pollack, *J. Exp. Med. 115*: 919–28 (1962).

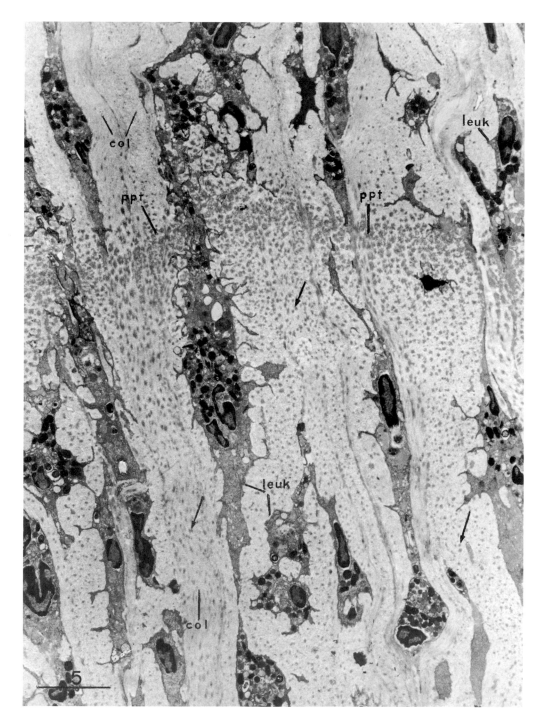

Fig. 12.13. Antigen–antibody reaction in avascular cornea. Low-power electron micrograph of similar 24-hour corneal lesion, elicited with BSA. The line of precipitate (ppt) is made up of small, electron-opaque particles which do not stop abruptly but become less dense (arrows) toward center of cornea (bottom of figure). The limitation toward the limbus (top) is more definite. The infiltrating leukocytes (leuk) are elongated and have many pseudopodia (col, collagen).

×3780. From Movat, Fernando, Uriuhara, and Weiser, *J. Exp. Med. 118*: 557–64 (1963).

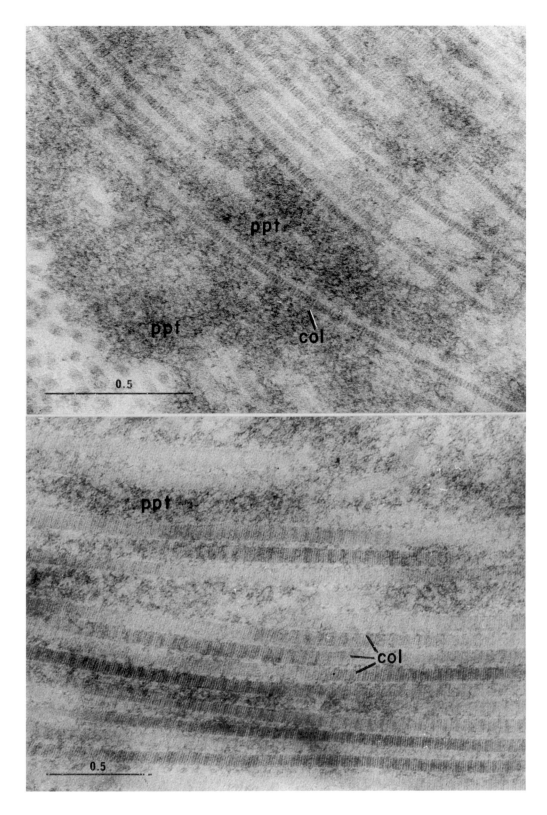

Fig. 12.14. (Above) Corneal lesion at 72 hours in leukopenic rabbit, showing several collagen fibrils (col) transversing masses of BSA–anti-BSA precipitate (ppt). Their periodicity is well preserved; ×76,000. (Below) Similar 24-hour lesion in sclera. The normal-appearing collagen fibrils, which are more robust than those of the cornea, are separated by aggregates of BSA–anti-BSA; ×57,000. From Movat, Fernando, Uriuhara, and Weiser, *J. Exp. Med. 118*: 557–64 (1963).

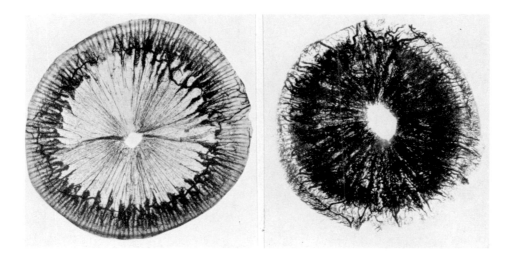

Fig. 12.15. "Serum disease" in the eye. Whole mounts of rabbit iris and ciliary body, removed within a few minutes after intracardiac injection of 50 ml India ink. (Left) Normal, showing direct connection between iris vessels and vessels of ciliary processes. (Right) Iris removed at height of uveitis, 9 days after intravitreous injection of 0.1 ml undiluted horse serum, shows tortuosity of vessels and intense hyperemia (disease onset at 7 days).

From Foss, *Acta Path. Microbiol. Scand.*, suppl. *81*: 1–128 (1949).

13. Systemic Phenomena of Arthus Type (Immune Complex Disease)

"Serum sickness" is the term originally used to describe the disease resulting from a massive dose of serum (usually horse serum, containing diphtheria or scarlet fever antitoxin) given to a human subject. Enough antigen remains in the circulation to give one or another type of hypersensitive reaction when the appropriate antibody (or cellular sensitivity) is formed 1–2 weeks after the original injection. Of the many antigens in horse serum, some give rise to cytotropic antibody, some to precipitating antibody, and some to cellular sensitivity; all are present in different concentrations and immunize with different degrees of efficacy. The disease therefore consists of simultaneous or sequential episodes of urticarial (anaphylactic) and Arthus-like lesions, of morbilliform (measles-like) rashes which are probably delayed reactions, and of other changes less readily classified—leukopenia, fever, painful nodes, enlarged painful joints, edema, albuminuria, and rarely bronchitis and bloody diarrhea. Any antigen given in sufficient dosage, e.g. penicillin, can produce part or all of this picture. The onset may be accelerated in subjects previously exposed to the same antigen(s), and there may be acute anaphylaxis in subjects who still have circulating antibody at the time antigen is given (Figs. 11.9,10).

In animals (rabbits, in most recent work) given one or more doses of a single foreign protein, *serum disease* is easily produced. Since rabbits readily produce large amounts of precipitating, complement-fixing γG-globulin antibody, most of the lesions have an Arthus mechanism. The best known are serum *arteritis* (Figs. 13.1,5), a lesion resembling human polyarteritis nodosa, *endocarditis* (Figs. 13.2,8), various types of *glomerulonephritis* (Figs. 13.2,6), *joint lesions*, and *hyperplasia of reticuloendothelial elements* in the lymph nodes and spleen of animals with chronic disease resulting from repeated antigen dosage (Figs. 13.3,4). Deposition of immune reactants in the portal tracts of the liver may lead to connective tissue formation and a type of *late cirrhosis*. Different antigens produce somewhat different effects: bovine serum albumin, for example, produces more arteritis and bovine γ-globulin more granulomatous lesions, and these differ in organ localization and time course.

The arteritis and glomerulonephritis have both been shown to result from secondary localization of antigen–antibody complexes preformed in the circulation. Both can be produced passively by infusion of sufficient quantities of immune complex into normal animals (Fig. 13.6). Very large amounts of complex produce arteritis and an *acute glomerulonephritis* by deposition in the arterial wall and in the glomerulus (Figs. 13.5,6). Small amounts of complex formed over a long period of time give rise to granular, irregular deposits on the outside of the glomerular basement membrane ("lumpy-bumpy" deposits) and a *chronic, membranous glomerulonephritis* (Figs. 13.7,12–15). Thus of animals given daily doses of antigen, those that form high titers of antibody tend to develop arteritis and those forming low levels of antibody develop chronic membranous glomerulonephritis instead.

The acute lesions correspond in histologic character and time course to the picture of the Arthus reaction: segmental fibrinoid vascular necrosis, followed by massive exudation of neutrophils and some eosinophils (Figs. 13.1,2). The deposition of immune complexes and the local fixation of complement have been demonstrated by immunohistochemical methods (Figs. 13.5–7). The remaining steps of lesion formation, i.e. chemotactic attraction of polys, phagocytosis of immune aggregates, discharge of lysosomal hydrolases, and vascular injury, are all comparable to those seen in the local Arthus. In the case of chronic membranous glomerulonephritis, however, immune complexes located outside the glomerular basement membrane are inaccessible to circulating leukocytes, and the final steps leading to an Arthus type of lesion are not initiated.

Chronic membranous glomerulonephritis in man (Fig. 13.10) and its exaggerated form, the "wire-loop" lesion seen in systemic lupus erythematosus (Fig. 13.10) and in NZB and NZB/NZW mice (Fig. 13.9), show lumpy-bumpy deposits which, in the case of lupus and the corresponding mice, have been shown to be deposited complexes of DNA or nucleoprotein with the corresponding autoantibody. A similar membranous glomerulonephritis develops in partially tolerant mice infected with lymphocytic choriomeningitis virus; these have high levels of both virus and antibody to virus in their circulation, and complexes of virus with antibody are deposited in their glomeruli.

Joint lesions occur commonly in human subjects and less frequently in rabbits with serum disease. A fulminating Arthus lesion is produced when protein antigen is injected directly into the joint of an immunized experimental animal (e.g. Fig. 16.14). However, with repeated antigen injections or with certain antigenic proteins such as fibrin, the joint lesion has a chronic course and histologically resembles the joint lesion of rheumatoid arthritis. In the latter disease, extensive production of autoantibody against γG-immunoglobulin (rheumatoid factor) results in formation of circulating immune complexes. Since, in addition, rheumatoid factor is synthesized by cells within the joint synovia (Figs. 6.11,12), large amounts of complex must be formed in the joint itself and may be responsible for lesion formation there.

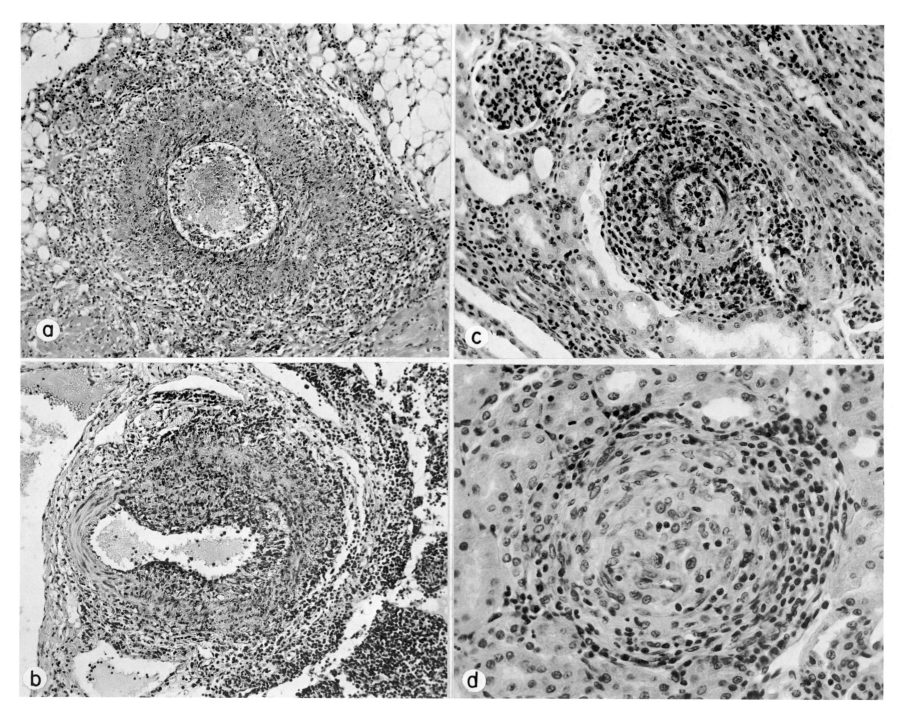

Fig. 13.1. Experimental serum arteritis in rabbits given multiple iv doses of bovine serum albumin and bovine γ-globulin. (a) Acute necrotizing coronary arteritis with early cellular reaction at 12 days (two injections of albumin and three of γ-globulin); ×123. (b) Partially healed, segmental, necrotizing arteritis with intimal proliferation in mesenteric lymph node at 24 days (five injections of albumin and five of globulin); ×148. (c) Necrotizing renal interlobular arteritis with mononuclear cell reaction and many plasma cells at 30 days (three injections of albumin and five of globulin); ×245. (d) Granulomatous renal arteritis, with formation of epithelioid cells at 35 days (six injections of albumin and four of globulin). Lumen of artery is still patent; ×395.

Hematoxylin-eosin. From Heptinstall and Germuth, *Bull. Johns Hopk. Hosp. 100*: 71–98 (1957).

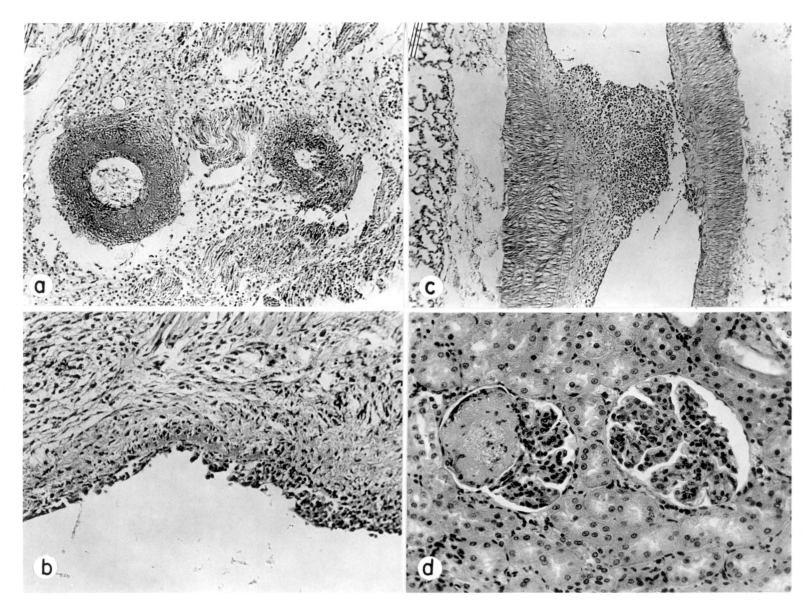

Fig. 13.2. Other lesions of serum disease in rabbits given bovine serum albumin or bovine γ-globulin iv. (a) Lesions produced passively in rabbit given 0.5 g albumin iv and continuous iv infusion of specific rabbit antibody (162 mg antibody N over 54 hours) and sacrificed at end of infusion. Fibrinoid necrosis and slight inflammation in and about medium-sized arteries in submucosa of stomach; × 136. (b) Surface lesion of mitral valve, with endothelial proliferation and subendothelial infiltration of mononuclear cells, in rabbit sacrificed after receiving four injections of bovine globulin in 34 days; × 202. (c) Intimal proliferation and subendothelial infiltration with mononuclears in segment of a branch of the pulmonary artery in rabbit given a single 0.5-g dose of albumin and sacrificed at 15 days. The media is edematous; × 96. (d) Focal necrotizing glomerulonephritis in rabbit dead on 10th day after receiving two injections of albumin and one of globulin; × 252.

Hematoxylin-eosin. (a) From Germuth and Pollack, *Bull. Johns Hopk. Hosp. 102*: 245–62 (1958). (b) From Germuth and Heptinstall, ibid., *100*: 58–70 (1957). (c) From Germuth, *J. Exp. Med. 97*: 257–82 (1953). (d) From Heptinstall and Germuth, *Bull. Johns Hopk. Hosp. 100*: 71–98 (1957).

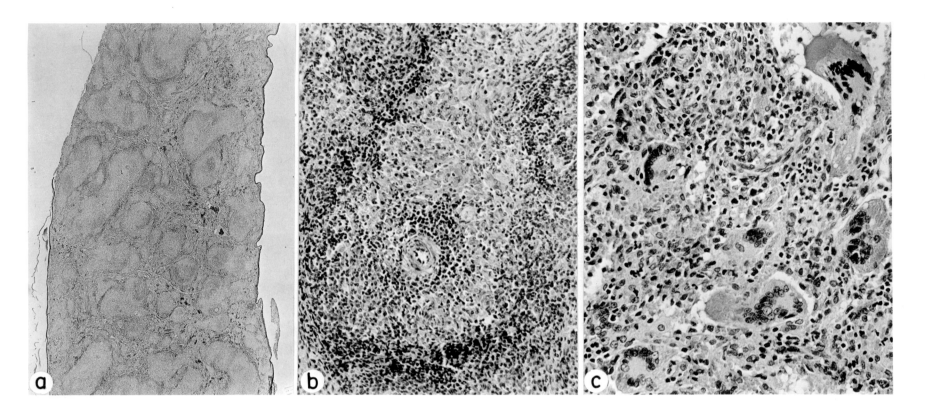

Fig. 13.3. Splenic changes in rabbits given a single large dose of foreign protein (0.5 g bovine serum albumin) iv. (a) Granulomatous change in splenic follicles of rabbit sacrificed at 8 days. (b) Higher-power view, showing extensive replacement of white pulp by rapidly proliferating epithelioid macrophages, in rabbit sacrificed at 12 days. (c) Granulomatous white pulp lesion, at 12 days, with large foreign-body giant cells and a few epithelioid cells.

(a) Wilder's reticulum stain; ×14.5 (b, c) Hematoxylin-eosin; ×195, ×295. From Germuth, *J. Exp. Med. 97*: 257–82 (1953).

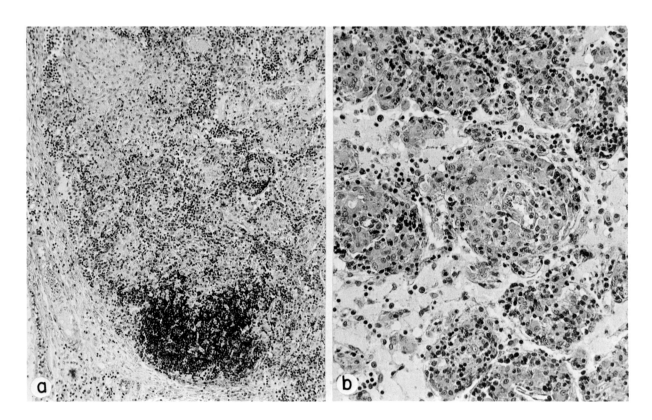

Fig. 13.4. Lymph node changes in rabbits given a single large dose iv of foreign protein (0.5 g bovine serum albumin) and sacrificed at 12 days. (a) Cortex of mesenteric node showing partial (below) and complete (above) replacement of follicles by epithelioid cells; ×115 (b) Medulla of same node showing more or less complete replacement of cords by aggregates of similar cells; ×220.

Hematoxylin-eosin. From Germuth, *J. Exp. Med. 97*: 257–82 (1953).

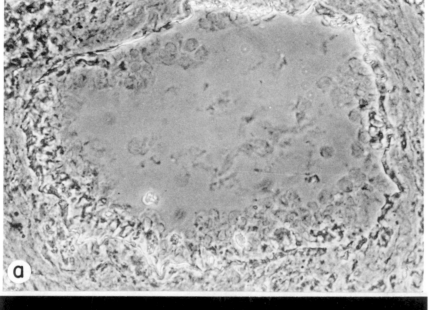

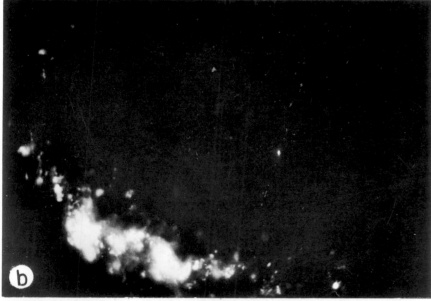

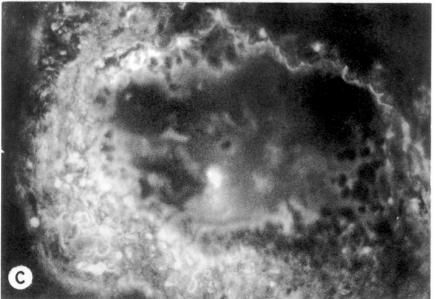

Fig. 13.5. Serum disease arteritis. Medium-sized coronary artery of rabbit actively sensitized with massive doses of BSA. (a–c) Same artery by phase microscopy and stained for BSA and for host γ-globulin respectively (fluorescence technique). Note that lesion corresponds to zone of deposition of antigen–antibody complexes. Nonspecific accumulation of γ-globulin is seen in wider zone.

From Dixon, Vazquez, Weigle, and Cochrane, *Arch. Path. 65*: 18–28 (1958).

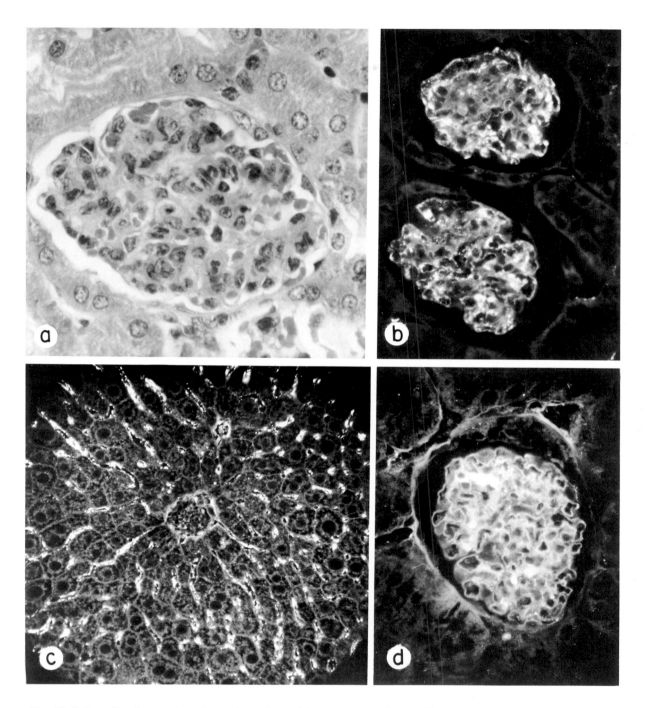

Fig. 13.6. Localization and pathogenic action of immune complexes. (a) Mouse injected with complexes of ovalbumin and mouse antibody three times in 24 hours and killed 1 day later. Glomerulus is swollen and hypercellular and contains a few polymorphs. Capillary lumina are almost entirely occluded. (b) Mouse similarly injected with doubly-labeled complexes of rabbit antibody and BSA. Fluorescence photograph shows uneven subendothelial deposition of complexes in glomeruli, giving characteristic beaded or lumpy appearance. (c, d) Localization of complexes containing rabbit antibody and labeled BSA in organs of mouse sacrificed 4 hours after last of multiple injections. Complexes are seen in lining of liver sinusoids and cytoplasm of Kupffer cells and in basement membrane of a glomerulus and of Bowman's capsule.

(a) Hematoxylin-eosin; ×650; (b–d) Fluorescence method; ×468, ×200, ×400. (a) Courtesy of Dr. R. T. McCluskey. (b) Courtesy of Dr. R. C. Mellors. (c, d) From Mellors and Brzosko, *J. Exp. Med.* *115*: 891–902 (1962).

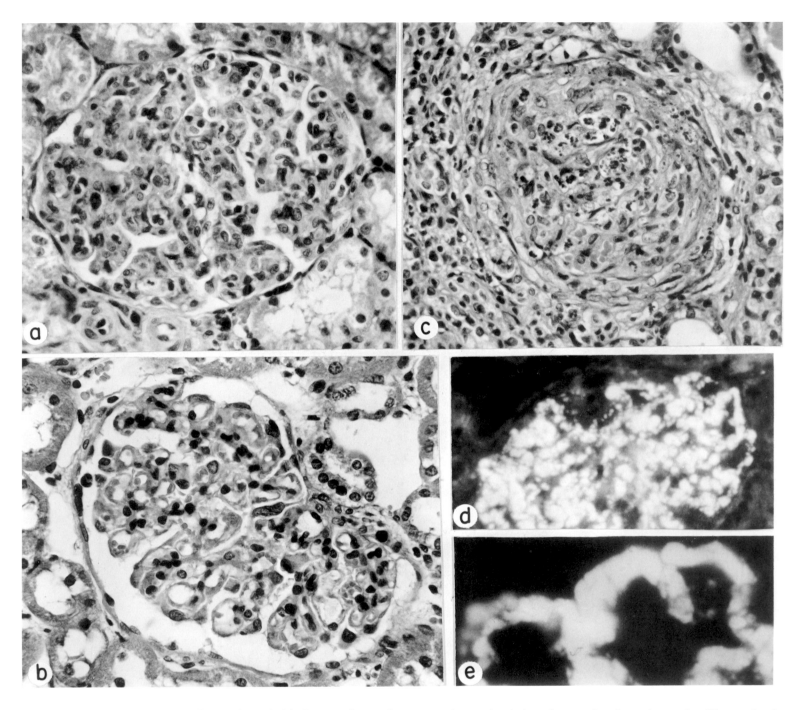

Fig. 13.7. Acute and chronic glomerulonephritis in experimental serum disease, produced in rabbits by repeated daily doses of protein antigen. (a) Acute lesion, second week of injections. Typical hypercellular glomerulus. Capillary lumina are almost filled by swollen, proliferating endothelial cells. Few leukocytes are seen in the occluded capillaries. (b) Chronic lesion, third month of severe proteinuria. Glomerulus shows markedly thickened basement membrane, moderate proliferation of glomerular cells, two early adhesions of capillary tufts to Bowman's capsule, and some distortion of glomerular architecture. (c) Severe lesion, second month of chronic proteinuria and uremia. Glomerulus is obliterated by proliferation, infiltration, and scarring. This degree of damage is common in rabbits dying of renal failure. (d, e) Chronic lesions, stained for antigen by fluorescence technique. Discrete antigen deposits are seen throughout basement membrane. Beaded or lumpy deposits of antigen–antibody complex are characteristic.

(a–c) Hematoxylin-eosin; ×305. (d) ×305, (e) ×915. From Dixon, Feldman, and Vazquez, *J. Exp. Med. 113*: 899–920 (1961).

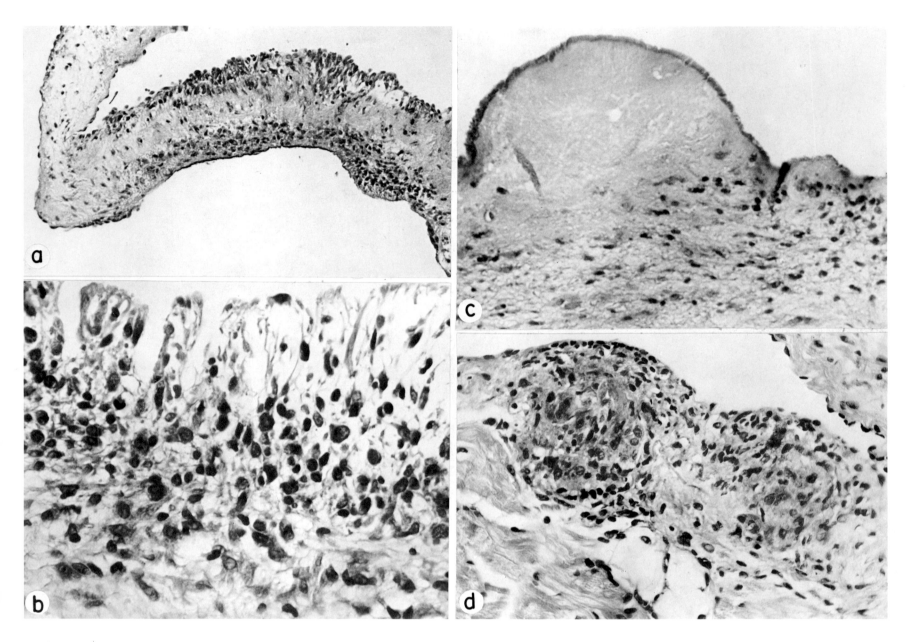

Fig. 13.8. Cardiac lesions in rabbits injected iv over several months with denatured autologous γ-globulin. (a) Mitral valve, showing endothelial proliferation and chronic inflammatory infiltrate in segmental distribution. (b) Higher power of same lesion showing subendocardial edema and infiltrate made up almost entirely of lymphocytes and histiocytes. (c) Verrucous vegetation on mitral valve, with degeneration, fibrinoid change, and swelling of subendothelial connective tissue and a few infiltrating mononuclears. (d) Two granulomatous foci in auricular endocardium, made up largely of reacting fixed tissue elements and a mononuclear infiltrate and showing little or no necrosis.

Hematoxylin-eosin: magnifications not given. From Dixon, Schultz, and Milgrom, *Lab. Invest. 14*: 2056–62 (1965).

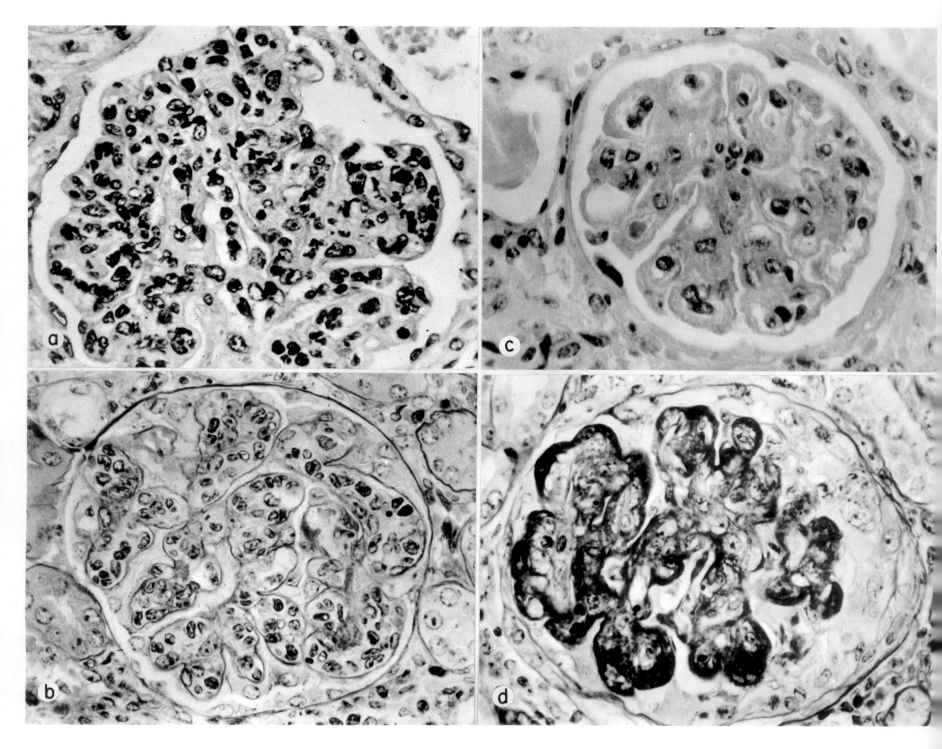

Fig. 13.9. Spontaneous renal lesions resembling those of lupus erythematosus in (NZB × NZW)F$_1$ mice. (a, b) Early proliferative lesions. (c, d) "Wire-loop" lesions seen at a later stage.

(a, c) Hematoxylin-eosin; (b, d) PAS–hematoxylin; all approximately × 825 Courtesy of Drs. B. J. Helyer and J. B. Howie.

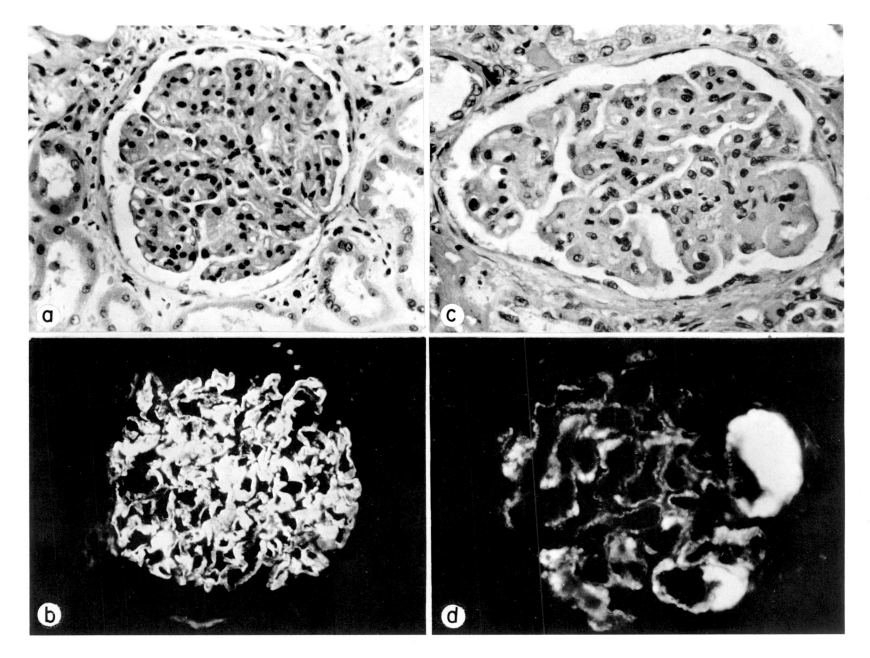

Fig. 13.10. Renal lesions in chronic membranous glomerulone-phritis (a, b) and systemic lupus erythematosus (c, d) in conventional hematoxylin-eosin stain (a and c) and stained by the fluorescence technique for human γ-globulin (b and d). Glomerulus in (a) shows diffusely thickened basement membrane. Glomerulus of lupus kidney (b) shows similarly thickened basement membrane, focally accentuated, with wire-loop lesion at 8 o'clock. Stain with fluorescent antibody shows γ-globulin localization in zone of thickening in both cases and in two wire-loop lesions at 7 and 10 o'clock (d).

(a) ×385, (b) ×335, (c) ×450, (d) ×570. From Mellors, Ortega, and Holman, *J. Exp. Med. 106*: 191–202 (1957).

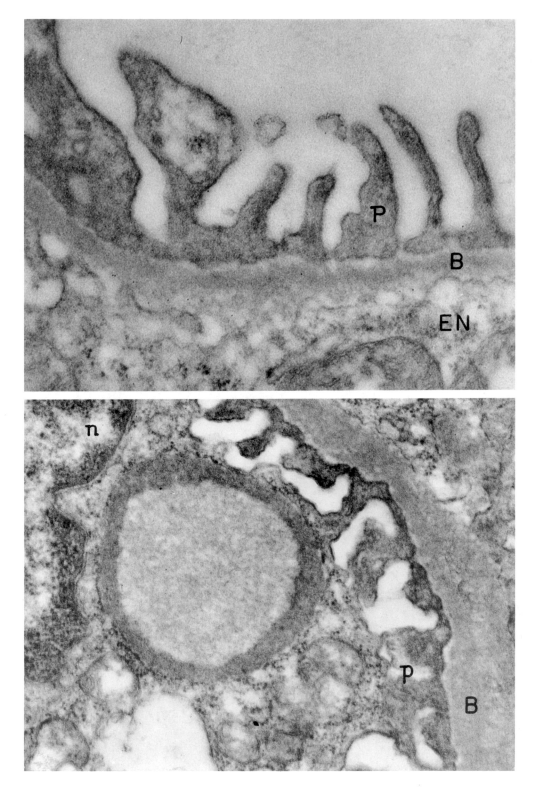

Fig. 13.11. Electron microscopic appearance of normal kidney of rat. Upper figure shows usual aspect of basement membrane (B), epithelial foot processes (P), and endothelial cytoplasm (EN). Lower figure shows epithelial nucleus at left (n) and, in center, a dilated cisterna of endoplasmic reticulum containing basement membrane-like material. To right are foot processes, basement membrane, and capillary endothelium.

Electron micrographs; ×63,000. From Andres, Morgan, Hsu, Rifkind, and Seegal, *J. Exp. Med. 115*: 929–36 (1962).

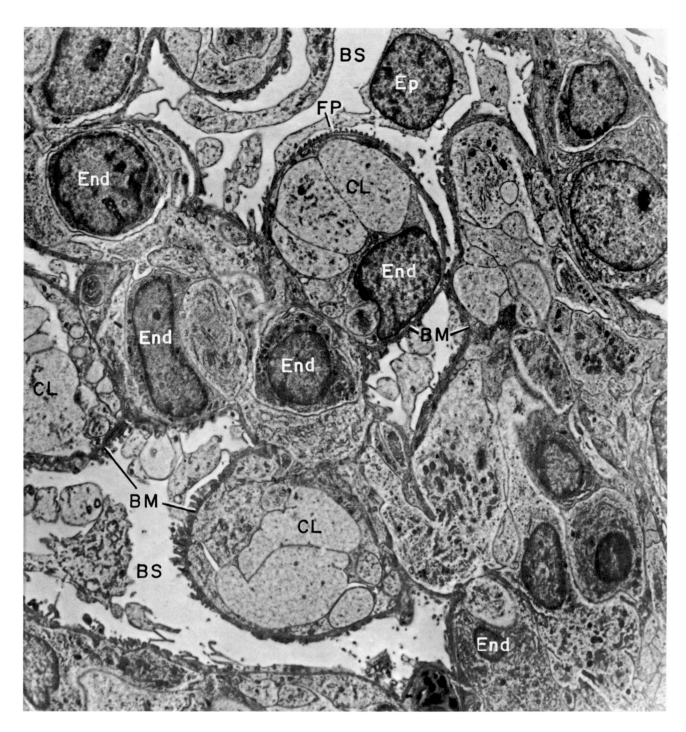

Fig. 13.12. Acute glomerulonephritis in experimental serum disease. Several loops of glomerulus from a rabbit injected with a single large dose of BSA iv. Electron micrograph of biopsy taken 18 days later reveals endothelial proliferation and swelling, characteristic of this lesion, and beginning resolution of the process. Capillaries (CL) are completely or partially filled with increased numbers of endothelial elements (End). Foot processes (FP) of epithelial cells (Ep) are infrequent; for the most part they are replaced by apposition of cytoplasm over the entire periphery of the basement membrane (BM). The basement membrane is of normal thickness and texture and is not involved in the lesion (BS, Bowman's space).

× 4,700. Courtesy of Dr. F. J. Dixon. See Dixon, Feldman, and Vazquez, *J. Exp. Med. 113*: 899–920 (1961).

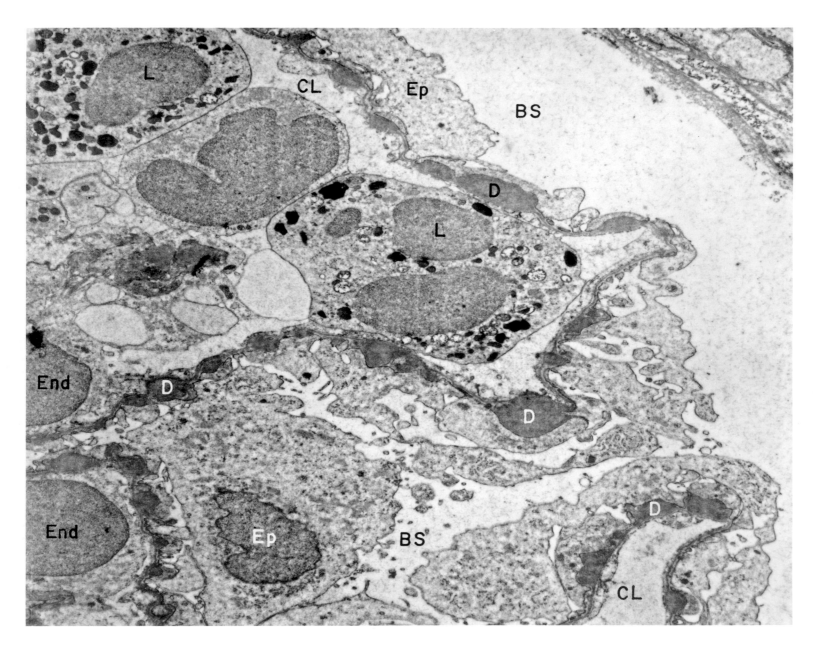

Fig. 13.13. Chronic glomerulonephritis in experimental serum disease. Portion of a glomerulus from a rabbit injected daily with BSA iv for 3 months. The basement membrane (BM) is beaded with dense deposits (D) of varying size, presumably antigen–antibody complex. Where the deposits are prominent, the epithelial cytoplasm (Ep) is smeared, lacking foot processes. Within the capillary lumens (CL) are leukocytes (L) and swollen endothelial cells (End); BS = Bowman's space.

×11,000. Courtesy of Dr. F. J. Dixon (see Dixon, Feldman, and Vazquez, *J. Exp. Med. 113*: 899–920, 1961).

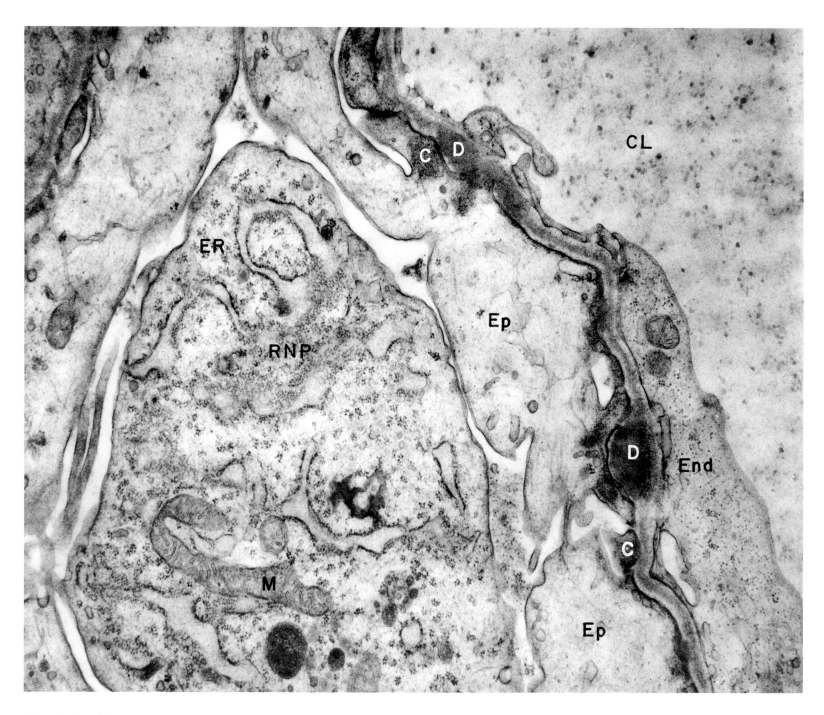

Fig. 13.14. Higher-power view of similar lesion from a rabbit injected daily with BSA for 7 weeks. The deposits (D) of dense material, presumably antigen–antibody complex, are easily seen at the basement membrane (BM). Epithelium (Ep) is smeared over the basement membrane and shows dense material (C) in its cytoplasm close to the basement membrane. Part of another epithelial cell shows a simple pattern of endoplasmic reticulum (ER), accumulation of ribonucleoprotein particles (RNP) mitochondria (M), and several droplets. The capillary lumen (CL) is patent and the endothelium (End) appears normal.

× 32,000. Courtesy of Dr. F. J. Dixon (see Dixon, Feldman, and Vazquez, *J. Exp. Med. 113*: 899–920, 1961).

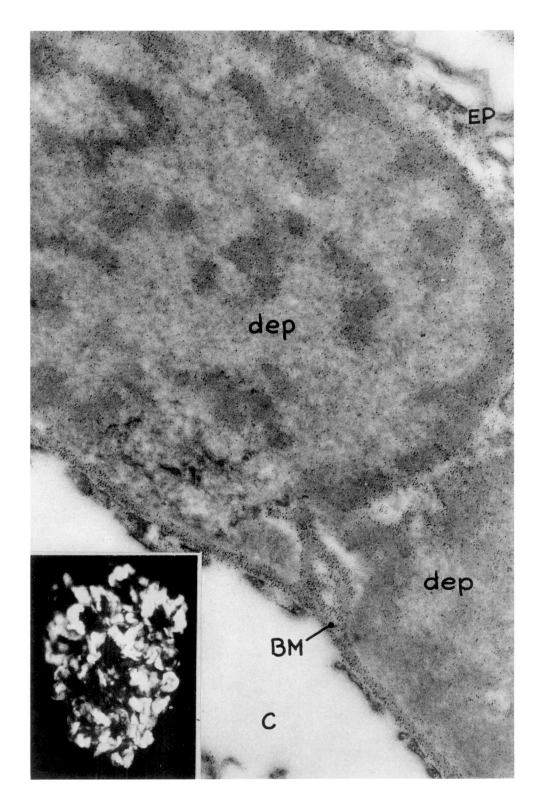

Fig. 13.15. Chronic glomerulonephritis with serum disease. Portion of a glomerulus from rabbit injected daily for 10 weeks with BSA (total dose 1.05 g). Large deposit (dep) between basement membrane (BM) and epithelial cytoplasm (EP). Staining with ferritin-labeled anti-BSA shows that denser component of deposit contains BSA, as does the basement membrane itself. Insert shows same glomerulus stained with same antibody against BSA, labeled with fluorescein. Beaded pattern of deposits is characteristic. (C, capillary lumen).

× 60,000, × 350. From Andres, Seegal, Hsu, Rothenberg, and Chapeau, *J. Exp. Med. 117*: 691–702 (1963).

14. Lesions Produced by Antibody against Extracellular Tissue Antigens: "Nephrotoxic" Nephritis

Lesions which share many or all of the features of Arthus reactions are produced by hetero- and autoantibody against vascular connective tissue or its components. With local introduction of heteroantibody against vascular basement membranes, such lesions may be elicited in the meninges, lungs, or other organs. However, when antibody is introduced into the systemic circulation, it affects primarily the renal glomerulus, producing so-called nephrotoxic or Masugi nephritis (Fig. 14.1). There is extensive cross-reactivity between vascular basement membranes in different tissues (Figs. 1.11; 14.1). However, circulating antibody reacts almost exclusively with the glomerular basement membrane, as shown with radiolabeled antibody (Fig. 14.2), by immunofluorescence (Figs. 14.3,4), or by electron microscopy (Figs. 13.11; 14.5). This may depend on its greater accessibility. The antibody is deposited in a continuous smooth pattern throughout the membrane (Figs. 14.3,5), in contrast to the lumpy-bumpy pattern characteristic of immune complex nephritis (Section 13). Occasionally, deposition of antibody in the vascular basement membrane of the lung may be sufficient to result in disease.

The actual production of disease after injection of nephrotoxic antibody follows one of two distinct immunologic sequences. With large amounts of complement-fixing antibody, an Arthus mechanism is triggered immediately, the steps corresponding to those described earlier. With small amounts of antibody or with non-complement-fixing antibody, no lesion is observed till the host forms antibody against the foreign protein present in the glomerulus (Fig. 14.3). In both cases, the participation of polys, platelets, and the clotting mechanism is obligatory (Fig. 14.4), and the resulting lesion is a fibrinoid vasculitis of the glomerulus. A similar lesion is produced by autoantibody. Certain cases of human glomerulonephritis have been shown to result from the formation and deposition of nephrotoxic autoantibody. In rare instances, a lesion is also produced in the lung, similar to that in the glomerulus, in both experimental animals and human subjects (Goodpasture's syndrome).

Antibody-mediated lesions in which the antigen is a component of connective tissue ground substance are suppurative. Presumably, leukocytes may be attracted to a site some distance from the vessels by mechanisms similar to those in the Arthus reaction, but the cathepsins which they release produce tissue damage that does not involve the vessel wall.

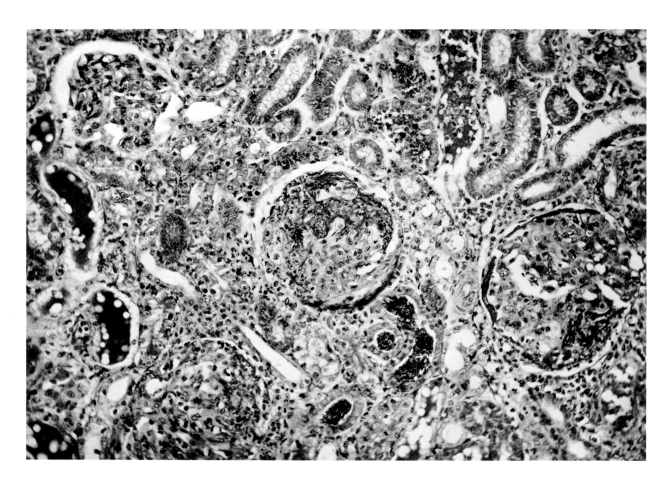

Fig. 14.1. Acute nephrotoxic nephritis. Section of dog kidney, removed 9 days after injection of nephrotoxic antiserum (rabbit antihuman glomerular basement membrane, 1.5 ml/pound of dog) shows severe exudative, necrotizing, and proliferative glomerulonephritis. There are varying degrees of glomerular damage, tubular degeneration, atrophy, and dilation, casts of various types and red cells in the tubules, as well as an interstitial mononuclear cell exudate. Production of lesion shows nonspecies specificity of basement membrane antigen.

Hematoxylin-eosin; ×250. From Stebley and Lepper, *J. Immunol. 87*: 636–46 (1961).

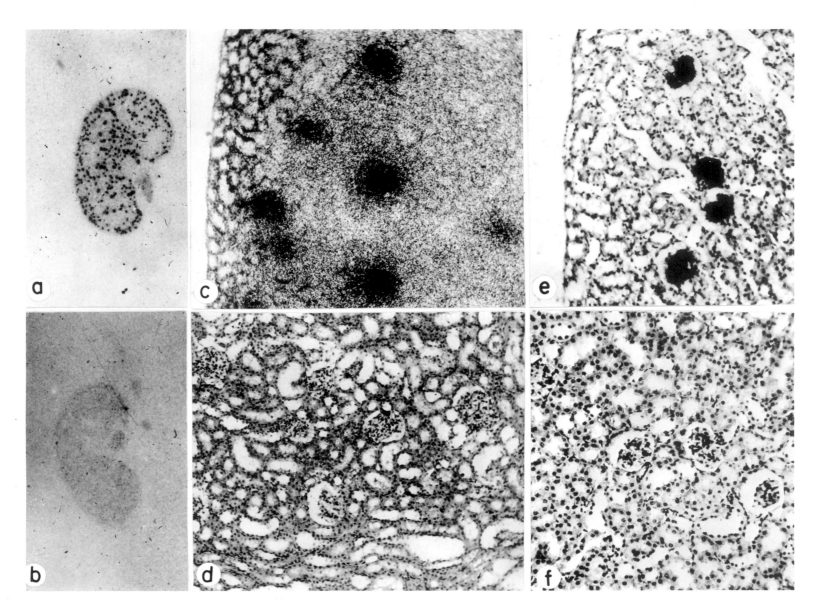

Fig. 14.2. Localization of nephrotoxic antisera. (a, b) Kidneys of mice injected with I[131]-labeled globulin fractions of rabbit antisera against mouse kidney and plasma respectively. (c, d) Kidney sections from rats injected with I[131]-labeled globulins from rabbit antisera against rat lung and ovalbumin, respectively, and sacrificed at 2½ hours. (e, f) Similar sections from rats injected with S[35]-labeled globulins prepared against rat kidney and ovalbumin. All show specific localization of nephrotoxic antibody in glomeruli and cross-reactivity of antilung antibody for glomerular basement membrane. Much better resolution is obtained in autoradiographs prepared with S[35] than with I[131].

Autoradiographs on "no-screen" X-ray plates, developed and then stained with metanil yellow and iron hematoxylin. From Pressman, Hill, and Foote, *Science 109*: 65–66 (1949); Eisen, Sherman, and Pressman, *J. Immunol. 65*: 543–58 (1950); and Pressman, Eisen, Siegel, Fitzgerald, Sherman, and Silverstein, ibid., pp. 559–69.

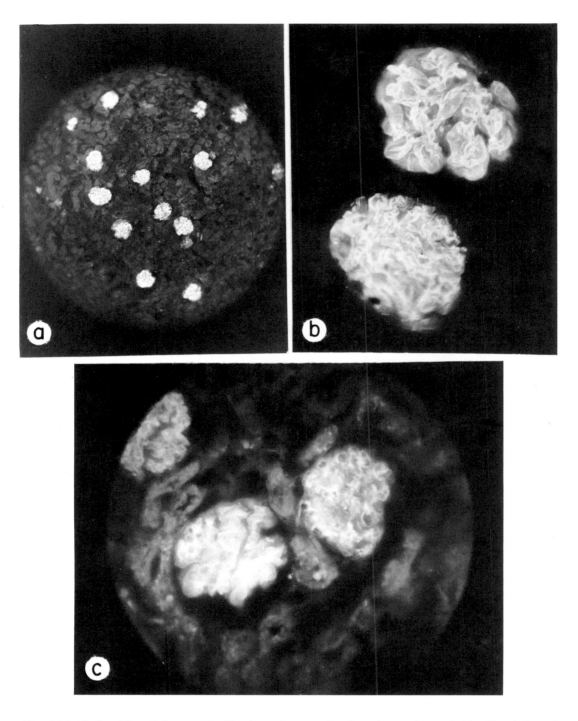

Fig. 14.3. Role of localizing antibodies in pathogenesis of nephrotoxic nephritis. Rat injected with rabbit–antirat kidney serum. (a) Six days. Stained with Goat–anti-Rab. This is the characteristic fluorescence pattern of all the nephritic kidney sections treated with this fluor; × 37. (b) Same at higher power. The tuft at the top shows predominantly membranous localization of nephrotoxic antibodies. The other tuft is partly out of focus and shows a crushing artefact; × 205. (c) Four weeks. Stained with Rab-anti-Rat. There is a predominantly membranous localization of autogenous antibodies. Note that both the injected heteroantibody, acting as antigen, and the autogenous antibody are deposited in a uniform manner in the basement membrane, in sharp contrast to the beaded, irregular deposition of antigen–antibody complexes in serum disease; × 210.

Fluorescence technique. From Ortega and Mellors, *J. Exp. Med. 104*: 151–79 (1956).

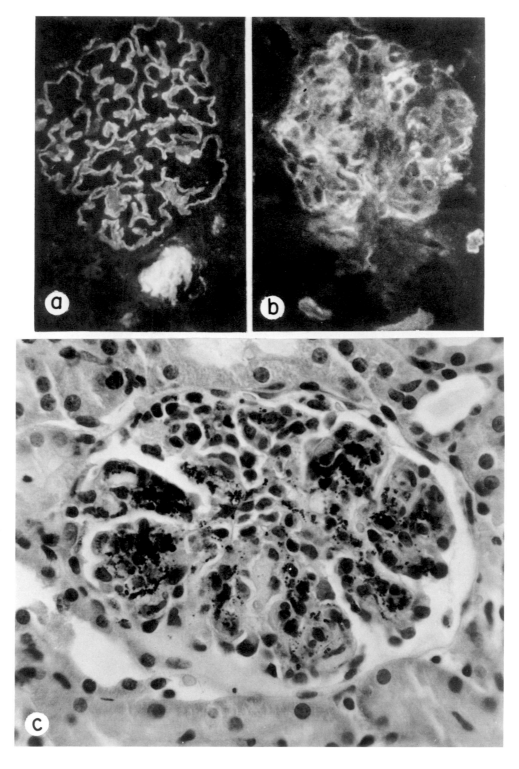

Fig. 14.4. Role of fibrin deposition in pathogenesis of nephrotoxic nephritis. Rabbit injected with sheep antirabbit kidney serum. (a) Stained with antirabbit γ-globulin. Uniform, membranous deposition, like that illustrated in Fig. 14.3, is seen in animals after fifth day. (b) Stained for rabbit fibrinogen or fibrin. Fluorescence is seen in cells and along basement membrane throughout glomerulus. (c) Renal glomerulus in similar rabbit injected with carbon iv. Carbon uptake (comparable to fibrin uptake) is seen in axial and endothelial cells.

(a, b) Fluorescence technique; ×400. (c) Hematoxylin-eosin; ×800. From Vassalli and McCluskey, *Ann. N.Y. Acad. Sci. 116*: 1052–62 (1964).

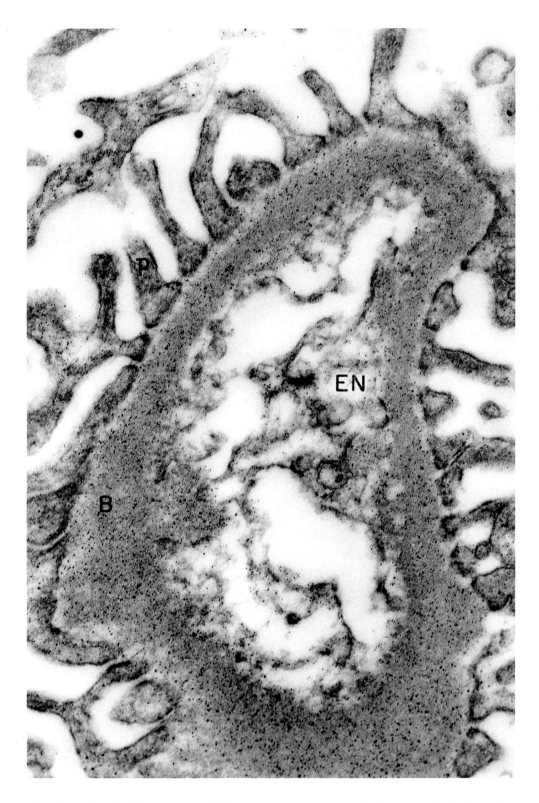

Fig. 14.5. Acute glomerulonephritis produced by nephrotoxic serum (rabbit antirat kidney) in rat, with sacrifice at 1 week. Electron micrograph, with staining by ferritin-labeled duck antibody against rabbit γ-globulin, shows diffuse localization of nephrotoxic antibody in basement membrane (B) with little in epithelium (P) or endothelium (EN).

×60,000. From Andres, Morgan, Hsu, Rifkind, and Seegal, *J. Exp. Med. 115*: 929–36 (1962).

15. Endotoxin and the Local and General "Shwartzman" Reactions

The Shwartzman reactions are hemorrhagic necrotizing lesions, first recognized in normal animals given two doses of endotoxin (cell wall lipopolysaccharides of Gram-negative organisms, e.g. the meningococcus, *E. coli*) spaced approximately 24 hours apart. They appear to be nonimmunologic.

Since endotoxins are components of organisms commonly found in the gastrointestinal flora, normal adults have both natural antibodies, largely γM, and cellular sensitivity against them. Injection of endotoxin in adult human or animal subjects (Fig. 2.8) elicits lesions which are in part toxic and in part immunologic. These include Arthus-like and delayed skin reactions (Fig. 15.1,13); direct damage of polys, leukopenia, and fever mediated by endogenous pyrogen released from the damaged leukocytes; damage of reticuloendothelial cells followed by compensatory hyperplasia; release of histamine, 5-HT, and thromboplastic substances from platelets; secondary release of catecholamines and kinins and vasomotor effects due to all the released mediators; and endotoxin shock, frequently fatal. The role of specific immunologic reactions in producing many of these effects is being elucidated by studies in neonatal and germ-free animals.

The *local Shwartzman reaction*, produced by giving the first dose of endotoxin intradermally and the second intravenously, is a hemorrhagic lesion at the prepared (intradermal) site, appearing 2–5 hours after the second (provocative) injection, reaching a maximum at 4–5 hours, and often giving a late slough (Fig. 15.2). The *prepared site* shows a local *increase in aerobic and anaerobic glycolysis*, reflecting local infiltration of leukocytes elicited by the first toxin injection (Fig. 15.13). Preparation may also be achieved by local injection of poly granules (lysosomes) or granules of peritoneal or alveolar macrophages. Other sites of intense aerobic glycolysis, notably tissues infected with bacteria, rapidly growing tumors, the decidual placenta, and reactions of cellular hypersensitivity (Figs. 15.4–6) are also prepared for a local Shwartzman.

The *provocative injection* of toxin produces *clumping of leukocytes and platelets*, their segregation in the viscera, and intravascular *accumulation at the prepared site* (Fig. 15.13). The provocative material need not be the same toxin injected for preparation. Indeed any of a wide variety of colloidal substances, including antigen–antibody aggregates, can cause poly–platelet clumping and will provoke the local Shwartzman reaction. The colloids commonly used—starch, agar, glycogen, and dextran—are thought to act by forming immune complexes with natural antibodies present in the test animal's circulation. A Shwartzman lesion may also appear in animals given just a single intradermal toxin injection if reticuloendothelial function is depressed by blockade, systemic infection, or treatment with corticosteroids. In this case, endotoxin escaping from the prepared site into the circulation is not destroyed and persists long enough to act as the provocative material.

The developing reaction shows prominent cellular (poly–platelet) and acellular thrombi (Figs. 15.4–6,13), extensive diapedesis of polys throughout the skin and subcutaneous tissues, vascular and ischemic necrosis, and hemorrhage. The clotting mechanism plays an as yet unknown role, and release of lysosomal hydrolases from polys is undoubtedly an essential feature of pathogenesis, as in Arthus lesions (Section 12). The relationship among increased glycolysis, ischemia due to thrombosis, and release of enzymes in lesion formation has not been fully clarified. The reaction is prevented by reducing the level of circulating leukocytes with X ray or nitrogen mustard, lowering the platelet count with specific platelet antisera, or preventing clotting with heparin or Dicumarol.

The *general Shwartzman reaction*, produced by successive doses of endotoxin given intravenously, is a generalized intravascular clotting, with infarction and hemorrhagic necrosis of various organs, the kidney in particular (Fig. 15.7). Histologically, one finds massive intravascular deposits of fibrinoid material and ischemic necrosis of the most severely involved tissues (Fig. 15.9). Later, the foci of fibrinoid necrosis may show a granulomatous cellular response. By immunofluorescence techniques and electron microscopy, the intravascular material is proven to consist largely or entirely of fibrin (Figs. 15.9,10).

The toxin produces a number of independent effects which may play a role in this reaction. First, as noted above, it damages leukocytes. A general Shwartzman reaction cannot be elicited in animals depleted of leukocytes by X ray or nitrogen mustard unless certain natural or synthetic polysaccharides (dextran, liquoid) are substituted for the second toxin dose. It is thought, therefore, that damaged polys may release a similar material in the elicitation step of the reaction. Toxin also produces an altered fibrinogen, which is readily precipitated by such polysaccharides as heparin or dextran. Further, it releases thrombopolastic substances from platelets, blockades or inhibits the RES, and causes stasis in certain vascular beds, notably in the renal glomerulus (Fig. 15.11). A single injection of endotoxin produces a general Shwartzman reaction in pregnant rabbits, rabbits with RES blockade, rabbits treated with cortisone, or rabbits with systemic infection. These are all situations in which RES function (and therefore endotoxin clearance) is compromised and in which there are localized zones of vascular stasis (Figs. 15.11,12) to which the distribution of elicited lesions corresponds. Conversely, as with the local Shwartzman reaction, lesion formation is prevented by leukopenic agents or agents which reduce clotting, such as heparin, warfarin, or streptokinase.

It appears clear that a general Shwartzman reaction results from deposition of fibrin in small vessels and will occur when one or more of the following conditions are met: (1) *decreased RE clearance of fibrin* due to toxin, blockade, cortisone, etc.; (2) *increased precipitation of fibrin*, by actual clotting or by precipitation with leukocytic mucopolysaccharide or injected materials such as liquoid; (3) *decreased fibrinolysis*: and (4) *embarrassment of local blood flow*. An extreme example of the concatenation of factors which can lead to a Shwartzman lesion is seen in pregnant rats (local vasodilatation in glomerulus and placenta) fed a diet containing certain oxidized lipids (which diminish RE function), in which the process affects both the kidneys and placenta and is thought to resemble toxemia of pregnancy in the human.

General Shwartzman reactions occur in human subjects with sepsis produced by Gram-negative organisms, e.g. after burns or peritonitis, and particularly when such infections occur in relation to pregnancy (septic abortions, abruptio placentae) or when the patient is under treatment with steroids. A classical Shwartzman lesion is the generalized hemorrhagic state seen in meningococcemia (Fig. 15.18), often accompanied by massive adrenal hemorrhage, the Waterhouse-Friderichsen syndrome.

The use of the fluorescent antibody technique permits specific staining of protein in tissue sections (immunohistochemistry). Study of the "fibrinoid" in a variety of conditions leads to distinction of two classes of lesions. Processes in which the fibrinoid contains γ-globulin include: experimental lesions such as the Arthus reaction, serum arteritis, acute and chronic glomerulonephritis, and amyloid; and human lesions such as glomerulonephritis, systemic lupus erythematosus, rheumatic fever, rheumatoid arthritis, polyarteritis nodosa, and amyloid. Processes in which the fibrinoid contains fibrin include: the experimental local and general Shwartzman reactions; and such human lesions as thrombotic thrombocytopenic purpura, bilateral renal cortical necrosis of pregnancy, malignant hypertension, and the renal lesions of scleroderma. The immunohistochemical findings alone do not provide a sufficient basis for regarding the former lesions as of Arthus type and the latter as Shwartzman type but offer a strong suggestion that this may be the case (Fig. 22.7).

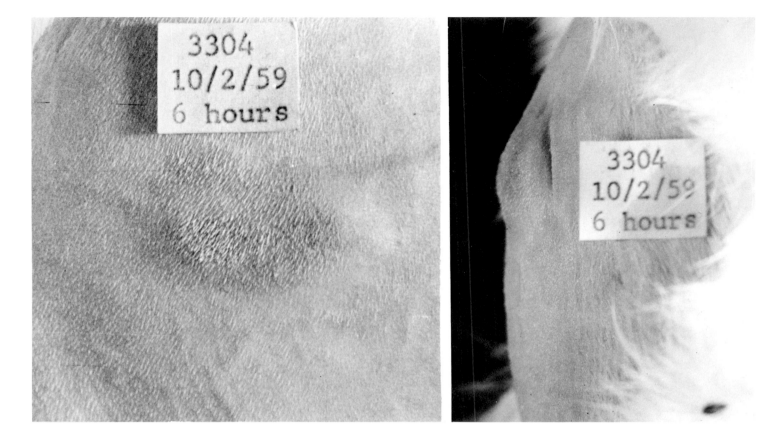

Fig. 15.1. "Accelerated" lesion (6 hours) produced by endotoxin. *E. coli* endotoxin given intradermally in a dose of approximately 100 μg in a rabbit which had received (2 days earlier) an iv injection of the same endotoxin in the same dosage. Normally by this time, after a single intradermal dose of toxin, there is only minimal or no induration or erythema.

Front and side views; × 1.45. Courtesy of Dr. L. Lee.

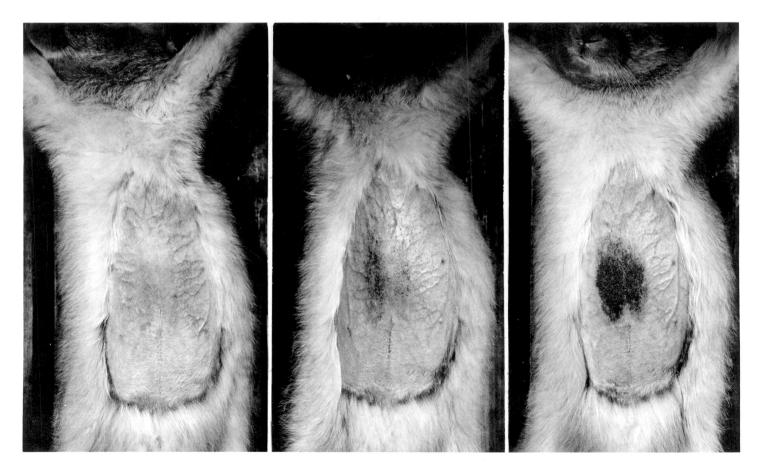

Fig. 15.2. Development of local Shwartzman reaction in rabbit skin. *Serratia marcescens* lipopolysaccharide, 50 μg injected intradermally at 10:00 a.m. and 100 μg of the same endotoxin injected iv 24 hours later. (Left) "Prepared" skin shows edema, induration, and erythema, immediately before iv challenge. (Middle) Early Shwartzman lesion 3 hours and 25 minutes later shows cyanotic skin area and beginning petechiae. (Right) Four hours after challenge, site shows complete area of hemorrhagic necrosis.

0.4 × natural size. Courtesy of Dr. C. A. Stetson.

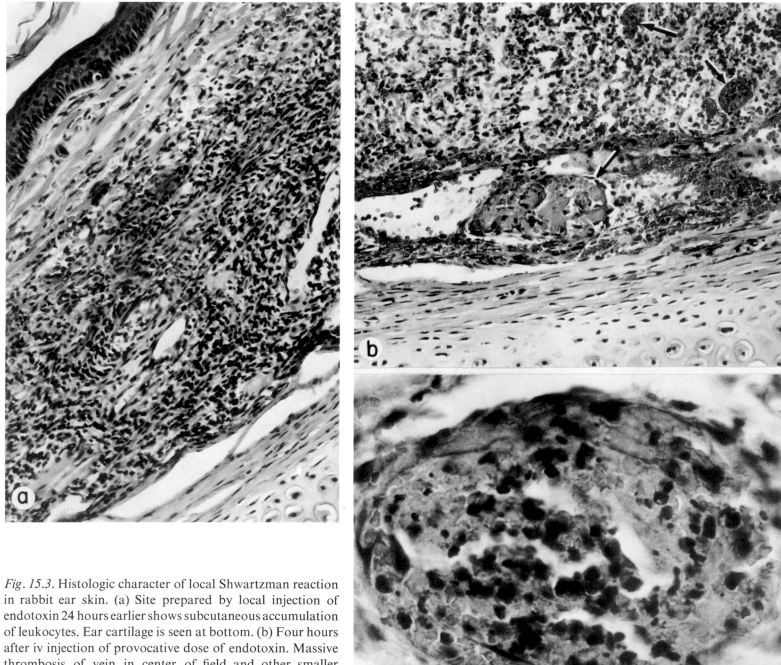

Fig. 15.3. Histologic character of local Shwartzman reaction in rabbit ear skin. (a) Site prepared by local injection of endotoxin 24 hours earlier shows subcutaneous accumulation of leukocytes. Ear cartilage is seen at bottom. (b) Four hours after iv injection of provocative dose of endotoxin. Massive thrombosis of vein in center of field and other smaller venules (arrows). (c) Thrombus in another vein, seen at higher power, contains mainly necrotic leukocytes and cellular debris.

Hematoxylin-eosin; magnifications not given. Courtesy of Dr. D. G. McKay.

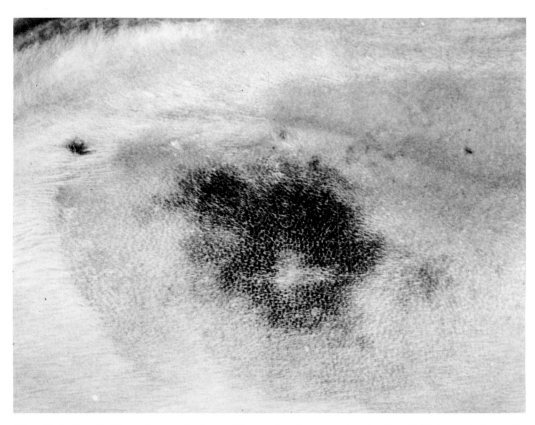

Fig. 15.4. Local Shwartzman lesions. Hemorrhagic necrosis at site of 24-hour tuberculin reaction (in BCG-vaccinated rabbit, skin tested with undiluted, dialyzed old tuberculin) 5 hours after iv injection of *E. coli* endotoxin, 100 μg. Animal died at this time. Delayed skin reaction is prepared site.

Courtesy of Dr. C. A. Stetson.

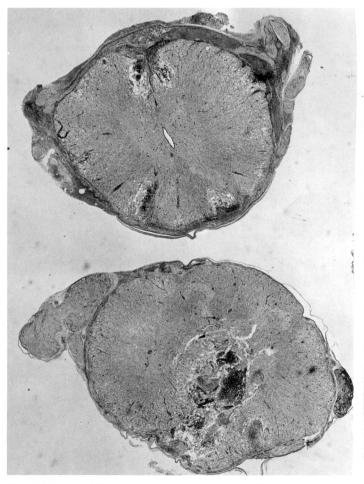

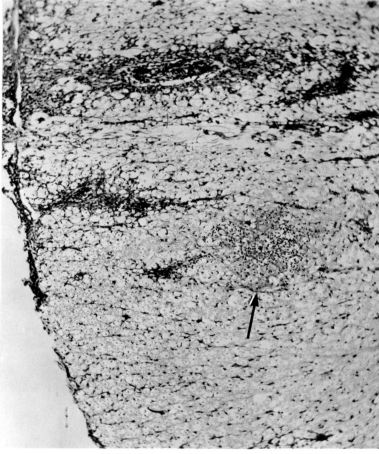

Fig. 15.5. Local Shwartzman lesions, in spinal cords of rabbits with autoallergic encephalomyelitis. (Left) Severe encephalomyelitis of 4 days' duration; two doses of meningococcal endotoxin (0.0008 ml/kg) 24 hours apart; sacrifice 31 hours after second dose; cerebrospinal fluid is bloody. Several areas of severe hemorrhagic necrosis are seen in both sections of cord, and there is massive hemorrhage in subarachnoid space. (Right) Spinal cord of rabbit with moderate encephalomyelitis of several days' duration; no toxin administered. An area of vascular necrosis, fibrin impregnation, and poly infiltration is seen (arrow) below and to right of typical perivascular and subpial encephalomyelitis lesions.

(Left) Hematoxylin-eosin; ×7. (Right) Cresyl- violet; ×125. From Waksman and Adams, *Am. J. Path. 33*: 131–53 (1957).

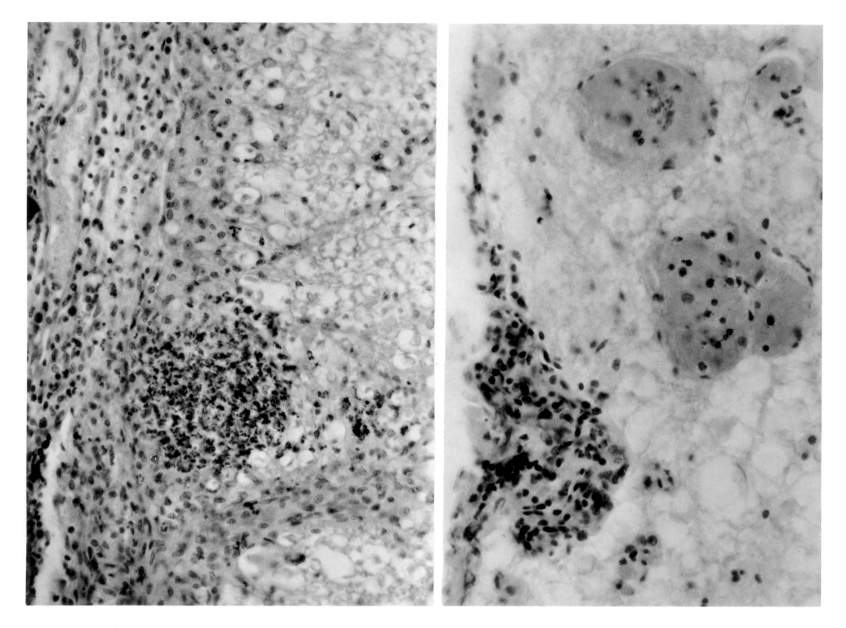

Fig. 15.6. Local Shwartzman lesions. Spinal cord of rabbits, with moderate to severe autoallergic encephalomyelitis, injected iv with meningococcal endotoxin (0.03 ml/kg) on day of onset of neurological symptoms. (Left) Sacrifice at 7 hours. Typical thrombotic mass of necrobiotic neutrophils plugging small vessel in the center of usual infiltrative mononuclear cell lesion of encephalomyelitis. Normal spinal cord white matter at right. Meninges filled with in-filtrating mononuclears to left; × 320. (Right) Death at 16 hours. Congested vessels near periphery of cord, adjacent to mild meningeal lesion, filled with fibrinoid material, erythrocytes, and a few leukocytes. Encephalomyelitis lesions act as prepared site for Shwartzman reaction; × 450.

Hematoxylin-eosin. From Waksman and Adams, *Am. J. Path.* *33*: 131–53 (1957).

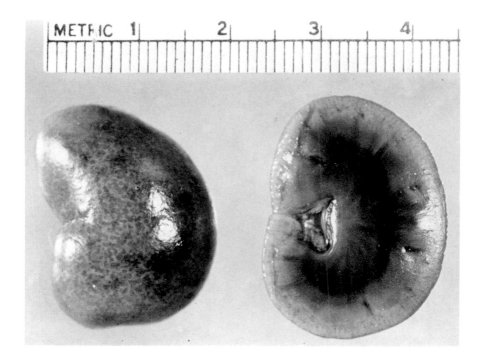

Fig. 15.7. Typical renal change seen in the general Shwartzman reaction, produced in the rabbit by two successive doses of lipopolysaccharide endotoxin 24 hours apart. After several hours, the cortex shows a striking mottled appearance, the light areas representing zones of necrosis and the dark areas zones of hemorrhage. In this specimen, with mild changes, the medulla remains uninvolved.

Courtesy of Dr. J. Brunson (see Thomas and Good, *J. Exp. Med. 96*: 605–24, 1952).

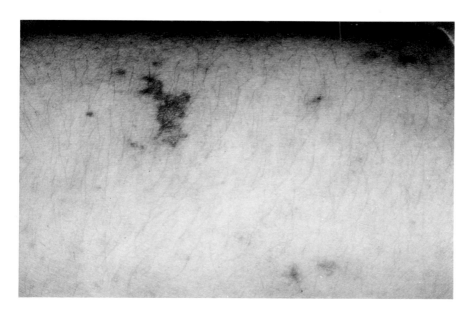

Fig. 15.8. Local petechial hemorrhages in the skin of a human subject with meningococcemia. This change is regarded as comparable to the generalized thrombotic and hemorrhagic lesions seen in the general Shwartzman reaction

Courtesy of Dr. I. Braverman.

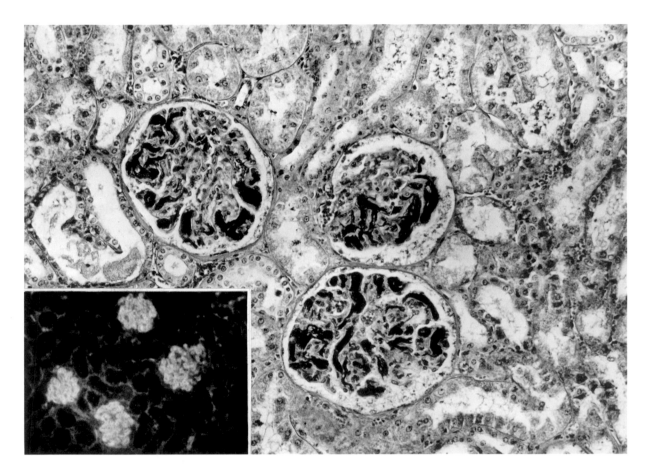

Fig. 15.9. General Shwartzman reaction in the rabbit produced by successive iv injections of *E. coli* endotoxin, given 24 hours apart. Characteristic renal lesion, shown here, consists of occlusion of glomerular capillaries by hyalin (fibrinoid) thrombi and more or less tubular necrosis. Insert shows fluorescence photomicrograph of similar kidney, stained with antibody specific for rabbit fibrinogen. Positive staining of deposits in glomeruli indicates presence of fibrinogen and/or fibrin. Similar thrombi and secondary infarct necrosis are common in various other organs, such as the liver, spleen, heart, etc.

Hematoxylin-eosin; insert, fluorescence technique. Courtesy of Dr. D. G. McKay. Insert, courtesy of Dr. J. Vazquez.

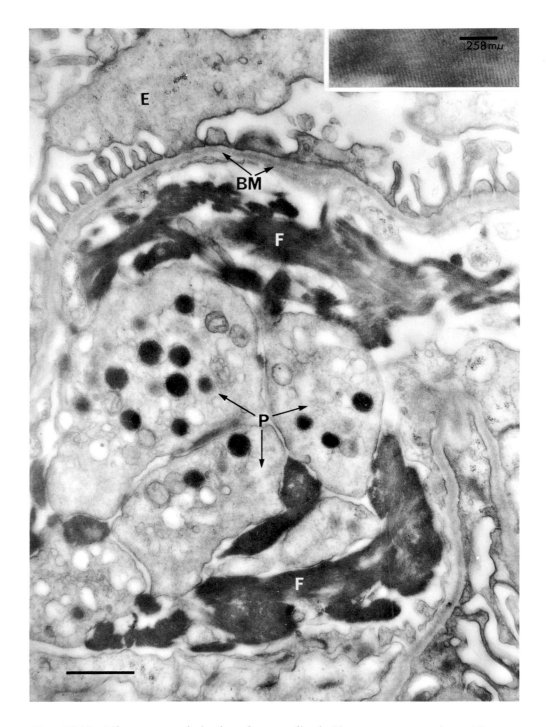

Fig. 15.10. Ultrastructural basis of generalized Shwartzman reaction. Electron micrograph of a single capillary loop in renal glomerulus of rabbit with generalized reaction, following activation of Hageman factor (by injection of ellagic acid), stimulation of α-adrenergic receptor sites, and inhibition of fibrinolysis. Lumen of vessel contains fibrin and platelet thrombi; ×17,000. The insert shows a high-power view of the fibrin, with its characteristic periodicity (215 Ångström units); ×38,850. BM, basement membrane; F, fibrin; P, platelets.

Courtesy of Dr. D. G. McKay (see McKay and Müller-Berghaus, *Fed. Proc. 27*: 436, 1968, abstr.).

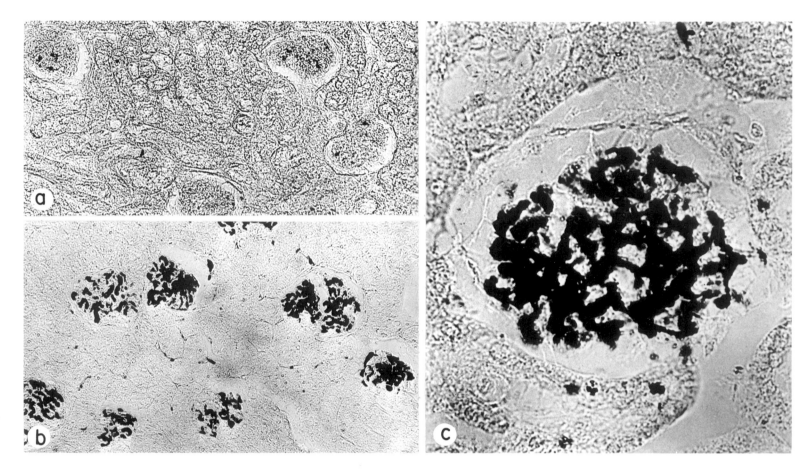

Fig. 15.11. Factors determining localization of general Shwartzman reaction. Vascular patterns in rabbits, demonstrated by intra-aortic injection of 10 ml. of 10 per cent suspension of India ink. Rabbits sacrificed immediately after injection. (a) Normal kidney. A few ink granules are present in the glomerular capillaries; ×88. (b) Four hours after second injection of bacterial endotoxin. The glomerular capillaries are dilated and filled with ink; ×98. (c) Higher power of glomerulus, 4 hours after endotoxin. This vasodilatation appears to determine the primary localization of fibrinous precipitate in the glomerulus as the lesion develops; ×390.

Unstained paraffin sections. (a, b) From McKay and Rowe, *Lab. Invest. 9*: 117–26 (1960). (c) From McKay and Merriam, *Arch. Path. 69*: 524–30 (1960).

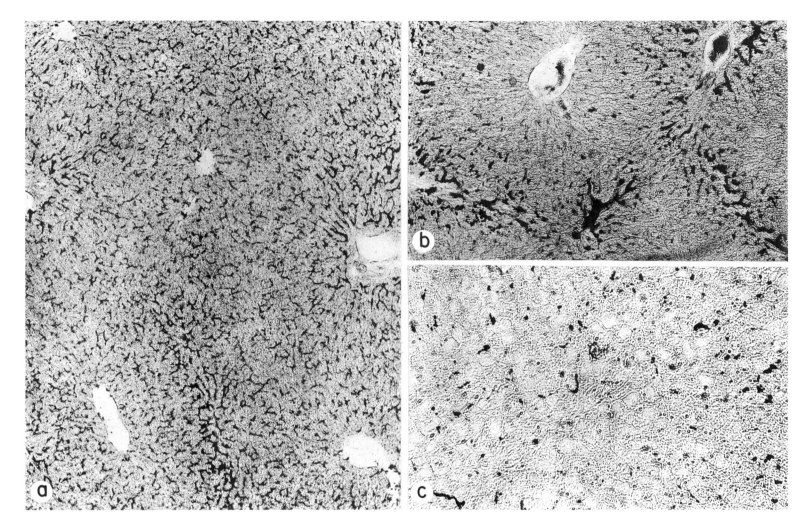

Fig. 15.12. Factors determining localization of general Shwartz-man reaction (as in Fig. 15.11). (a) Normal liver. The ink has reached every sinusoid and appears evenly distributed through all portions of the lobule; ×42. (b) Liver, 4 hours after endotoxin injection. Ink has been virtually excluded from the centers of the lobules and has accumulated in the dilated peripheral sinu-soids; ×42. (c) Liver of cortisone-treated animal 4 hours after endotoxin; the redistribution of blood 4 hours after endotoxin does not occur in animals prepared by cortisone; ×190.

Unstained, 30 μ paraffin sections. (a, b) From McKay and Rowe, *Lab. Invest. 9*: 117–26 (1960). (c) From McKay and Merriam (*Arch. Path. 69*: 524–30 (1960).

16. Local Reactions Due to Delayed or Cellular Hypersensitivity

A large group of immunologic phenomena is mediated by antibody bound to circulating lymphocytes, so-called sensitized cells, and cannot be shown to have any relation to humoral antibody. This category includes (1) *bacterial or infectious allergy*, of which tuberculin sensitivity is the prototype, usually expressed as the delayed reaction to skin test with the specific antigen (Fig. 16.9); (2) delayed skin *reactivity to purified proteins or protein conjugates* with simple haptens, commonly studied experimentally; (3) certain *disseminated lesions produced by microbial* or other *antigens* (Fig. 17.1); (4) *contact allergy*, elicited by application of a reactive chemical allergen to the surface of the skin or mucous membrane (Fig. 16.15); (5) *rejection of homografts (allografts)* of solid, vascularized tissues such as skin (Fig. 19.1); (6) *graft-vs.-host (GVH) reactions* produced by grafting immunologically competent lymphocytes (blood, spleen, lymph node) to hosts unable to destroy the grafted cells (Figs. 20.9,16); (7) the experimental *autoallergies* produced by immunization with ocular lens, myelin, thyroglobulin, etc. (Figs. 21.1,16,17); and (8) certain poorly understood *granulomatous processes*, of which zirconium granuloma may be taken as a prototype (Fig. 17.11). These are referred to collectively as involving "cellular immunity" or the "delayed type of hypersensitivity."

The *distribution of lesions* in phenomena of this type is quite precisely determined by the *distribution of eliciting antigen* (Fig. 16.1). In cases (1) and (2) above, intradermally injected protein or conjugate diffuses to blood vessels and lymphatics throughout the dermis and may remain attached to collagen fibers of the dermal connective tissue for some time (Fig. 1.16). Specific lesions occur throughout the zone of diffusion (Figs. 16.7,8) Similar lesions may be elicited in any organ where antigen is injected (Figs. 16.13,14). Even in the avascular cornea, antigen diffusing to the limbal vessels elicits a reaction with secondary changes in the cornea itself (Figs. 16.11,12). In (3) and (8) there may be a similar distribution within the vessels or connective tissue of any organ to which antigen penetrates (Fig. 17.2). In (4), complete antigen is formed by combination of allergen with protein constituents of epidermis (Figs. 1.17,18) and sometimes with serum proteins as well. Here the reaction involves only the uppermost layers of the dermis, adjacent to the epidermis in which antigen is formed (Figs. 16.16,17). In (5), the transplantation antigens are constituents of all nucleated cells of the graft (Fig. 3.13), and the reaction affects predominantly cellular elements, notably the blood vessels themselves or the epidermis and hair follicles (Figs. 19.4–9). The lesions in (6) are comparable and may be local, if cells are introduced locally (Figs. 20.10–13), or systemic, affecting lymphoid organs, such parenchymatous organs as liver and kidney, and the joints and skin (Figs. 20.2–8). Finally, in (7) antigen is a constituent of parenchymal cells or such tissue elements as myelin and thyroglobulin (Figs. 1.5,9), and the geography of the lesion reflects the geography of the affected tissue. Thus perivascular lesions occur in white matter, where the eliciting antigen surrounds vessels throughout the nervous system (Fig. 21.1), and interstitial inflammatory lesions occur in the testis or thyroid, where islands of antigen-containing parenchyma are surrounded by mesenchyme and vessels (Figs. 21.16,17, 22–24).

A restriction is placed on the distribution of lesions by the *character of the vascular network* in areas where eliciting antigen is found. The lesions (see below) are perivenous and can occur only where there are small to medium-sized veins. Thus delayed skin reactions in the rat are largely deep or even subcutaneous, and contact reactions cannot be elicited since few or no vessels of venous type are found in the upper dermis of flank skin in this species (Fig. 16.2). Disseminated lesions tend to occur in areas where there are venous plexuses, in joint synovia and ciliary body of the eye in particular (Fig. 17.9). The distribution of autoallergic lesions in the peripheral nervous system, testis, and adrenal is clearly related to the presence of veins (Figs. 21.11–13,28).

The lesions themselves are *perivenous infiltrates of mononuclear cells* (the "perivascular island" reaction).

which increase in number and size over a period of hours to a day or two, in reactions to diffusible, easily catabolized antigens, or over several days in cases involving noncatabolizable exogenous substances, as in zirconium granuloma, or substances which are tissue constituents present in large supply (grafts and the autoallergies) (Figs. 16.7,8; 17.2; 21.1). A *zone of parenchymal damage* (the "invasive–destructive" lesion) is seen which corresponds closely to the zone of cellular infiltration about vessels. It is particularly obvious in the autoallergies where the antigen is part of a parenchymal constituent such as myelin (Figs. 21.2,3). It is a major element of lesion formation in grafts, where the parenchymal element affected may be vascular endothelium and where many or most of the pathologic changes are secondary to vascular destruction (Figs. 19.4–9). It is also a major element of contact reactions, in which epidermal damage and vesiculation are the principal elements of clinical disease (Figs. 16.16–19). *Vasodilatation and a mild increase in vascular permeability* parallel the cell infiltration.

Three other elements are not infrequently observed in lesions of cellular hypersensitivity. Extremely intense lesions, particularly in certain species, may show a *"vasculonecrotic" change*, with edema, impregnation of vessel walls by serum proteins, secondary accumulation of polymorphonuclears, and hemorrhage (Fig. 21.6). Certain lesions, e.g. the tuberculin reaction in the guinea pig, may show central vascular stasis and *gross central necrosis* (Fig. 16.21); in some instances, this may result from a local Shwartzman event (Fig. 15.4). Gross necrosis is particularly common in relatively avascular tissues such as the white matter of the spinal cord (Fig. 16.21) and the cornea (Figs. 16.11,12), when their vascular supply is compromised by the inflammatory lesion. Finally *plasma cell accumulations* or even *germinal centers* may be seen, as the lesion ages (Fig. 21.7). These appear late and may be some distance from the actual site of elicitation. They resemble the "progressive immunization reaction" occurring in response to exogenous antigen in isolated organs such as the eye (Fig. 5.23).

These lesions, wherever they occur, differ strikingly from the lesions that result from trauma, toxic substances, or other agents, including circulating antibody against tissue elements, which produce primary damage of the tissue itself (Section 23). Where damage of parenchymal elements, such as the Schwann cell of peripheral nerve or the myocardial cell, is primary, there may be a reaction of polymorphonuclears if the reaction is acute and intense (Fig. 23.1) or a mild histiocytic reaction if the lesion develops slowly (Fig. 23.2). Even with extensive tissue damage or necrosis, the inflammatory changes are limited to a transient increase in vascular permeability, an early massive poly response, and a minimal histiocytic reaction (Figs. 16.17; 23.6). Nothing morphologically comparable to a delayed reaction has been produced by tissue injury. With virus infection, one finds viral inclusions in infected cells and evidence of cell damage, but the secondary inflammation again is limited to polymorphs, in acute reactions, and minimal histiocytic activation in more chronic lesions (Figs. 23.3,4).

The *infiltrating cells* in the early perivascular island reaction have been described as lymphocytes varying from less than 8 to 11 μ in diameter (Figs. 16.9; 21.16). They are pleomorphic (i.e. highly motile), slightly basophilic, and phagocytic. In lesions of more than a few hours' duration, the majority of these cells finally assume the aspect of typical histiocytes. However in certain cases, the contact reaction for example, they may continue to resemble lymphocytes even in advanced lesions (Figs. 16.18,19). In others they may form masses of epithelioid and even giant cells, as in GVH reactions (Figs. 20.10–13) and certain granulomas (Fig. 17.11). The infiltrating cells, though they resemble medium-sized lymphocytes in conventional stained preparations when they first appear, apparently *correspond to circulating monocytes* or "prehistiocytes," since they are phagocytic (Fig. 21.3) and possess enzymes such as acid phosphatase and esterase, which are characteristic of reticuloendothelial cells (Figs. 19.13,14). Their perivascular location suggests that they come from the blood stream. This possibility is supported by passive transfer studies which have shown that essentially comparable lesions are elicited by systemic (intravenous) transfer of "sensitized cells" and an intradermal test dose of antigen, by local injection of cells and intravenous antigen, or indeed by intradermal injection of mixtures of cells with antigen. Their hematogenous origin has been firmly established by labeling studies with tritiated thymidine (H³T). In a variety of experiments involving delayed skin reactions (Fig. 16.10), adjuvant arthritis, autoallergic encephalomyelitis and thyroiditis (Figs. 21.4,5,18), and skin homografts, it has been shown by the use of H³T that most or all of the infiltrating cells are hematogenous, that they come from a population of continuously dividing cells, that they continue to divide in the lesions, and that they actually are transformed from "lymphocytes" to typical histiocytes over several hours. These events account for the increase in number and size of lesions and for their changing histological character.

Experiments in which passive transfer of tuberculin-type sensitivity with lymphoid cells is combined with H³T labeling of donor or recipient show that a *small proportion of cells at the reaction site are specifically sensitized*, i.e. bear cell-bound antibody, while the overwhelming *majority are nonspecific*, presumably being brought to the site by a specific trigger mechanism (Fig. 16.20). The presumption is strong that the former come from specific blast-like precursors in the lymph node cortex (Figs. 6.18–20), these in turn being derived from immunocompetent small lymphocytes which originate in the thymus and recirculate in the peripheral pool of uncommitted small lymphocytes (Section 6). The latter have been shown, by the combined use of passive transfer and fluorescent labeling with antisera against cellular transplantation antigens (Fig. 3.13), to come directly from the bone marrow and thus to resemble closely the mononuclear cells appearing at sites of nonimmunologic irritation in the skin or in peritoneal exudates elicited nonspecifically (Fig. 2.13). Agencies that deplete the pool of immunocompetent small lymphocytes, among them X-irradiation, cyclophosphamide, thoracic duct drainage, antilymphocyte serum, and neonatal thymectomy (Figs. 5.6–12), prevent sensitization of the delayed type, and the defect which such agencies produce is immediately corrected by infusion of a sufficient number of competent cells (Fig. 16.4). Such agencies as antilymphocyte sera also act to suppress pre-existing sensitization by removing either the sensitized cells or the nonspecific monocytes (Figs. 16.5,6).

After a local delayed reaction has waned, a few small nests of cells with the morphology of lymphocytes remain at the reaction site. If the original antigen is now readministered locally or systemically, there is a flare-up at the site which differs from the original delayed reaction in time course and in histologic and physiologic character. The lesion shows edema and erythema, reaching a peak at 12 hours, and striking local infiltration of eosinophils (Fig. 11.12). It appears to result from the anamnestic formation of antibody (of unknown immunoglobulin class) by those cells remaining after subsidence of the original lesion and which must therefore be regarded as a type of memory cell.

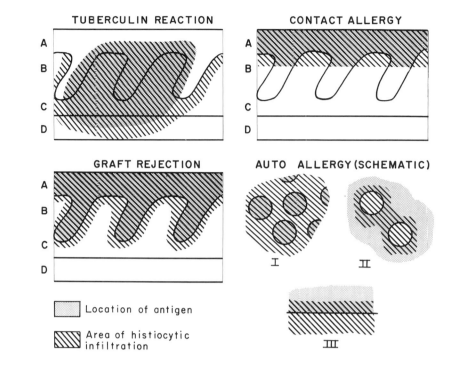

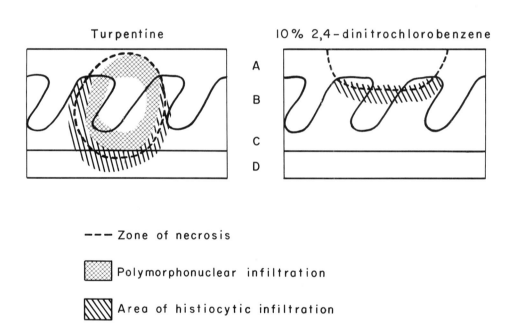

Fig. 16.1. Delayed or cellular sensitivity. (a) Relationship between tissue location of antigen (as far as known at present) and areas in which mononuclear cell infiltration and the invasive–destructive type of lesion occur. A, Surface epidermis; B, follicles and upper dermis; C, deeper dermis; D, subcutaneous fat and muscle. I, Islands of antigen-containing parenchyma, e.g. in testis or thyroid; II, islands of mesenchymal tissue surrounded by antigen-containing parenchyma, e.g. in central nervous system; III, parallel or interpenetrating arrangement, e.g. in adrenal, peripheral nerve, uvea, meninges. (b) Relationship between primary tissue injury or necrosis produced in normal skin by nonspecific "irritants" and areas of cellular inflammation.

From Waksman In CIBA *Foundation Symposium on Cellular Aspects of Immunity*, G. E. W. Wolstenholme and M. O'Connor, eds., Churchill, London, 1960, pp. 280–322.

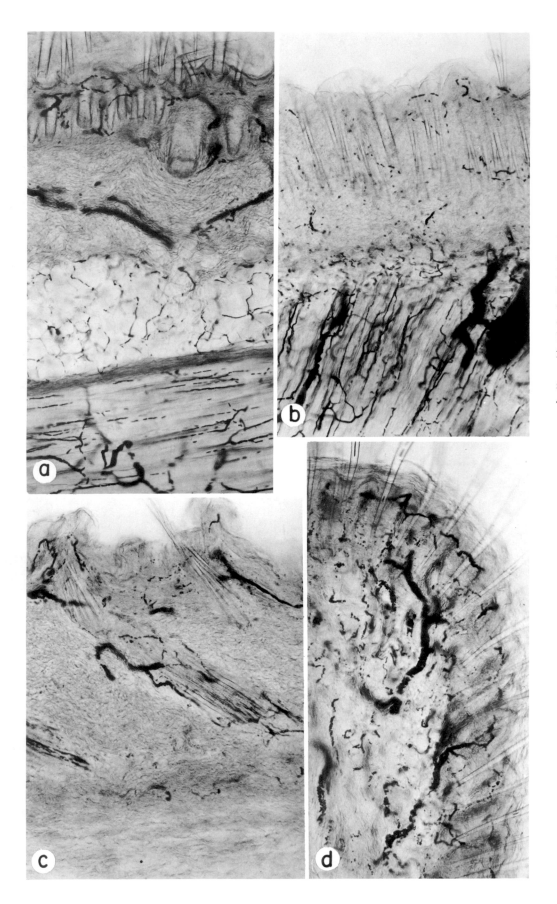

Fig. 16.2. Comparison of vascular pattern in several types of skin. (a) Guinea pig flank skin, showing large veins in dense dermal connective tissue and venules in upper zone of dermis between follicles, as well as veins in underlying panniculus. (b) Rat flank skin, showing large veins in panniculus and at base of dermis but almost total absence of veins in dermis proper or in subepidermal region. (c) Rabbit flank skin, showing vascular pattern similar to that of guinea pig with, however, fewer veins in dense dermis. (d) Rat ear, showing venules between follicles and larger veins throughout deeper connective tissue. Location of veins, shown here, determines possibility of eliciting delayed skin reactions, e.g. tuberculin reactions, in the dermis of guinea pigs and rabbits but only in deeper layers of rat skin. Contact reactions, elicited by surface application of allergen, requires superficial veins like those in guinea pig skin.

Frozen sections, 250 μ. Pickworth benzidine stain; ×80. From Waksman, *Lab. Invest. 12*: 46–57 (1963).

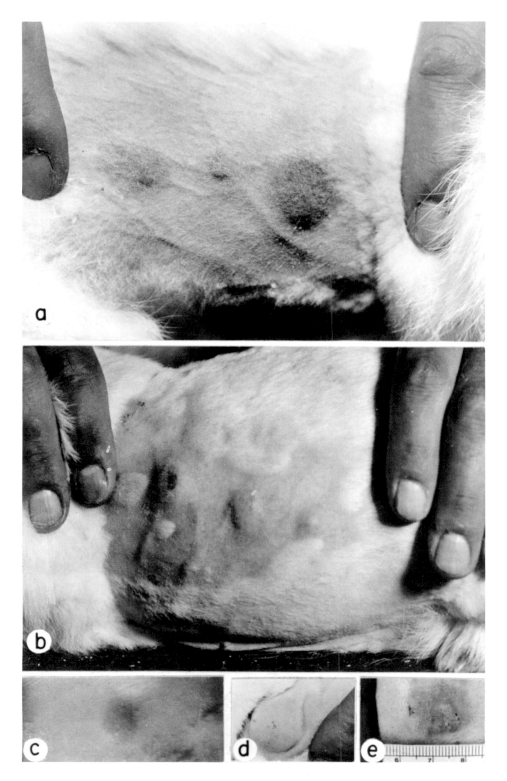

Fig. 16.3. Classical skin reactions of delayed (tuberculin) type. (a) Rabbit inoculated with BSA, 25 mg in complete adjuvant in footpads, and skin tested at 14 days with old tuberculin 1:100, BSA (6.5 μg) and BSA (65 μg). Reactions photographed at 48 hours show typical induration and dark red erythema. (b) Rabbit similarly inoculated with total "lipide" extract of bovine white matter plus adjuvant and skin tested at 10 days with saline emulsion of same preparation (equivalent to 25, 11.2, and 5 per cent white matter). Reactions at 72 hours show massive induration, central necrosis, and relative lack of erythema characteristic of reactions elicited with poorly soluble antigen. Encephalomyelitis appeared at 11 days. (c) Rabbit inoculated with rabbit spinal cord and adjuvant and tested at 14 days with 10 per cent rabbit cord homogenate in saline. Reaction, 5 days later, is torpid, indurated erythematous nodule. Onset of encephalomyelitis at 17 days. (d) Rat sensitized with BSA and adjuvant in footpad and tested at 14 days with BSA (30 μg). 24-hour reaction shows deep induration and minimal erythema. (e) Reaction at 48 hours to 5 μg PPD in rat sensitized with adjuvant alone 14 days earlier. Erythema and mild induration.

(a, c–e) Approximately natural size; (b) 3/4 natural size. (a) From Leskowitz and Waksman, *J. Immunol. 84*: 58–72 (1960). (b) From Waksman, *J. Infect. Dis. 99*: 258–69 (1956). (c) From Waksman and Adams, *J. Infect. Dis. 93*: 21–27 (1953). (d) From Flax and Waksman, *J. Immunol. 89*: 496–504 (1962). (b, c) Reproduced by permission of the University of Chicago Press.

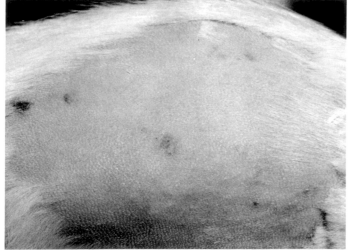

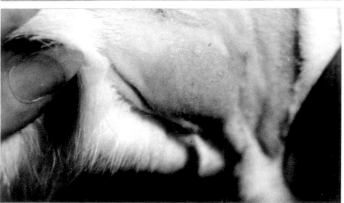

Fig. 16.4. Essential role of small lymphocytes in the cellular type of sensitization. 48-hour skin reactions to BSA (30 μg) in rats sensitized 14 days earlier with BSA and adjuvant. (Above) Neonatally thymectomized rat shows no sign of reaction at skin test site. (Below) Littermate, also thymectomized at birth but supplied with 10^9 small lymphocytes on days 0, 1, and 2 of sensitization period, shows indurated reaction (12 × 14 mm) indistinguishable from reactions obtained in sham-operated (nonthymectomized) controls. Lymphocytes were obtained from lymph nodes of syngeneic normal donors. Blood lymphocyte count of animal shown in (a) was less than half the normal value.

× 1.3. From Isaković, Waksman, and Wennersten, *J. Immunol.* **95**: 602–13 (1965).

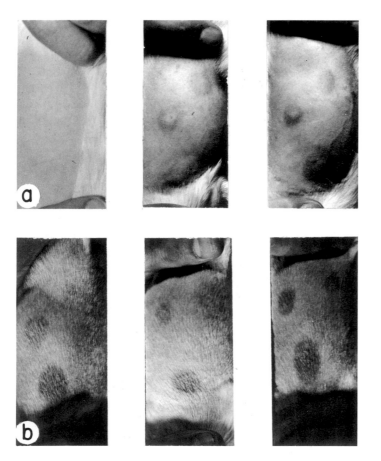

Fig. 16.5. Suppression of delayed skin reactions by lymphopenic agents. (a) Reactions (24-hour) to old tuberculin 1:20, 1:100, and 1:500 in tuberculin-sensitive guinea pigs treated with rabbit sera directed against guinea pig lymphocytes, guinea pig polymorphonuclears, and adjuvant respectively. Sera, injected 21 and 3 hours before skin test, produced lymphopenia, agranulocytosis, and leukocytosis, respectively, at time of test. Tuberculin reactions are completely suppressed in the first animal but expressed normally in others. (b) PCA reactions elicited in the same three animals, immediately after reading of tuberculin sites, show no suppressive effect by any of the three sera. Sensitization 24 hours earlier with rabbit antibody (1.0, 0.2, and 0.04 μg N); elicitation with 1.0 mg of antigen (ovalbumin) plus Evans blue iv; reading at 15 minutes.

Half normal size. From Waksman, Arbouys, and Arnason, *J. Exp. Med.* **114**: 997–1022 (1961).

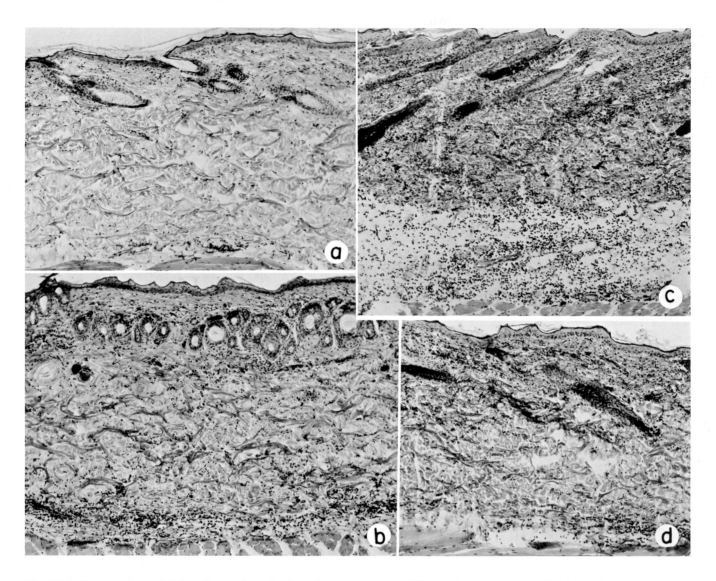

Fig. 16.6. Suppression of delayed reactions by lymphopenic agents. Histologic appearance of tuberculin skin reactions in guinea pigs shown in Fig. 16.5. (a) Reaction elicited with OT 1:20 in lymphopenic animal. (b) Reaction to OT 1:500 in agranulocytic animal. (c, d) Reactions to OT 1:20 and 1:500 in animal given control serum. Response is completely suppressed by treatment with antilymphocyte serum and unaffected by antipoly serum.

Hematoxylin-eosin; ×60. From Waksman, Arbouys, and Arnason, *J. Exp. Med. 114*: 997–1022 (1961).

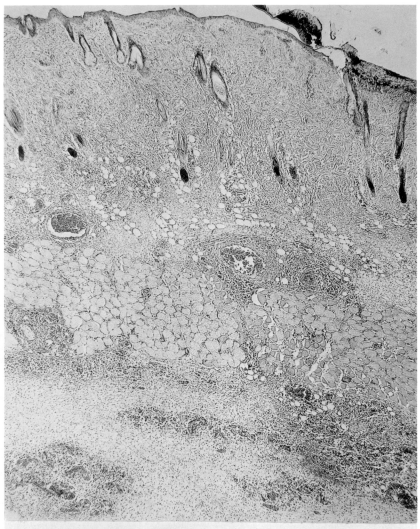

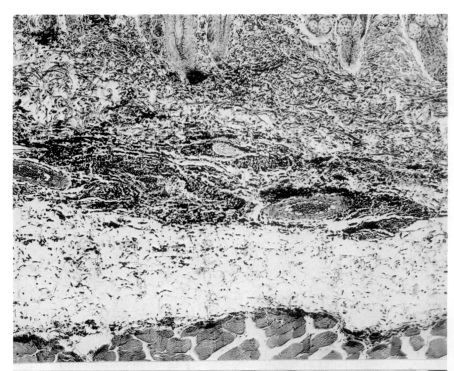

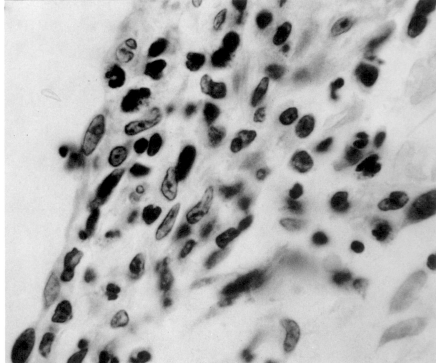

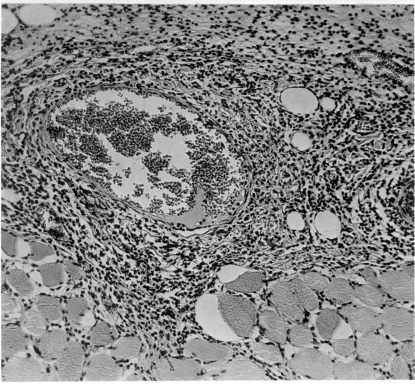

Fig. 16.7. Classical skin reactions of delayed hypersensitivity. Rat skin reaction at 48 hours to BSA (30 μg), comparable to that shown in Fig. 16.3(d). Perivascular infiltrates, made up almost entirely of mononuclear cells, are seen in deep dermis and in and beneath the muscle layers of the panniculus.

Hematoxylin-eosin; ×36, ×125. From Flax and Waksman, *J. Immunol.* *89*: 496–504 (1962).

Fig. 16.8. Classical skin reactions of delayed hypersensitivity. (Above) Skin reaction (24-hour) to 10 μg BSA in sensitized rabbit. Massive infiltration of mononuclear cells is seen about deep dermal vessels and a more moderate infiltrate in mid-dermis, near the hair follicles. (Below) Similar 24-hour reaction to PPD in tuberculin-sensitive rabbit. On left is lumen of small vein in deep dermis. Endothelial cells, lymphocytes, histiocytes, and rare polymorphonuclear leukocytes are clearly distinguishable.

Hematoxylin-eosin; ×80, ×1,100. From Leskowitz and Waksman, *J. Immunol.* *84*: 58–72 (1960).

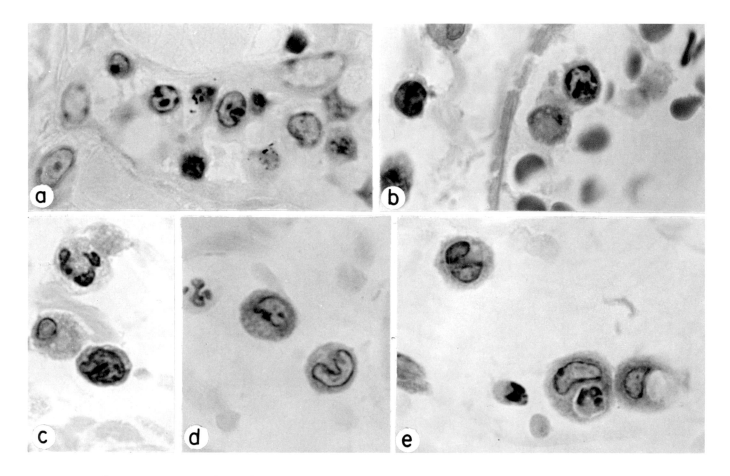

Fig. 16.9. Cell types characteristic of classical delayed skin reactions. From perivascular infiltrates, in skin reactions of various durations, in tuberculin-sensitized guinea pigs tested with PPD. (a) Small to medium-sized lymphocytes with smooth nuclei. (b, c) Medium "lymphocytes" with highly irregular (pleomorphic) nuclei. (d) Another medium "lymphocyte" and a monocyte. (e) Monocyte and histiocyte (macrophage). Erythrocytes and polymorphonuclear leukocytes permit an estimate of relative size.

Methacrylate embedding, thin sections (1–2 μ), stained with May-Grünwald–Giemsa; $\times$1,500. From Kosunen, Waksman, Flax, and Tihen, *Immunology 6*: 276–90 (1963).

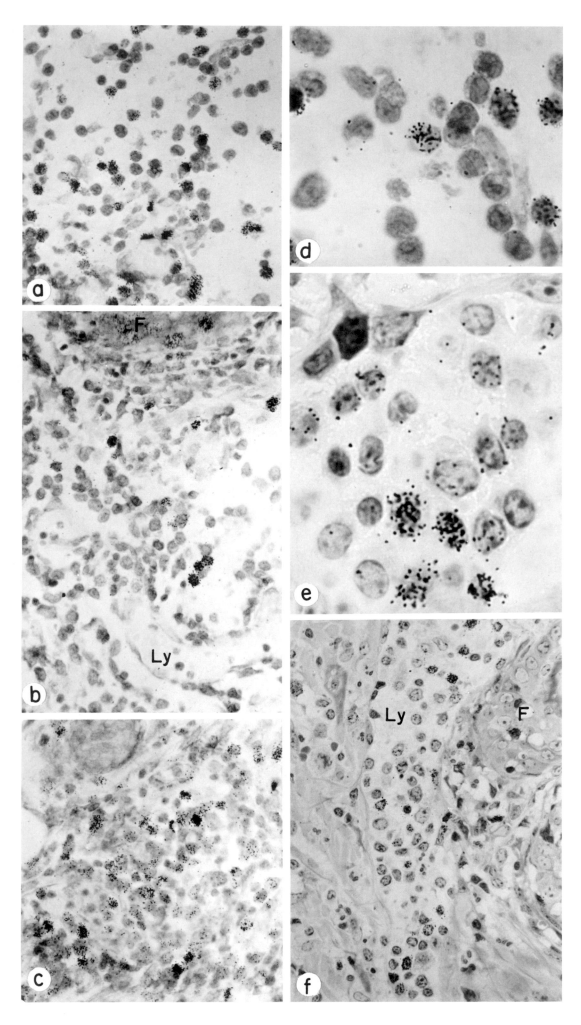

Fig. 16.10. Origin of cells in delayed reactions, shown by labeling experiments with H³-thymidine. Tuberculin reactions elicited by 25 μg PPD in sensitized rats (a–d) or guinea pigs (e, f) given label (1 μc/g) iv. All figures show cell infiltrate in dermis near follicles, 12 hours after skin testing (a, d), 18 hours (b), and 48 hours (c, e, f). In (b) follicle epithelium (F) is shown above and a large lymphatic (Ly) below. In (f) a similar lymphatic is filled with cells leaving the site as the reaction subsides (48 hours). (a, d) Thymidine given ½ hour before testing; 12-hour infiltrate shows labeling of about 30 per cent of cells in the infiltrate, mainly small to medium-sized cells of lymphocytic character. (c, e, f) Similar labeling; 48-hour infiltrate shows labeling of higher proportion of cells, now mainly histiocytic, with decreasing grain count. (b) Thymidine ½ hour before sacrifice, labels 5–10 per cent of infiltrating cells. Thus cells are seen to be hematogenous, to come from a dividing cell population, and to divide in the lesion itself.

(a–d) Paraffin sections, 6–8 μ. (e, f) Methacrylate sections, 1–2 μ. All are stripping-film autoradiographs developed at 3–6 weeks and stained with Giemsa; (a–f) ×500, (d) ×1,150, (e) ×1,400. From Kosunen, Waksman, Flax, and Tihen, Immunology 6: 276–90 (1963).

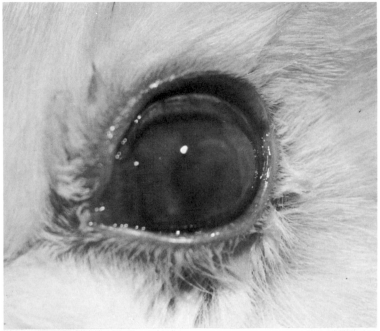

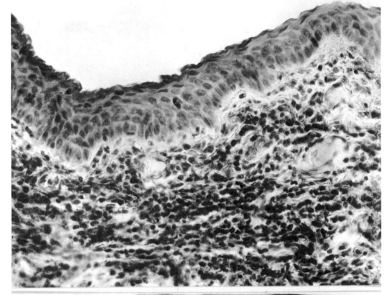

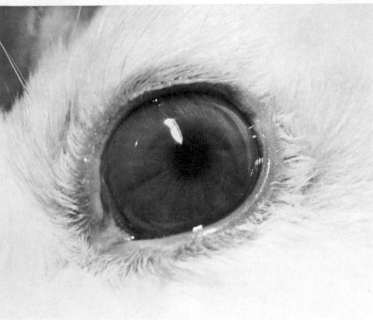

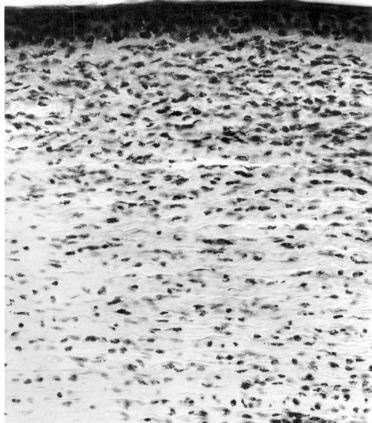

Fig. 16.11. Corneal reactions to BSA (2 μg N) injected intra-corneally in rabbits sensitized 14 days earlier with BSA in adjuvant. (Above) Moderate reaction, with general corneal clouding and partial ring of antigen–antibody precipitate. (Below) Mild reaction, with slight peripheral clouding only. From Leskowitz and Waksman, *J. Immunol.* **84**: 58–72 (1960).

Fig. 16.12. Histologic evolution of corneal reaction seen in delayed hypersensitivity. Corneal reactions to BSA, comparable to those shown in Fig. 16.11. (Above) Limbus at 6 hours shows typical delayed reaction, i.e. massive mononuclear cell infiltrates with few or no polymorphonuclears. (Below) Cornea at 26 hours shows heavy infiltration of both mononuclears and polys. Central cornea at this time shows mild infiltration, mainly of polys.

Hematoxylin-eosin; ×235. Waksman, unpublished.

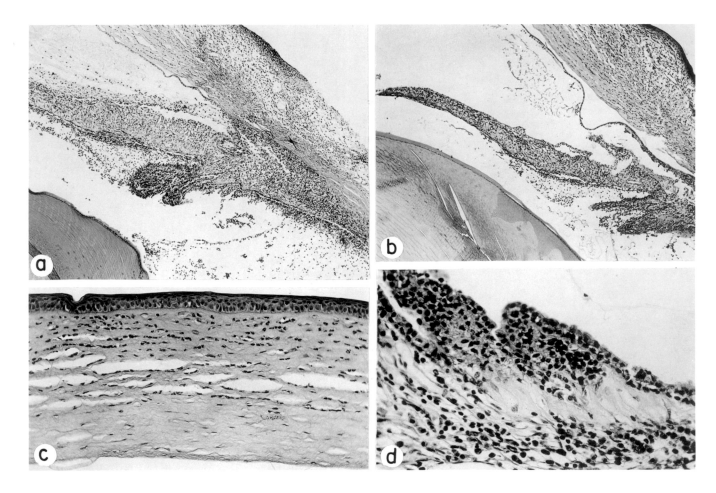

Fig. 16.13. Delayed reactions in guinea pig eye. (a) Ocular reaction, 24 hours after injection 0.5 μg tuberculoprotein (PPD) into vitreous of tuberculin-sensitive guinea pig: anterior uveitis with massive infiltration of the iris, ciliary body, choroid, and even the cornea by a mixed population of lymphocytes and polymorphonuclear cells; ×52. (b) Similar reaction after injection of 3 μg BSA into vitreous of guinea pig sensitized to BSA: the iris, ciliary body, and corneal limbus are massively infiltrated by mononuclear cells, with cells and protein in the anterior and posterior chambers; ×33. (c) Cornea in similar reaction elicited by 3 μg ovalbumin in guinea pig sensitized by the specific precipitate technique: diffuse polymorphonuclear infiltration between corneal lamellae; ×155. (d) Ciliary body 2 weeks after acute reaction; lymphocytic infiltrate has given way to marked plasmocytosis here, as well as throughout the uveal tract; ×285.

Hematoxylin-eosin (AFIP negs. 59–3637, 59–3168, 59–3169, 59–3162). From Silverstein and Zimmerman *Am. J. Ophthal. 48*: Part II, 435–47 (1959).

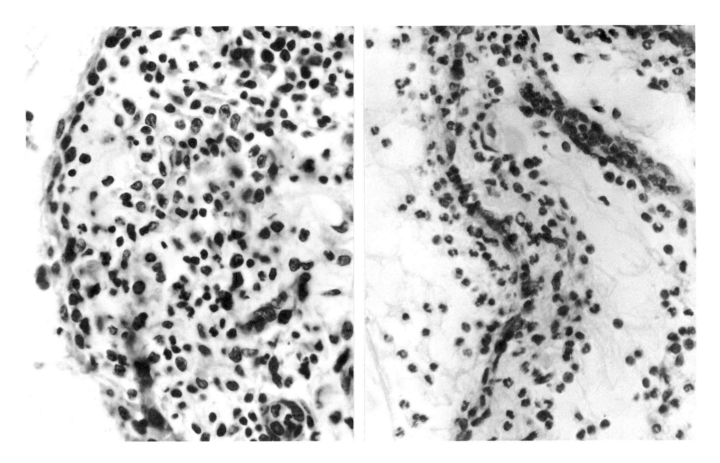

Fig. 16.14. Pure delayed and Arthus reactions elicited by specific antigen in knee joints of guinea pigs, actively sensitized with allotypic γ-globulin and passively sensitized with iv injection of antibody against BSA. (Left) Delayed reaction, 24 hours after intra-articular injection of antigen, shows typical lymphohistiocytic infiltrate and complete absence of polymorphonuclear leukocytes. (Right) Arthus reaction, at 4 hours, shows exudation of plasma protein and massive infiltration with neutrophils, both beneath the synovial lining and in the joint space at left. These may be regarded as prototypic lesions, obtainable under rather artificial experimental conditions. Lesions elicited in actively sensitized animals with usual antigens are frequently of mixed type.

Hematoxylin-eosin; magnifications not given. Courtesy of Dr. R. T. McCluskey (see *Fed. Proc. 20*: 17, 1961, abstr.).

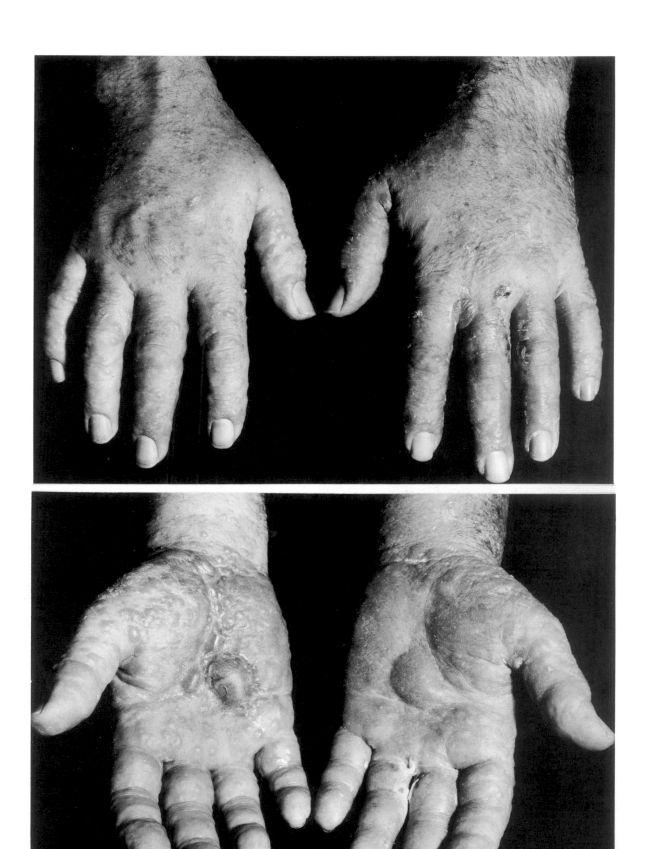

Fig. 16.15. Typical contact reaction in human subject, elicited by exposure to poison ivy allergen (urushiol), to which subject is intensely sensitive. General inflammatory lesion with striking epidermal vesiculation (corresponding to spongiosis illustrated in Figs. 16.16, 18, 19) and formation of large, fluid-filled bullae.

Courtesy of Dr. A. M. Kligman.

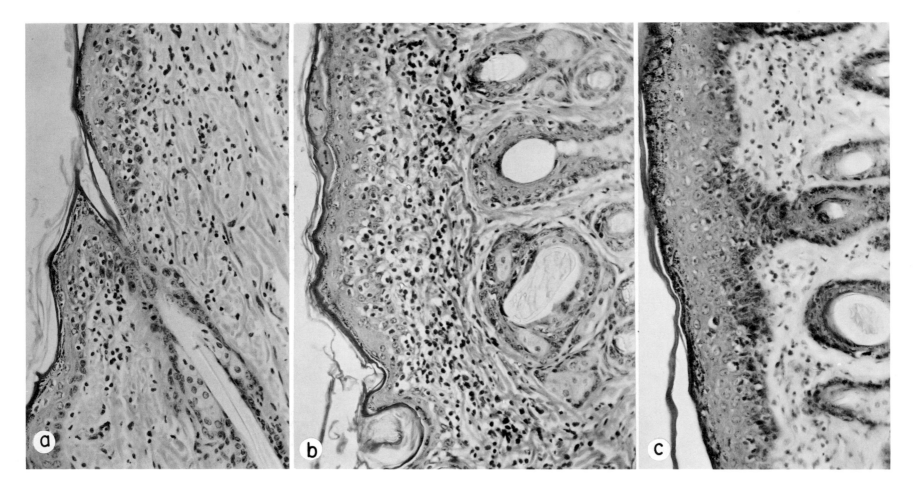

Fig. 16.16. Histologic character of contact reaction. Sensitized guinea pig tested with 2,4-dinitrochlorobenzene, 0.1 per cent in acetone. (a–c) Reactions at 6, 24, and 48 hours, showing appearance of mononuclear cell infiltrate in upper dermis, invasion of epidermis containing antigen by mononuclears, and epidermal spongiosis about the infiltrating cells. Reaction has begun at 6 hours, is very intense at 24 hours, and is resolving at 48 hours. Note epidermal thickening resulting from (nonimmunologic) irritant effect of allergen.

Hematoxylin-eosin; × 235. From Waksman, in CIBA *Foundation Symposium on Cellular Aspects of Immunity*, G. E. W. Wolstenholme and M. O'Connor, eds., Churchill, London, 1960, pp. 280–322.

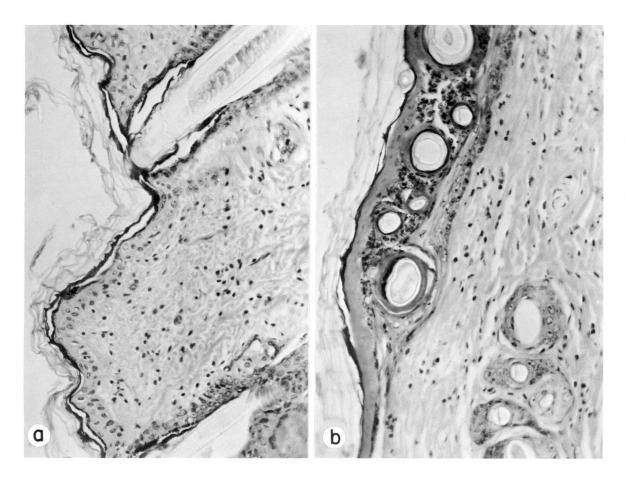

Fig. 16.17. Irritant effect of high concentrations of allergen on normal skin. (a, b) Effect produced by 2,4-dinitrochlorobenzene, 5 per cent in acetone, at 6 and 48 hours. Epidermal damage is shown early by shrinkage of nuclei and pink, homogeneous staining of epidermal cytoplasm. At 48 hours, necrotic epidermis is cast off and formation of a layer of new epidermis is in progress beneath. Note almost total absence of inflammatory cell response at both times.

Hematoxylin-eosin; × 235. From Waksman, in CIBA *Foundation Symposium on Cellular Aspects of Immunity*, G. E. W. Wolstenholme and M. O'Connor, eds., Churchill, London, 1960, pp. 280–322.

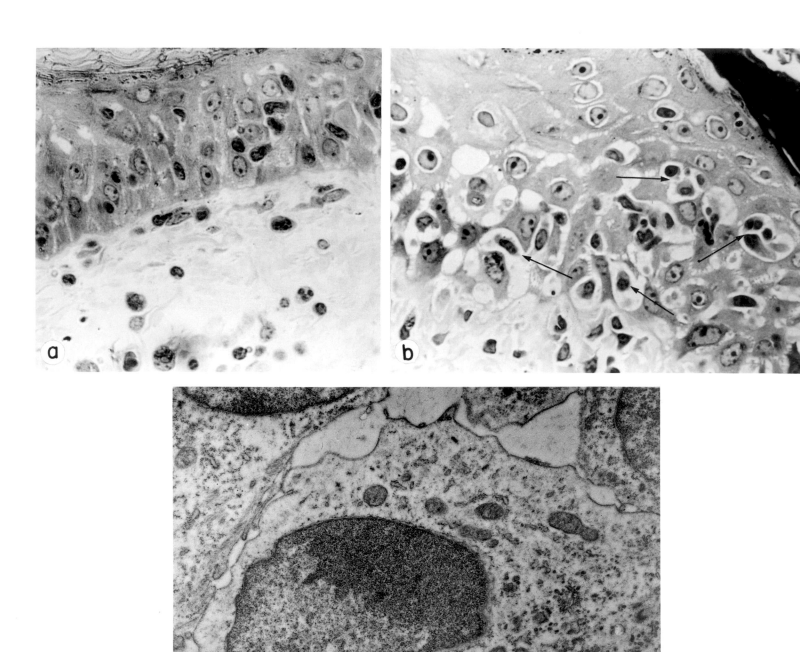

Fig. 16.18. Histologic character of contact reaction. Reactions to 2,4-dinitrochloroben-zene in guinea pigs sensitized 8 days earlier. Reaction starts at 5–6 hours with appearance of mononuclear cell infiltrate. By 8–10 hours there is extracellular edema (spongiosis) adjacent to infiltrating cells which have entered the epidermis. (a, b) 12 hours. Thin sections showing extensive infiltration of epidermis by mononuclear cells with morphologic aspect intermediate between lymphocytes and histiocytes (arrows). Large extracellular spaces primarily surround the invading cells. The total epidermal thickness is increased. (c) 24 hours. Mononuclear cell shows increased size with duration of the lesion. The cytoplasmic volume is greater and the cytoplasmic organelles become more numerous.

Osmium tetroxide fixation; methacrylate embedding. (a, b) Giemsa; ×425, ×625. (c) Electron micrograph; ×14,000. From Flax and Caulfield, *Am. J. Path. 43*: 1031–53 (1963).

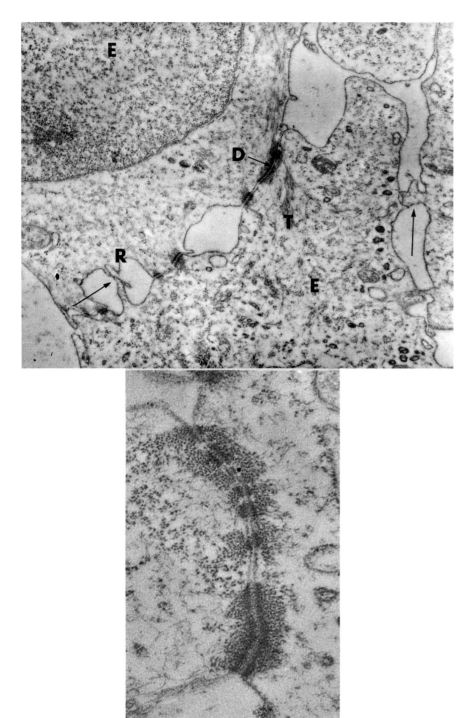

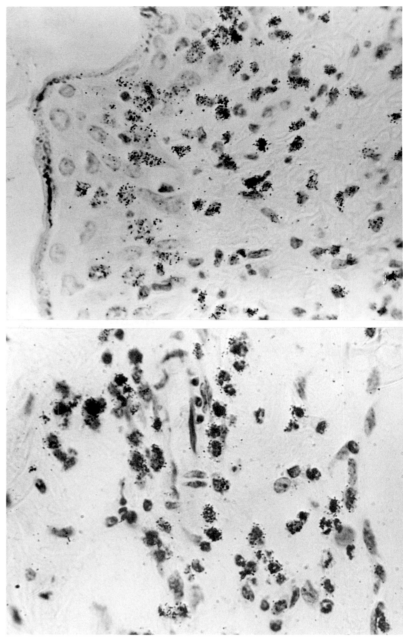

Fig. 16.19. Histologic character of contact reaction. Electron micrographs of epithelium 10 and 12 hours after test with 2,4-dinitrochlorobenzene, showing nature of spongiosis. (Above) Epithelial cells (E) are widely separated. The desmosomes (D) are reduced in number, and there is a diminution in the number of tonofilament packets (T). Though desmosomes are not apparent, there is still evidence of cellular cohesion in some areas (arrow). In the absence of desmosomes, however, the intercellular adherence is soon lost; ×15,300. (Below) A single desmosome. The normal insertion of tonofilaments into the desmosome is disrupted, and the alternating light and dark zones of the desmosome itself are not clearly defined; ×54,000.

From Flax and Caulfield, *Am. J. Path. 43*: 1031–53 (1963).

Fig. 16.20. Origin of cells in delayed reactions, studied by combined passive transfer and labeling techniques. Both photographs show contact reactions elicited by specific allergen in guinea pigs sensitized passively to p-chlorobenzoyl chloride. H³-thymidine was given to each recipient (six doses over 2 days, total dose 1 μc) *prior* to transfer of lymph node cells from sensitized donor. An area of maximal infiltration is shown 24 hours after application of test dose of allergen (2 per cent PCBC in 20 per cent olive oil in acetone). Most infiltrating mononuclears in upper dermis and epidermis (68–91 per cent in different areas) are labeled and must therefore be of recipient origin, i.e. nonspecific participants in reaction. Other labeling experiments suggest their origin from the bone marrow.

Autoradiograph prepared with 5-μ paraffin sections and NTB3 nuclear track emulsion, exposed 6 weeks, developed, and stained with Bullard's hematoxylin; ×600. Courtesy of R. T. McCluskey (see *J. Immunol. 90*: 466–77, 1963).

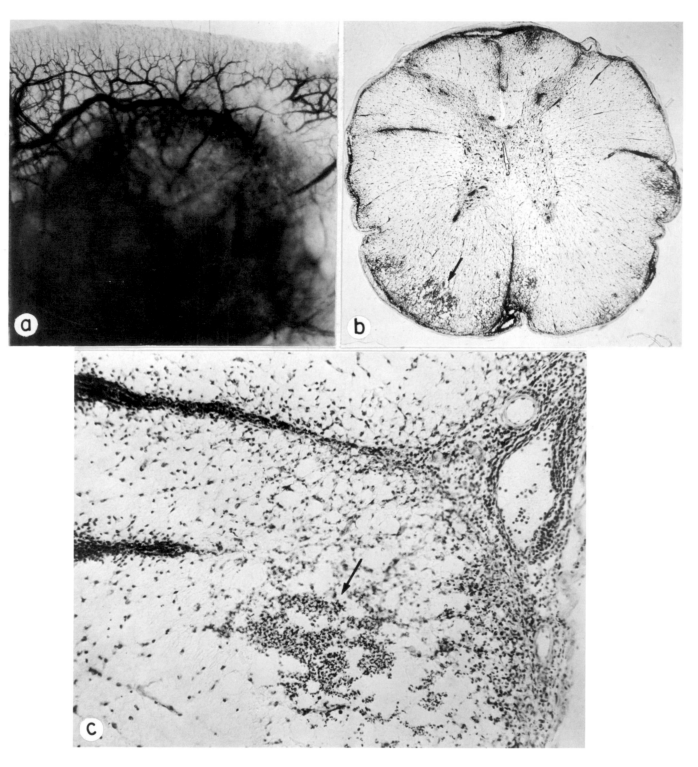

Fig. 16.21. Necrosis in reactions of cellular hypersensitivity. (a) Guinea pig ear: intense 17-hour reaction to old tuberculin (0.02 ml, 1:10), photographed 1 minute after iv injection of Evans blue dye. Central area of complete vascular stasis, indicated by failure of vessels to fill with dye, corresponds to zone of necrosis. Leakage of dye from vessels in surrounding zone indicates vascular injury. (b) Spinal cord with intense autoallergic encephalomyelitis lesions. Focus of necrosis (arrow) in white matter in lower left quandrant of cord may be the consequence of ischemia due to involvement of most adjacent vessels by the disease. (c) Higher power of lesion shows necrosis of glia, vacuolation of parenchyma, and collection of necrobiotic polymorphs.

(a) Approximately × 5.9; (b, c) cresyl violet, × 11.9, × 79.5. From Waksman, in *Mechanism of Cell and Tissue Damage Produced by Immune Reactions*, Benno Schwabe, Basel, 1962, pp. 146–60.

17. Disseminated Lesions Due to Cellular Hypersensitivity

A systemic delayed reaction is produced by parenteral injection of a large dose of antigen in the sensitized animal. Reaction of the antigen with "sensitized" lymphocytes in the circulation leads to their segregation in the lungs, other viscera, and skin (with resultant *lymphopenia*); their diapedesis, with the formation of *perivascular infiltrates of mononuclear cells* like those seen in local delayed reactions; and sometimes a grossly visible papular *rash*. Release of endogenous pyrogen (from reticuloendothelial cells, participating secondarily?) results in a characteristic *febrile response*. The lesion may be mimicked with an injection of antilymphocyte serum, which reacts with lymphocytes in the circulation and also leads to their segregation and diapedesis.

It is highly probable that the transient morbilliform rash and fever of serum disease in man (with protein antigens and drugs) represent systemic reactions of cellular hypersensitivity, and the granulomatous lesions of experimental serum disease, illustrated in Section 13, may also have this mechanism. As noted earlier, however, the renal and joint lesions and the arteritis are manifestations of immune complex disease and depend on circulating humoral antibody. The rash and fever of virus exanthemata such as measles were attributed by von Pirquet to a mechanism comparable to that of serum disease and there is evidence in favor of this suggestion. Measles virus disappears from its site of proliferation in the respiratory tract and lymphoid tissues when the rash appears, and the rash is lacking and virus persists in patients with lymphomas, who show depressed immunologic reactions. In some virus diseases, of which smallpox is an example, the skin lesion is a combination of that produced by viral growth following hematogenous dissemination and that resulting from the hypersensitivity reaction. The same concept is applicable to disseminated skin lesions (known as *ids*) appearing in tuberculosis, syphilis, and the mycoses. These have been inadequately studied from the immunologic standpoint. They may be comparable to the skin lesions produced in animals sensitized to bacterial antigens (see below). There are other lesions called ids, notably the acneiform and vegetative lesions occurring with excessive intake of bromides or iodides, which may have nothing to do with hypersensitivity.

With disseminated antigens other than soluble proteins and viruses, cellular hypersensitivity results in disease having a prolonged time course, often measured in weeks or longer. Several experimental conditions involving bacterial antigens have been well studied. The best known is *adjuvant disease*, produced in rats by intradermal or footpad injection of killed mycobacteria or *Nocardia* in oil (Figs. 17.1–7) and a similar process produced in guinea pigs by the same technique (Fig. 17.11). Both are *disseminated lesions* appearing in organs which possess a rich venous network, notably the *joint synovia* (Fig. 17.2), *eye* (Fig. 17.5), well-vascularized *skin* such as that of the ear (Fig. 17.1) and genitalia, and *mucous membranes* (Fig. 17.7). The rat lesions are perivascular mononuclear cell infiltrates, frequently accompanied by exudation of serum proteins and the appearance of fibrin and granulocytes in the joint space and the anterior and posterior chambers of the eye (Figs. 17.2,5). The derivation of the mononuclear cells, as shown in labeling studies with tritiated thymidine, is like that of cells in conventional delayed reactions. They produce a striking invasive–destructive lesion of bone and cartilage (Fig. 17.3), and there is a chronic proliferative response of bone (Fig. 17.2) or of other tissue elements close to the site of infiltration (Fig. 17.6). Passive transfer experiments have established the relation of the lesions to the cellular hypersensitivity mechanism (Fig. 17.8). The antigen appears to be an insoluble constituent of the injected bacteria, since passive lesions can be produced by intravenous transfer of sensitized lymphocytes mixed with very small amounts of bacillary material. It may be the lipopolysaccharide, wax D. The role of the vascular network (Fig. 17.9) in determining lesion localization may be to trap disseminated organisms, or, more probably, disseminated cells activated by antigen, as in systemic delayed reaction with soluble protein antigens. Lesion formation is greatly enhanced by local trauma or irritation. Adjuvant disease closely resembles Reiter's syndrome in man, with involvement of joints, spine, eye, skin, gastrointestinal tract, and the genitourinary system. Reiter's syndrome frequently follows urethral infections with mycoplasmas or the gonococcus and may well have a similar immunologic mechanism, elicited by antigens of these organisms. It also has morphologic features reminiscent of erythema nodosum, rheumatoid arthritis, arthritis with ulcerative colitis, and arthritis with psoriasis, but these may depend on other types of antigen, autoantigens for example, or in some instances may indeed be nonimmunologic.

The guinea pig lesion produced by adjuvant is *granulomatous* in character (Fig. 17.11). The infiltrating mononuclears become large pale histiocytes or reticular cells and may form epithelioid masses with occasional giant cells. On the other hand, the more acute features of adjuvant disease seen in the rat, notably "fibrinoid" and infiltration of polymorphonuclears, are lacking. These features of the lesion are thought to depend on insolubility or long persistence of the antigen and resemble what is seen in local and systemic graft-vs.-host lesions (Section 20), where there is a continuing supply of antigen. The proof of immunologic mechanism and the identification of the antigen are both incomplete in this case. The disease provides a possible model for the local *zirconium* and *beryllium granulomas* in man and for *chronic berylliosis*, a disseminated lesion affecting the lungs in particular (the allergen—beryllium oxide, phosphor, etc.—is inhaled and forms deposits remaining in the lungs for years). These processes are well correlated with delayed hypersensitivity elicited by intradermal or patch testing. The disease also provides a model for sarcoid-like lesions produced occasionally in human subjects by the tubercle bacillus, cryptococcus, histoplasma, etc. These cases may also involve sensitization to poorly catabolized constituents of the causative organisms. It is tempting to ascribe a similar mechanism to *Boeck's sarcoid*, but in this disease no antigen has been identified. Wegener's granulomatosis and similar diseases show both acute and chronic features reminiscent of several of the lesions described here.

One other experimental disease is illustrated, since it may well prove to have the same mechanism: the constellation of *cardiac and other lesions* appearing in rabbits after *repeated focal streptococcal infection* (Fig. 17.10). These lesions too are mononuclear cell infiltrates, accompanied by fibrinoid vascular necrosis and a destruction of myofibers. The muscle cells have a characteristic "owl-eyed" nucleus (the Anitschkow myocyte), and aggregates of regenerating, proliferating myocytes and multinucleated cells derived from them form bodies comparable to the *Aschoff bodies* of rheumatic fever which follows throat infections with hemolytic streptococci. The resemblance between animal and human disease parallels the resemblance between adjuvant disease and Reiter's syndrome, but in this case there is no evidence whatever regarding immunologic mechanism or identity of the antigen. One may say only that the lesion is most readily produced under circumstances that would be expected to lead to elicitation of cellular hypersensitivity lesions by cellular components of the streptococcus. It may, however, have an entirely different basis in the cross-reactivity between streptococcal and heart antigens (cf. Fig. 21.29) .

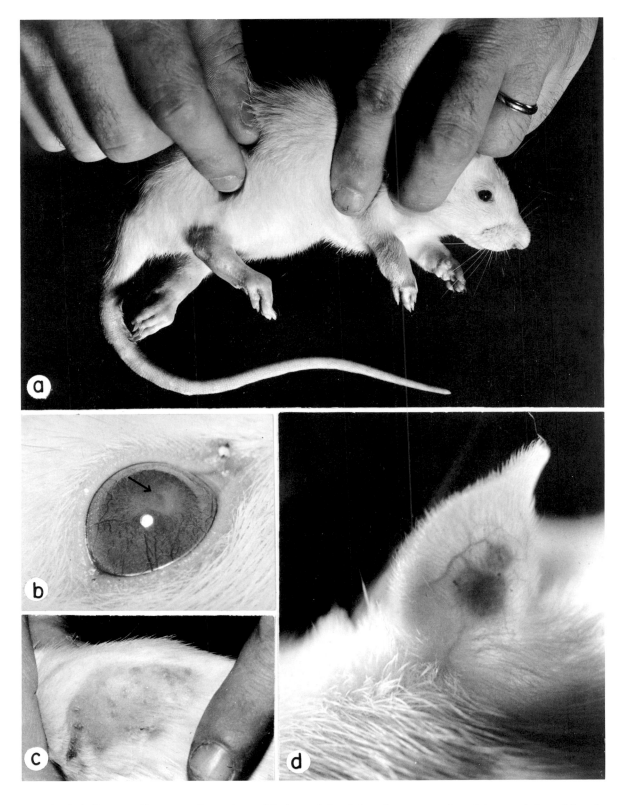

Fig. 17.1. Adjuvant disease, a disseminated lesion of the delayed type, produced in rats injected by the intradermal or footpad route, with mycobacteria or similar organisms in oil. (a) Rat with maximal disease of small joints in the extremities and tail, 20 days after injection of *Nocardia asteroides* in oil in one hind footpad. Note severe symmetrical involvement of wrists and ankles and metacarpophalangeal and metatarsophalangeal joints. (b) Right eye of rat receiving footpad injection of tubercle bacilli in oil. Moderate arthritis and severe iridocyclitis appeared at 9–10 days. Eye at 17 days shows dilated, tortuous iris vessels and a white fibrinous exudate, which partially fills the pupil (arrow). The ciliary body is seen as a light band behind the iris. (c) Papular rash at onset of arthritis, 15 days after *Nocardia* injection. Area was shaved 4 days earlier. (d) Ear nodules of 2 days' duration, one showing central ischemia, photographed 14 days after adjuvant injection.

(a) From Flax and Waksman, *Int. Arch. Allergy 23*: 331–47 (1963). (b) From Waksman and Bullington, *Arch. Ophthal. 64*: 751–62 (1960). (c, d) From Pearson, Waksman, and Sharp, *J. Exp. Med. 113*: 485–510 (1961).

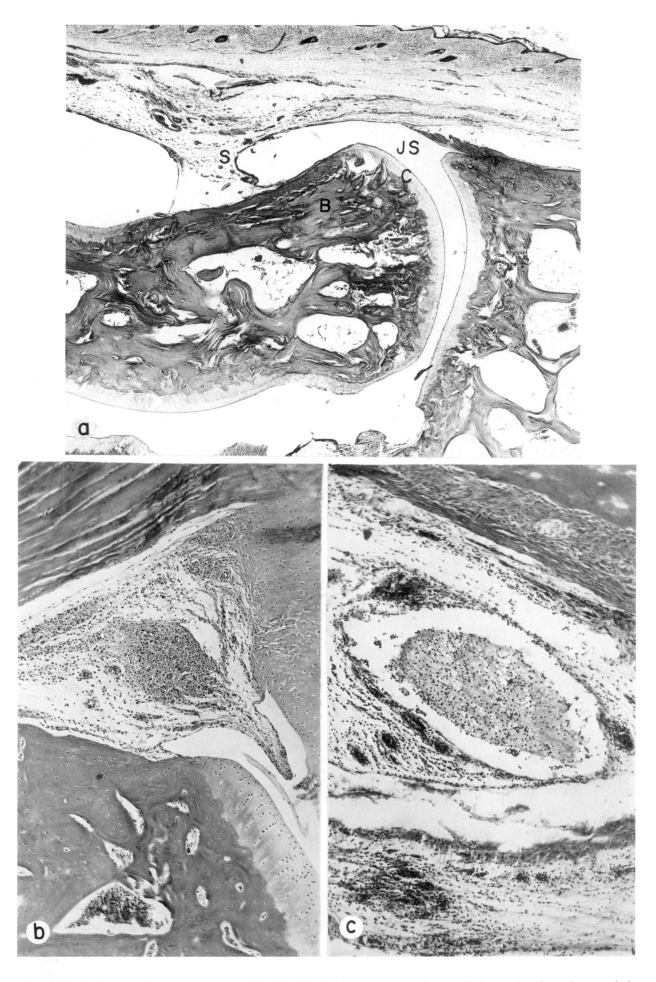

Fig. 17.2. Adjuvant disease in the rat. (a) Histological appearance of normal foot, showing characteristic bone (B), cartilage (C), joint space (JS), and synovia (S), with no sign of inflammation. Skin, above, shows thin epidermis and normal array of hair follicles; ×37. (b, c) Arthritis and tenosynovitis in rat sacrificed at onset of acute disease at 10 days; ×80. (b) Large perivascular infiltrate of mononuclear cells and polys in synovia of otherwise normal joint. (c) Several small perivascular infiltrates of the same type are seen in synovia of tendon sheath.

Hematoxylin-eosin. Waksman, unpublished photographs.

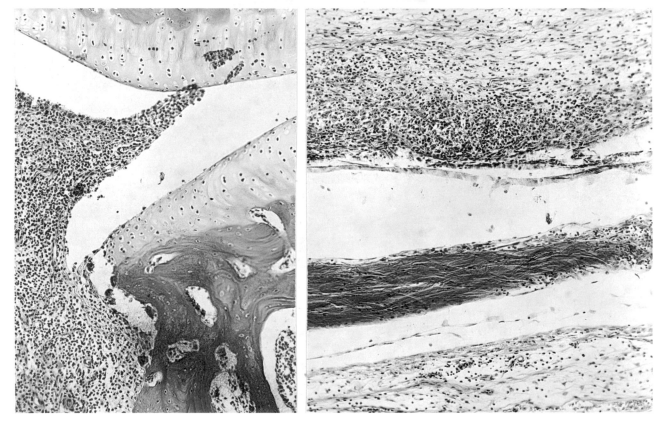

Fig. 17.3. Adjuvant disease in the rat. (Left) Arthritis of 3 day's duration; rat sacrificed at 13 days. Synovial and periosteal lesions, characterized by almost pure mononuclear cell infiltrates. Note appearance of osteoclasts and beginning erosion of bone. Cartilage and joint space are unaffected. (Right) Tenosynovitis at 19 days in rat with disease of 6 days' duration. Similar mononuclear infiltrates are present in the tendon sheath, and some inflammatory cells are seen on surface of tendon.

Hematoxylin-eosin; ×100. Waksman, unpublished photographs.

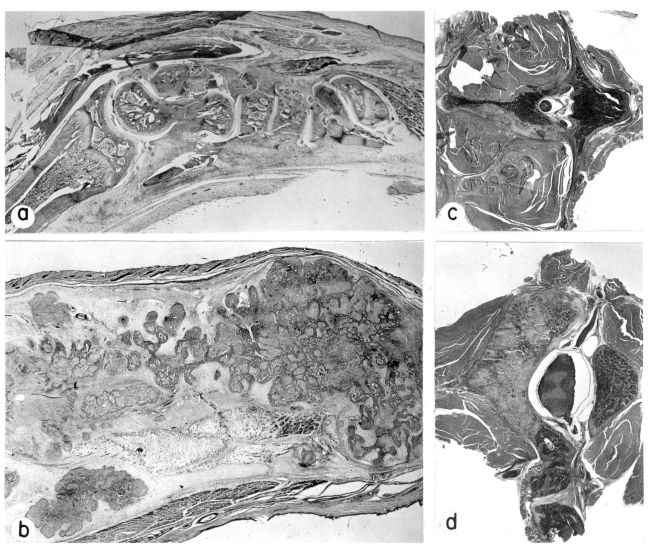

Fig. 17.4. Adjuvant disease in the rat. (a) Right ankle and foot with acute synovitis and tenosynovitis of 3 days' duration, in rat given tubercle bacilli in oil in left hind foot 13 days earlier. (b) Chronic damage in right hind foot of similar rat inoculated at 0 and 32 days and autopsied at 52 days. Normal architecture of foot is completely lost and there are extensive areas of fibrosis and new bone formation. (c, d) Same rat showing formation of granulomatous lesions with loss of normal bony structure in vertebral arches at different levels of spine (dorsal and cervical).

Hematoxylin-eosin; ×9. Waksman, unpublished photographs.

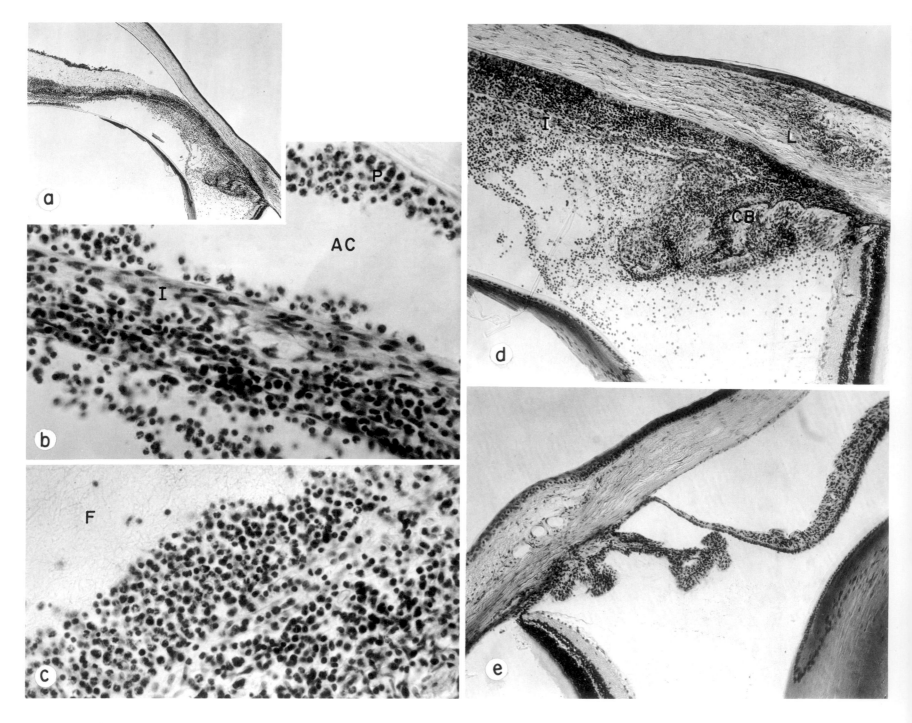

Fig. 17.5. Adjuvant disease in the rat. Acute iridocyclitis of less than 24 hours' duration in rat sacrificed 13 days after adjuvant injection. Eye disease in left eye (a–d) appeared 1 day after arthritis while right eye (e) remained entirely normal. (a) Left eye shows acute cellular inflammation affecting the ciliary body (CB) iris (I), and limbal area (L). The anterior chamber (AC) contains a mass of fibrin (F) and many cells, and there are cellular "precipitates" (P) on the posterior surface of the cornea and anterior suface of the lens; ×34. (b, c) the iris infiltrate is made up entirely of histiocytes, lymphocytes, and some plasma cells, while the cells in the anterior chamber and the keratitic precipitates are entirely polymorphonuclears. This separation of cell types is characteristic of delayed lesions involving serous spaces such as the joints or the eye; ×410. In (d, e) the affected and normal eyes are compared at intermediate power; ×115.

Hematoxylin-eosin. From Waksman and Bullington, *Arch. Ophthal. 64*: 751–62 (1960).

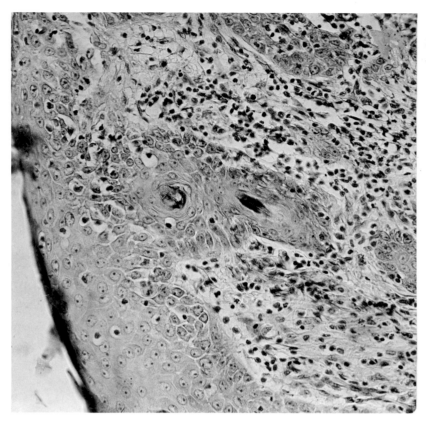
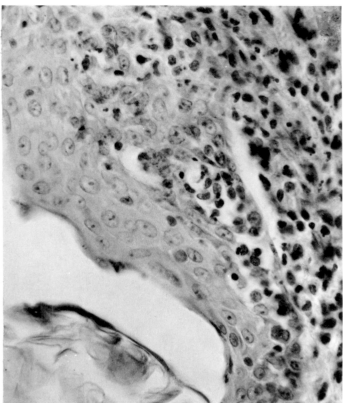

Fig. 17.6. Adjuvant disease in the rat. (Left) Neck skin from animal autopsied at 35 days. Note inflammatory infiltrate in upper dermis, acanthosis, spongiosis of basal layers of epidermis, and invasion of epidermis by mononuclear cells with beginning vesicle formation; ×250. (Right) Cheek skin of rat autopsied at 50 days. Onset of + + skin disease at 40 days. Formation of large multilocular vesicle and destruction of basal layer of epidermis by inflammatory infiltrate; ×450.

Hematoxylin-eosin. From Pearson, Waksman, and Sharp, *J. Exp. Med. 113*: 485–510 (1961).

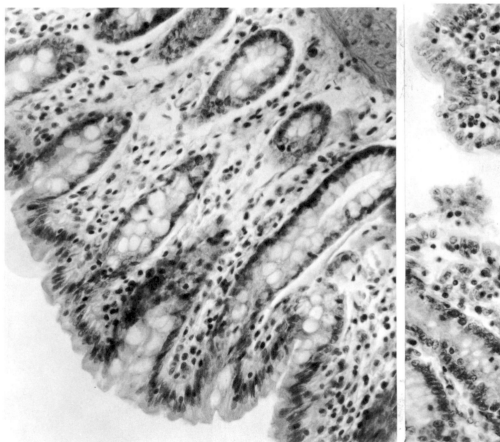
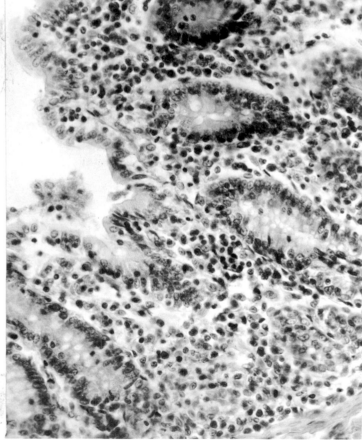

Fig. 17.7. Adjuvant disease in the rat. Descending colons of rats autopsied 33 (left) and 28 days (right) after adjuvant inoculation, showing normal appearance and moderate infiltration with mononuclear cells.

Hematoxylin-eosin; ×250. From Pearson, Waksman, and Sharp, *J. Exp. Med. 113*: 485–510 (1961).

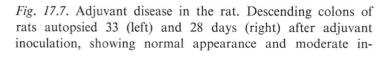

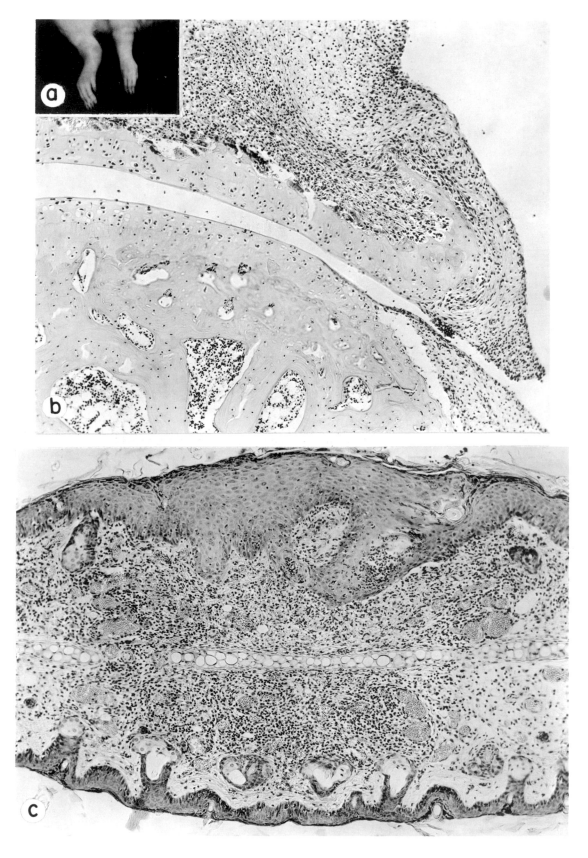

Fig. 17.8. Adjuvant disease in the rat. Passive transfer of arthritis in inbred (Lewis) rat by iv injection of 8.6×10^8 lymph node cells, taken at 10 days from nodes draining sites of footpad inoculation. Onset of disease in recipient 6 days after cell transfer. (a) Recipient's ankles 8 days after onset, showing + + + arthritis, bilaterally symmetrical. (b) Arthritis in joint biopsied at 22 days, showing preservation of cartilage, extensive destruction of bone, and early pannus formation. (c) Ear nodule from same rat 5 days after onset. Mononuclear infiltration, acanthosis of overlying epidermis, and microabscess formation.

(b, c) Hematoxylin-eosin; ×110. From Waksman and Wennersten, *Int. Arch. Allergy 23*: 129–39 (1963).

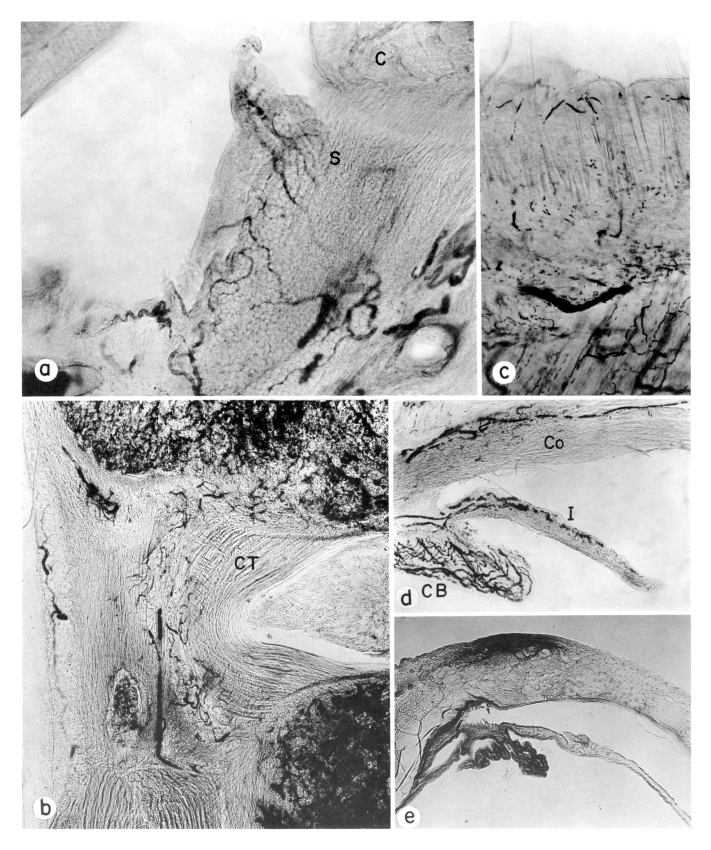

Fig. 17.9. Venous plexuses determining localization of lesions in adjuvant disease of the rat, a disseminated lesion of cellular sensitivity. (a) Synovia (S) of ankle joint. Some tortuous veins are seen, extending even into small synovial villus. Unvascularized joint cartilage (C) is above to right. (b) Tail joint, showing extensive venous plexus outside the joint capsule of dense connective tissue (CT). Large subdermal veins are seen at left. Dark areas above and below represent marrow. (c) Flank skin, showing large veins in subdermal connective tissue. (d) Extensive venous plexus in ciliary body (CB) and iris (I) of the rat eye. Large veins are also seen above in peripheral zone (limbus) of cornea (C) (e) Similar field showing eye of guinea pig, sacrificed 40 minutes after iv injection of Niagara sky blue 6B. Intense staining of limbus, base of iris, ciliary body, and choroid plexus corresponds to distribution of veins illustrated in (d).

(a–d) Frozen sections, 250 μ; Pickworth benzidine stain. (e) Carnoy's fixative; paraffin section, 32 μ. (a, c) ×79, (b, d, e) ×35. (d, e) From Waksman, *Am. J. Path. 37*: 673–93 (1960). Others unpublished.

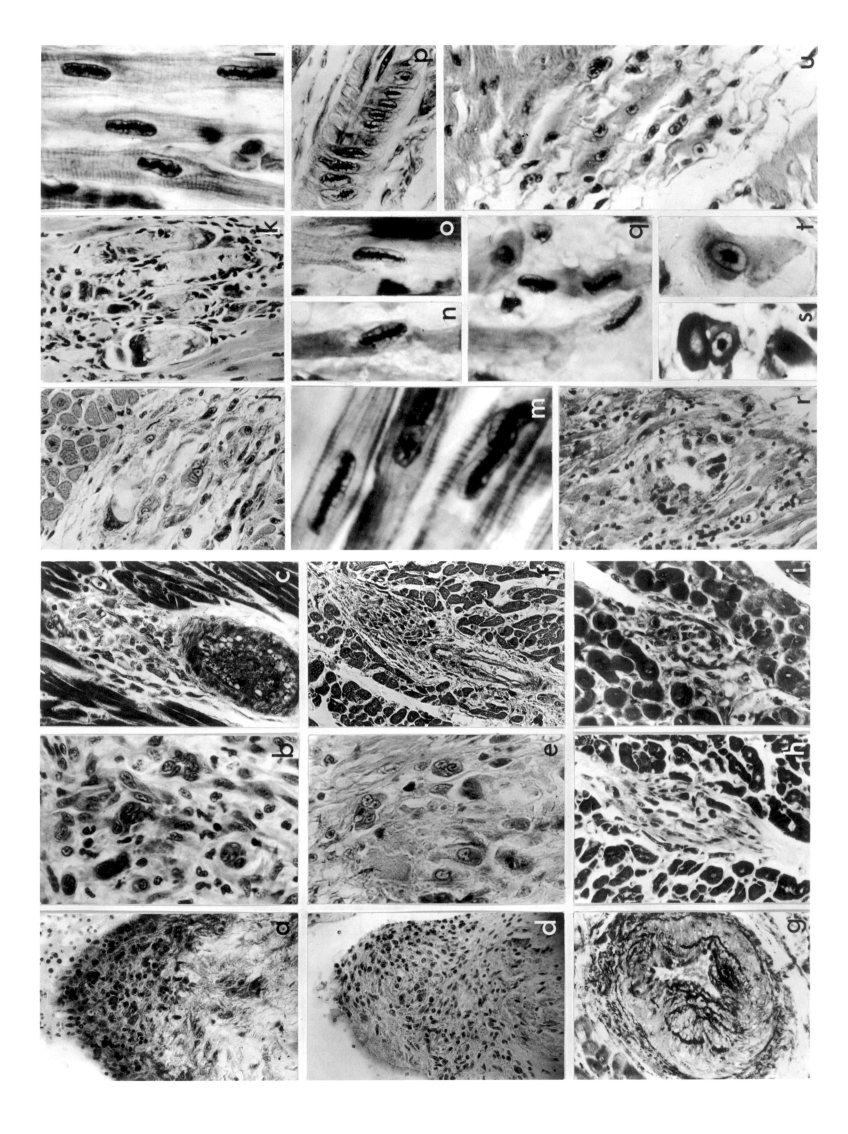

Fig. 17.10. Comparison of heart lesions in rabbits subjected to repeated focal infection with group A streptococci and in human subjects with rheumatic fever. While many features of both processes suggest an immunologic basis, this etiology has not been proven unequivocally, and the mechanism remains speculative. The histologic character of the lesions, mononuclear cell infiltration and damage of myofibers in zone of infiltration, is consistent with the cellular sensitivity mechanism. (a) Tip of trabecula carnea of a rabbit that died with irregular cardiac rhythm 8 days after the last of five focal infections with group A streptococci produced over a period of 9 months. Proliferation of endo- and subendo-cardial mono- and multinucleated cells. Note close resemblance to human rheumatic lesion in (d). Lesions in (b) and (p) are from the same rabbit heart. Giemsa; ×218. (b) Mitral valve ring of same rabbit heart. Mono- and multinucleated cells like those in human aortic valve ring shown in (e). Hematoxylin and eosin; ×443. (c) Interventricular septum of a rabbit that died 8 days after the last of eight focal infections with group A streptococci produced over a period of 14 months. Myocardial lesion adjacent to a myocardial artery. Note resemblance to the human Aschoff body adjacent to an artery shown in (f). Masson trichrome; ×220. (d) Tip of trabecula carnea of a 10-year-old boy who died 3 months after onset of first evident attack of rheumatic fever. Proliferation of endo- and subendo-cardial mono- and multinucleated cells. Lesions in (e) and (r) are from the same heart. Masson trichrome; ×194. (e) From aortic valve ring of same human heart. Mono- and multinucleated cells in mitral valve ring. Weigert–hematoxylin and eosin; ×443. (f) Left ventricular myocardium of a 7-year-old girl who died during an attack of acute rheumatic fever. Aschoff body adjacent to a myocardial artery. Hematoxylin-eosin; ×215. (g) Myo-cardial artery of a rabbit sacrificed 11 days after the last of eleven focal infections with group A streptococci. Laminated intimal musculo-elastic hyperplastic changes with splitting of internal elastica and narrowing of lumen. Weigert–hematoxylin and eosin; ×208. (h) Left ventricular myocardium of a 19-year-old man who died during the second recognized attack of rheumatic fever. Aschoff body apparently derived from heart muscle fibres sectioned obliquely or longitudinally. Masson trichrome; ×250. (i) Left ventricular myocardium of a rabbit sacrificed while very sick 10 days after the last of six focal infections with group A streptococci produced over a period of 16 months. Lesion appears to be derived from cardiac muscle fibers sectioned transversely. Note resemblance to the human Aschoff body in (h). Hematoxylin-eosin; ×316. (j) Left ventricular myocardium of a 14-year-old boy who died 3 months after onset of first recognized attack of rheumatic fever. Aschoff body, that has arisen from heart muscle fibers sectioned longitudinally. Lesion shown in (s) is from this heart. Giemsa; ×320. (k) Left ventricular myocardium of a rabbit sacrificed while very sick 12 days after onset of the second focal infection with group A streptococci. Although in an earlier stage, this lesion closely resembles the human Aschoff body in (j). Note the disintegrating muscle fibers and the basophilic, multinucleated masses—like the human one in upper left portion of (j)—occurring as caps at one pole of disintegrating muscle fibers. Giemsa; ×320. (l) Myocardium of a 3-year-old-boy who died 2 weeks after onset of the first known attack of rheumatic fever. Within heart muscle fibers are nuclei with caterpillar-like chromatin pattern characteristic of Anitschkow cells. Masson trichrome; ×124. (m) From the same myocardium. Caterpillar-like chromatin pattern in nuclei of heart muscle fibers. Masson trichrome; ×1,920. (n) Myocardium of a 10-year-old boy who died during a recurrent attack of rheumatic fever. Within a heart muscle fiber undergoing disintegration is a nucleus with caterpillar-like chromatin pattern. Cells in each are from the same myocardium. Hematoxylin-eosin; ×1,024. (o) Myocardium of a 14-month-old female infant who died 3 weeks after onset of a first attack of rheumatic fever. A nucleus with caterpillar-like chromatin pattern is escaping from a disintegrating heart muscle fiber. Hematoxylin-eosin; ×124. (p) Myocardial artery referred to in (a) and (b). Medial smooth muscle nuclei with caterpillar-like chromatin pattern. Masson trichrome; ×800. (q) Three caterpillar nuclei are shown. The one at the lower left and that in the upper center are emerging from fragmenting heart muscle fibers. The third caterpillar nucleus is within a heart muscle fiber fragment. Hematoxylin-eosin; ×1024. (r) From the 10-year-old boy referred to in (d) and (e) who died during an attack of rheumatic fever. Aschoff body, containing mono-, multi-, and non-nucleated heart muscle fiber fragments. Nuclei with caterpillar-like chromatin pattern or owl-eye appearance occur in some of these and in some of the adjacent muscle fragments. Weigert–hematoxylin and eosin; ×300. (s) From heart referred to in (j). Heart muscle nucleus with owl-eye appearance. Masson trichrome; ×800. (t) Myocardium of 25-year-old woman who died with active rheumatic disease. An obliquely sectioned heart muscle fragment contains a nucleus with owl-eye appearance. Hematoxylin-eosin; ×1,024. (u) Myocardium of a 3-year-old girl who died during a first attack of rheumatic fever. Aschoff body, comprising fragments of obliquely sectioned heart muscle fibers in several of which are nuclei with caterpillar-like chromatin pattern or owl-eye appearance. Hematoxylin and eosin; ×480.

(i) From Murphy and Swift, *J. Exp. Med. 89*: 687–98 (1949). (a, b, d, e, g) From Murphy and Swift, ibid., *91*: 485–98 (1950). (h, j, k) From Murphy, ibid., *95*: 319–32 (1952). (c, f) From Murphy, *Medicine 39*: 289–383 (1960). (p, s) From Murphy, ibid., *42*: 73–117 (1963). (l, o, q, r, t, u) From Murphy and Becker, *Am. J. Path. 48*: 931–57 (1966).

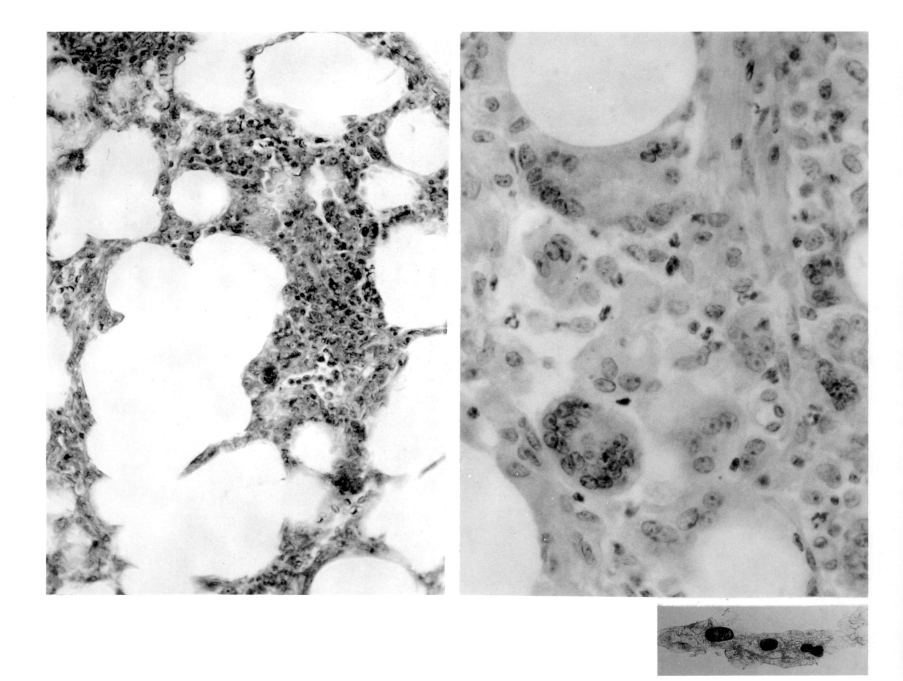

Fig. 17.11. Disseminated granulomatous lesions commonly observed in guinea pigs after intramuscular injection of killed mycobacteria in an oily vehicle. Apparently spontaneous lesions are observed at 2–5 weeks around joints and in highly vascular areas of the paragenital skin. Later, lesions appear at sites of skin injury produced by mechanical or chemical trauma (e.g. cantharidin) or reactions of specific hypersensitivity (as to picryl chloride or tuberculoprotein). In the latter instance, they appear during the repair process as nodules starting at the periphery of the healing lesion, as solid cords of tissue along draining lymphatics, and as distant nodular accumulations of cells. Genetic factors play a large role, as does sex, in determining the percentage of animals involved. (Left) Lung of guinea pig sacrificed 50 days after sensitization procedure and 15 days after cutaneous patch test (negative) with citraconic anhydride. Lesions were present in both paragenital and skin test areas at time of sacrifice. Lung shows giant cell formation and extensive granulomatous change reducing the respiratory surface. (Right) Skin nodule in guinea pig sensitized 3 months earlier and skin tested with citraconic anhydride (positive) 58 days before sacrifice. Additional skin tests were made at various times with picryl chloride, to which animal was not sensitive, and to PPD. Multiple nodular lesions appeared and grew around and between the skin test sites over the succeeding month. Lesion shown here is approximately 20 days old. In consists almost entirely of epithelioid macrophages and giant cells, formed by the fusion of these, in subcutaneous fat near a skin test site. The fat cells (clear spaces) are completely surrounded by the sheet of infiltrative cells. Insert shows a similar lesion from the inguinal area in another sensitized animal at low power. Subcutaneous fatty connective tissue with several lymph nodes and the extensive cellular infiltrates make up a bulky mass.

(Left) Acetic-Zenker fixation, Giemsa staining. (Right and insert) Bouin fixation, hematoxylin-eosin. Magnifications not given. Courtesy of Dr. M. W. Chase. See Chase in *Mechanisms of Hypersensitivity*. J. H. Shaffer, G. A. LoGrippo, and M. W. Chase, eds., Little, Brown, Boston, 1959, pp. 673–78.

18. Reactions of "Sensitized" Cells *in Vitro*

The actual events occurring in delayed reactions have been elucidated by recent *in vitro* studies. (1) *Sensitized lymphocytes* in lymph nodes (regional to the site of immunization) and the blood are able to *combine specifically with antigen* (Fig. 18.1). This finding has been established in a variety of immunologic systems involving soluble protein antigen, transplantation antigen, and autoantigen. (2) They then *undergo transformation to large basophilic, replicating cells* (Fig. 4.2). In tissue culture studies, the number of such transformed cells is usually less than 10 per cent of those surviving in culture over several days. (3) They *release* a substance, *migration inhibitory factor* (MIF), which has a number of effects on other cells in the close vicinity. It causes *macrophages* (or their monocyte precursors, such as are found in peritoneal exudates) to *become "sticky,"* as shown by their inability to migrate from a packed mass in a capillary tube (Figs. 18.3–6) and to undergo proliferation and rapid maturation to an *activated* form (Fig. 18.2). On both macrophages and fibroblasts, it may cause a *direct cytotoxic effect* resulting in cell death (Fig. 18.7). This cytotoxic effect itself appears to be the extreme result of activation (Fig. 18.7). MIF may damage epithelial cells without killing them, and its effect on endothelium remains unknown. The reacting sensitized lymphocytes may release other substances, among them "transfer factor," cytophilic antibody, a chemotactic factor distinct from MIF, a mitogenic factor, and interferon. (4) When antigen is a component of the target cells themselves, as in homograft immunity, tumor immunity, and the autoallergies, there is "contactual agglutination" of sensitized lymphocytes with the target cells and subsequent damage or killing (Figs. 18.8–11), apparently involving the same mechanism. (5) Activated *macrophages* themselves *exert a cytotoxic effect* on various target cells nonspecifically. The reaction of sensitized lymphocytes with antigen, by triggering activation of macrophages, confers on them the ability to damage or destroy other cells with which they come in contact, and this effect may be enhanced by the presence of cytophilic antibody which brings macrophages into intimate contact with target cells (Figs. 10.4; 18.4). (6) Lymphocytes, even cells of the uncommitted peripheral lymphocyte pool, may enter and move about within target cells such as thyroid follicle epithelium or synoviocytes, "emperipolesis" (Figs. 18.12,13). This phenomenon is not known to be related to the specific events described above. (7) Sensitized lymphocytes exposed to soluble antigen may be damaged ("lympholysis") (Fig. 10.16). This appears to be a case of complement-mediated immune lysis and unrelated to the problem of delayed hypersensitivity. (8) RNA extracted from sensitized lymphocytes can convert normal lymphocytes to the specifically sensitized form.

These findings appear to explain events *in vivo* satisfactorily, since it is probable that the sensitized lymphocytes which give reactions (1, 2, 3) above correspond to the circulating mediators of delayed or cellular hypersensitivity, and the macrophages which have been used to elucidate reactions (3) and (5) were obtained from peritoneal exudates and are thus similar in origin to the nonspecific cells found in delayed reactions. The trigger event *in vivo*, elicited by the presence of antigen, corresponds to reactions (1, 2, 3). It results in the local accumulation of sticky, activated macrophages, which pass through the vessel wall and produce damage or destruction of susceptible parenchymal elements in their immediate vicinity (5). Reactions (3, 4) may contribute to this parenchymal damage. In a reaction of sufficient intensity, there may be endothelial damage as well, with leakage of serum proteins, attraction of polys, and secondary changes resembling those occurring in Arthus reactions (basement membrane damage, hemorrhage) (Figs. 12.5–7). The contribution of reactions (6, 7, 8) to *in vivo* events remains problematical.

The blast transformation of lymphocytes resulting from their reaction with specific antigen and their cytotoxic effect on target cells to which they adhere are mimicked by the effect on uncommitted lymphocytes of such materials as phytohemagglutinin, staphylococcal toxin, and streptolysin S (Fig. 4.2); these may act on the lymphocyte surface or initiate a discharge of hydrolases from lysosomes within the cell. The damage of target cells, *allogeneic inhibition*, by these transformed lymphocytes may require the existence of a genetic difference between the participating cells. *Cellular immunity* against bacteria such as the brucella organism and the tubercle bacillus, manifested by suppression of intracellular multiplication of virulent organisms in macrophages of specifically "sensitized" hosts (Fig..18.15), has not as yet been shown to involve a two-cell mechanism. It may in time prove to be similar to the phenomena described above, involving macrophage activation secondary to antigen–lymphocyte interaction. The activated macrophages also produce interferon, which is responsible for cellular immunity against viruses, and an endogenous pyrogen, which is responsible for the fever of systemic delayed reactions.

Further experimental details concerned more directly with the homograft reaction, GVH lesions, and the experimental autoallergies are given in subsequent sections.

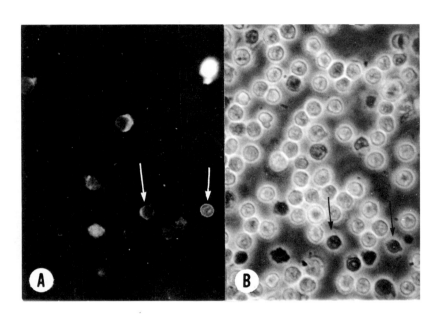

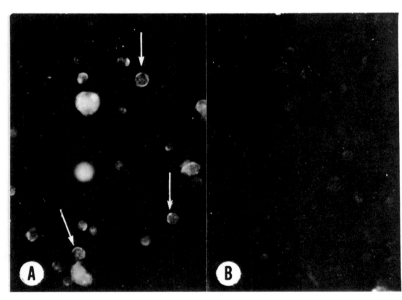

Fig. 18.1. Specific uptake of antigen by sensitized lymphocytes in cellular sensitivity. Cells from lymph nodes draining inoculation site in guinea pigs developing autoallergic encephalomyelitis after intradermal injection of neural antigen (100 μg KCl extract of bovine white matter) plus adjuvant. Cells have been allowed to react with encephalitogenic protein, followed by fluorescein-labeled rabbit antiserum against the same antigen. Upper figure: (A) Cell suspension viewed with fluorescence microscope. Arrows indicate specific antigen uptake as a "halo" effect on certain cells. (B) Phase contrast view of same field. Arrows point to cells marked in (A). Of the total cells in lymph node 5–10 per cent react in this manner, mostly small lymphocytes and occasional medium lymphocytes. Lower figure: (A) Similar preparation contrasted with control preparation (B) in which normal lymph node cells were exposed to antigen and fluorescent antiserum.

From Rauch and Raffel, *J. Immunol. 93*: 960–64 (1964).

Fig. 18.2. Stimulation of macrophage maturation by tuberculoprotein in cultures of peritoneal exudate cells from tuberculin-sensitized guinea pigs. All cells are from exudates harvested 5 days after ip injection of sodium caseinate. (a, b) Living mononuclear cells, vitally stained with neutral red, show either a small rosette of stained phagocytic vacuoles ("monocyte" pattern) or multiple vacuoles varying in size and distribution (typical macrophage). Single unstained cell is a small lymphocyte. An erythrocyte is shown to permit comparison of size. (c, d) Similar exudate, fixed and stained with May-Grünwald–Giemsa, shows two mononuclears and a larger serosal cell. Note horseshoe-shaped nucleus and basophilia (and shrinkage due to fixation). (e, f) Similar cells from sensitive donor, exposed in culture for 18 hours to control medium containing glycerol, show little or no morphologic change. (g–i) Sensitive cells, cultured with OT 1:300 for 48 hours, show marked increase in cytoplasm and loss of basophilia. These are typical macrophages. Little further change occurs with longer culture. (j, k) Sensitive cells, with OT 1:75, 48 hours. Same. (l) Sensitive cell, cultured with PPD 67 μg/ml, 48 hours. Same. (j, k, l) Stained with Wright's stain.

All ×1,100. From Waksman and Matoltsy, *J. Immunol 81*: 220–34 (1958).

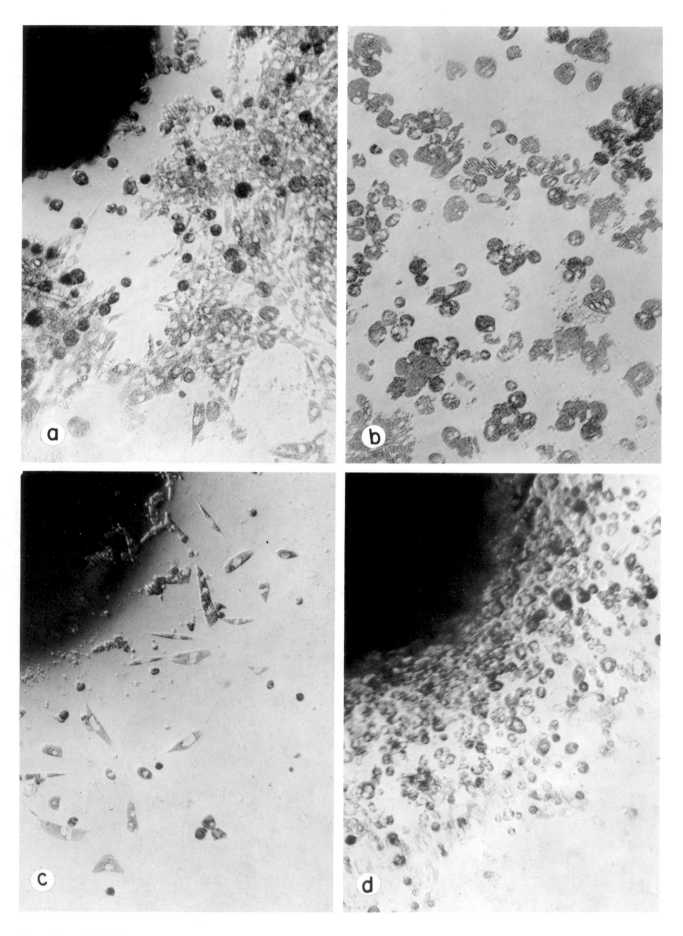

Fig. 18.3. Inhibition of macrophage migration (Rich phenomenon) by tuberculoprotein in cultures of spleen from tuberculin-sensitized guinea pigs. Photographs show 2-mm spleen fragments and living cells, photographed after 3 days of culture in plasma clot (medium 40 per cent horse serum and 7.5 per cent chick embryo extract). (a, b) Normal spleen, with and without added old tuberculin 1:144. (c, d) Sensitized spleen, with and without OT. Migration of sensitive macrophages is completely inhibited in presence of specific antigen. In other cultures, macrophages show granulation typical of old cultures but are otherwise healthy. Fibroblast migration appears greater in presence of tuberculin, from both sensitive and control spleens.

× 400. Waksman, unpublished.

Inhibition of macrophage migration in capillary tube cultures as a measure of cellular (delayed) hypersensitivity. All photographs are of living cultures of peritoneal exudate cells, after 24 hours in presence or absence of specific antigen.

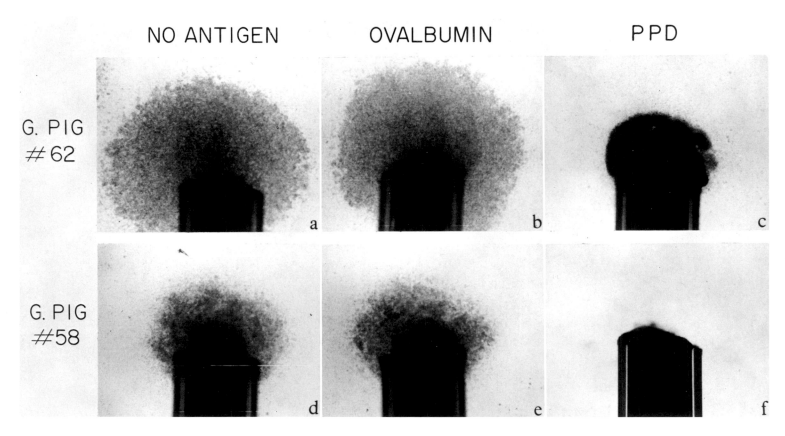

NO ANTIGEN   OVALBUMIN   PPD

G. PIG #62

G. PIG #58

a   b   c

d   e   f

Fig. 18.4. Reactions in cultures of cells from two guinea pigs with strong delayed sensitivity to tuberculin, actively engaged in producing antibody against ovalbumin but having no delayed sensitivity to this antigen (after intravenous and intramuscular injection of ovalbumin). Macrophage migration is inhibited by PPD but not by ovalbumin.

From David, Al-Askari, Lawrence, and Thomas, *J. Immunol. 93*: 264–73 (1964).

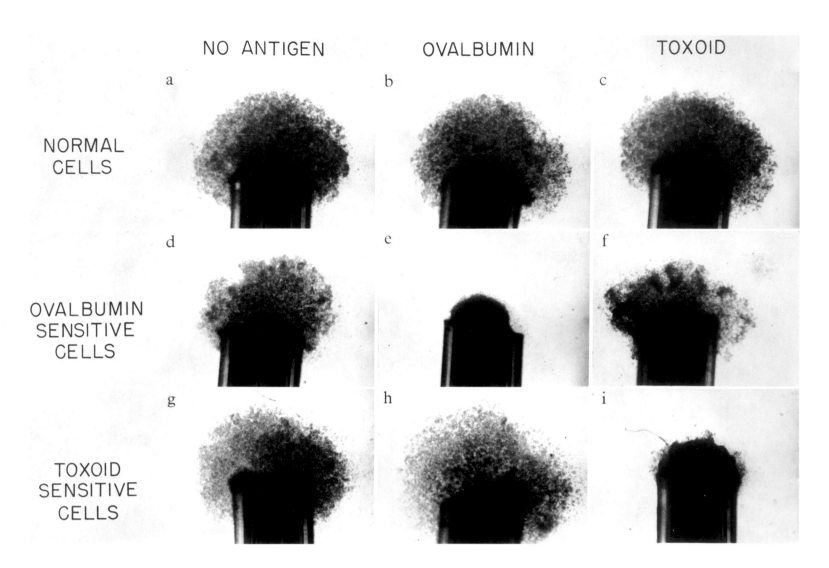

NO ANTIGEN   OVALBUMIN   TOXOID

NORMAL CELLS

OVALBUMIN SENSITIVE CELLS

TOXOID SENSITIVE CELLS

Fig. 18.5. Specificity of reactions in cultures of cells from normal guinea pigs and guinea pigs exhibiting delayed hypersensitivity to ovalbumin and diptheria toxoid respectively. In each case, only the specific antigen inhibits macrophage migration

From David, Al-Askari, Lawrence, and Thomas, *J. Immunol. 93*: 264–73 (1964).

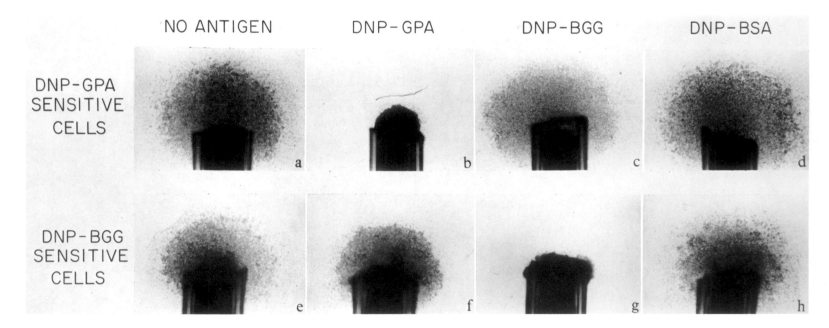

NO ANTIGEN   DNP-GPA   DNP-BGG   DNP-BSA

DNP-GPA SENSITIVE CELLS

DNP-BGG SENSITIVE CELLS

Fig. 18.6. Demonstration that reaction of macrophage inhibition shows antigen specificity comparable to that observed in studies of delayed skin reactivity. Reaction is not elicited by conjugates prepared with the specific hapten (dinitrophenyl) unless conjugate also contains the same carrier protein used in sensitization. Thus reaction shows both hapten and carrier specificity.

From David, Lawrence, and Thomas, *J. Immunol. 93*: 279–82 (1964).

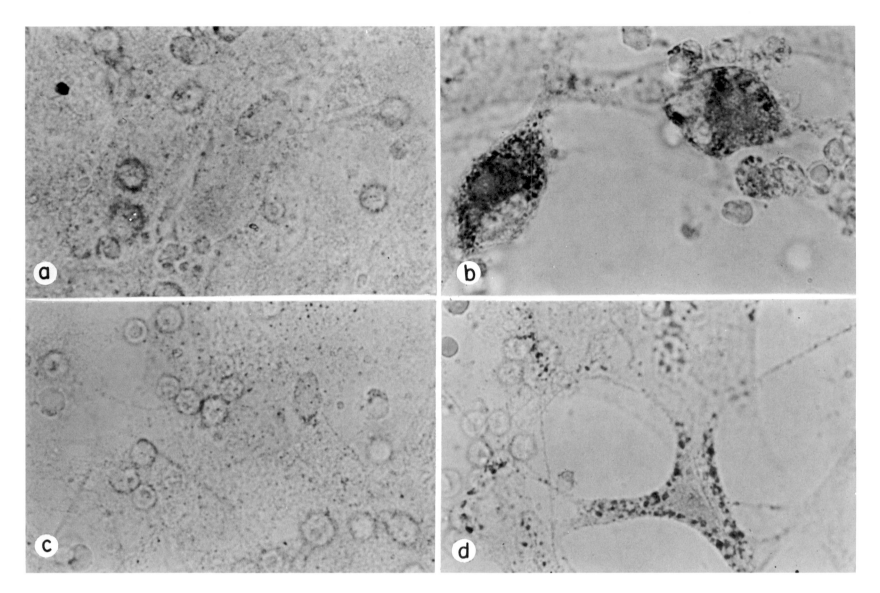

Fig. 18.7. Effect of interaction of tuberculin-sensitized lymphocytes with specific antigen (tuberculoprotein) on "innocent bystander" cells. Cultures of lymph node cells from normal (a, b) and sensitized (c, d) Lewis rats on monolayers of Lewis embryo fibroblasts in the presence of PPD, 12.5 μg/ml, after 48 (a, c) and 72 (b, d) hours. Acid phosphatase stain indicates amount of lysosomal enzyme in the cells and provides some measure of their degree of activation. Little or no enzyme appears in either lymphocytes or fibroblasts in culture of un-sensitized cells. Sensitized lymphocytes show limited amount of enzyme at 48 hours. However, the target fibroblasts in the sensitized cultures are full of enzyme at this time and dead by 72 hours. Early activation corresponds to activation of macrophages seen morphologically (Fig. 18.2) and to stickiness and inhibition of macrophage migration from capillary tube cultures (Figs. 18.4–6).

Courtesy of Dr. N. Ruddle.

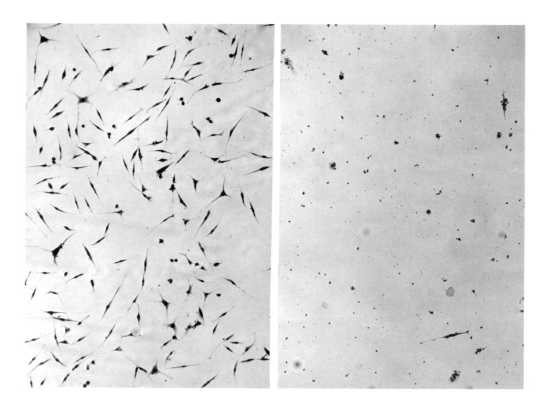

Fig. 18.8. Cytotoxic effect of sensitized mononuclear cells on specific target cells. Effect of BALB/c mouse lymphocytes from sensitized and unsensitized donors on antigenic mouse L cells serving as target. (Left) Nonsensitized lymphocytes, 48 hours. (Right) Sensitized lymphocytes, 48 hours. Marked destruction of the L cells is apparent.
× 68. From Rosenau and Moon, *J. Nat. Cancer Inst. 27*: 471–86 (1961).

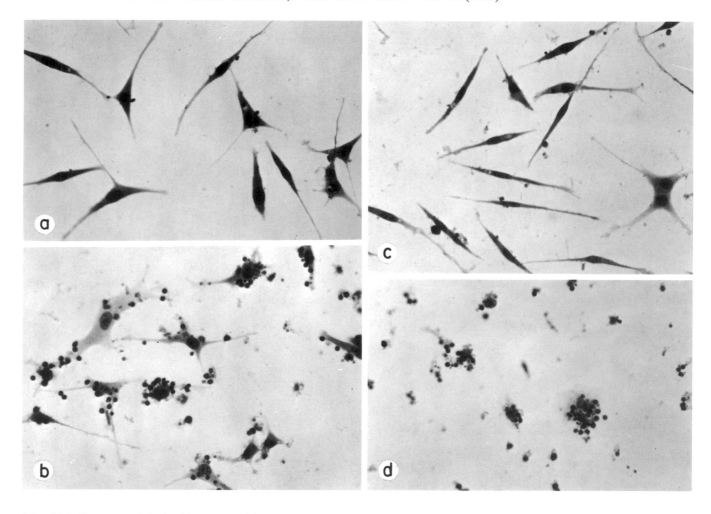

Fig. 18.9. Same as 18.8. (a, b) Nonsensitized and sensitized lymphocytes, 18 hours. The latter show marked clustering ("contactual agglutination"), and early cytotoxic changes are seen in the L cells. The normal lymphocytes do not show clustering and produce no damage in the target cells. (c, d) Similar preparations at 48 hours. There is still no change in the culture containing nonsensitized lymphocytes. In the culture with sensitized lymphocytes, there is lysis of almost all the L cells and only remnants remain.
All × 255. From Rosenau and Moon, *J. Nat. Cancer Inst. 27*: 471–86 (1961).

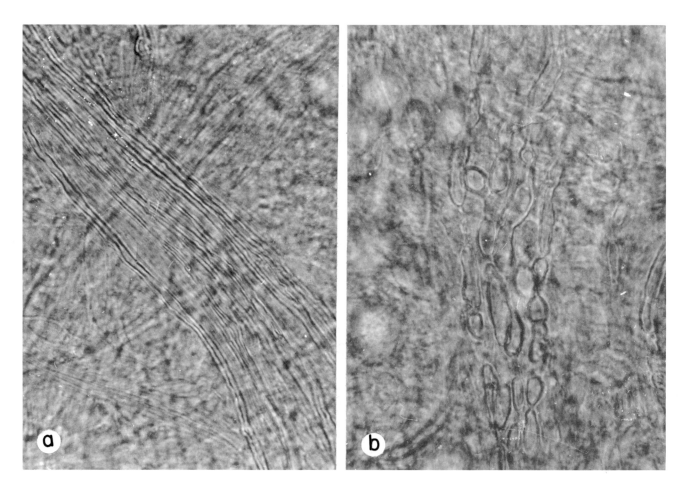

Fig. 18.10. Cytotoxic effect of sensitized mononuclear cells on specific target cells. (a) Living culture of fetal rat trigeminal ganglion, maintained over several weeks and containing fully myelinated peripheral nerve fibers. (b) Similar culture to which lymph node cells, taken from rats 10 days after footpad inoculation of rabbit sciatic nerve plus Freund adjuvant, were added 48 hours earlier. The myelin has broken into irregular ovoid masses of varying size and in some areas is no longer recognizable. No myelin change is seen in cultures containing lymph node cells from rats given adjuvant alone.

Phase contrast; ×640. See Winkler, *Ann. N.Y. Acad. Sci. 122*: 287–96 (1965).

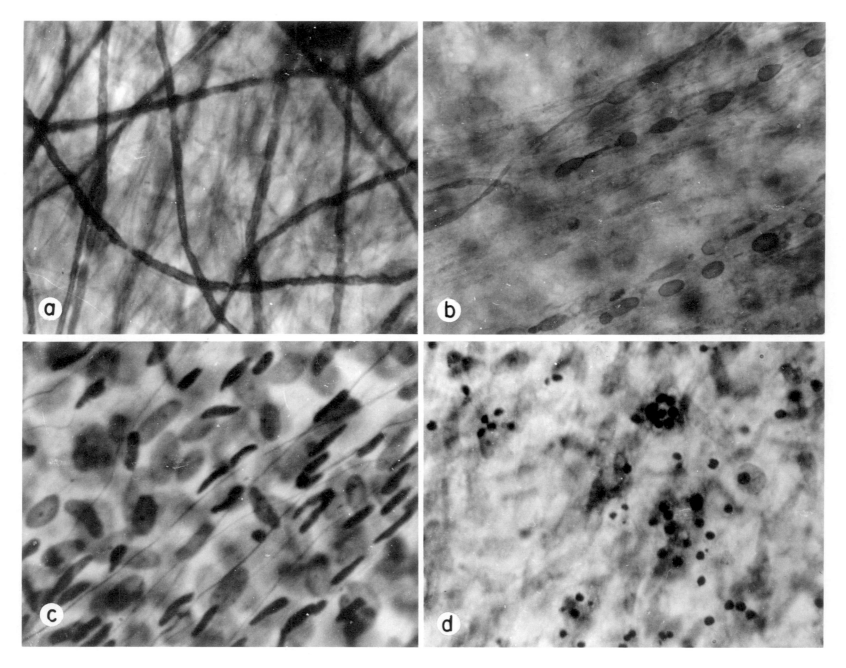

Fig. 18.11. Same as 18.10 (a, b) Preparations comparable to 18.10 (a, b), stained for myelin (Sudan black B). Myelin destruction by sensitized lymphocytes at 48 hours is striking. (c, d) Preparations similar to (b) stained for axis cylinders (Bodian) and cells (May-Grünwald–Giemsa) respectively. Clusters of lymphocytes are seen adherent to underlying cultured tissue elements.

×680. See Winkler, *Ann. N.Y. Acad. Sci. 122*: 287–96 (1965).

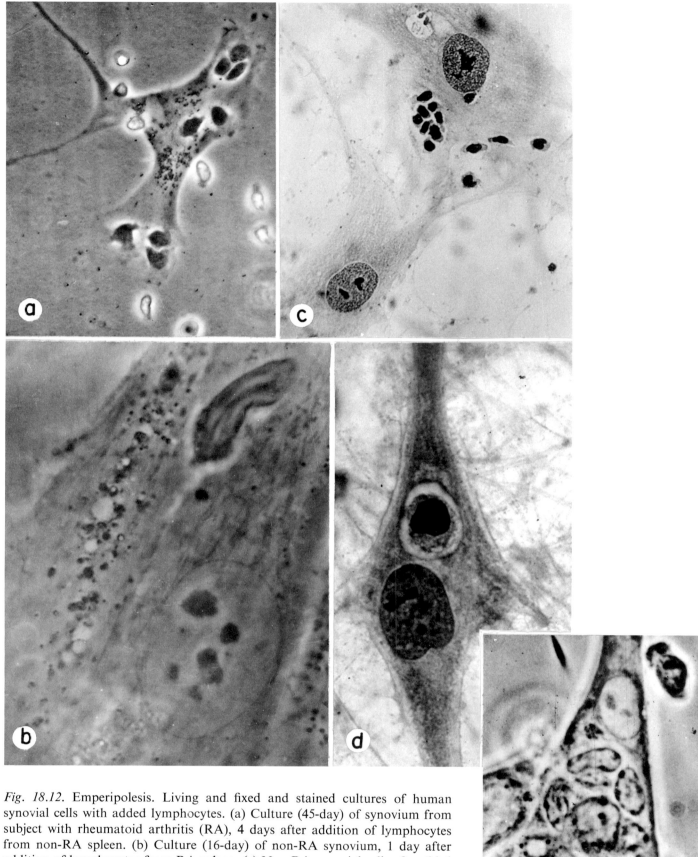

Fig. 18.12. Emperipolesis. Living and fixed and stained cultures of human synovial cells with added lymphocytes. (a) Culture (45-day) of synovium from subject with rheumatoid arthritis (RA), 4 days after addition of lymphocytes from non-RA spleen. (b) Culture (16-day) of non-RA synovium, 1 day after addition of lymphocytes from RA spleen. (c) Non-RA synovial cells after third transfer in culture, 4 days after "challenge" with non-RA buffy coat lymphocytes. (d) Non-RA cells transferred once, 4 days after addition of RA buffy coat lymphocytes. All show intracellular lymphocytes of entirely normal appearance.

Insert shows emperipolesis in living culture of thyroid affected by Hashimoto's disease (chronic thyroiditis). Lymphocytes are those present in the diseased gland itself. Phase microcinematography.

(a, b) Phase contrast; ×578, ×1,022. (c, d) Jacobson's stain; ×460, ×1,230.

(a–d) From Stanfield, Stephens, and Henthorn, *Tex. Rep. Biol. Med. 23*: 110–21 (1965). See also *Current Concepts in Rheumatoid Arthritis*, C.A.L. Stephens, Jr., and A. B. Stanfield, eds., Thomas, Springfield, pp. 155–77. Insert, courtesy of Dr. I. Roitt.

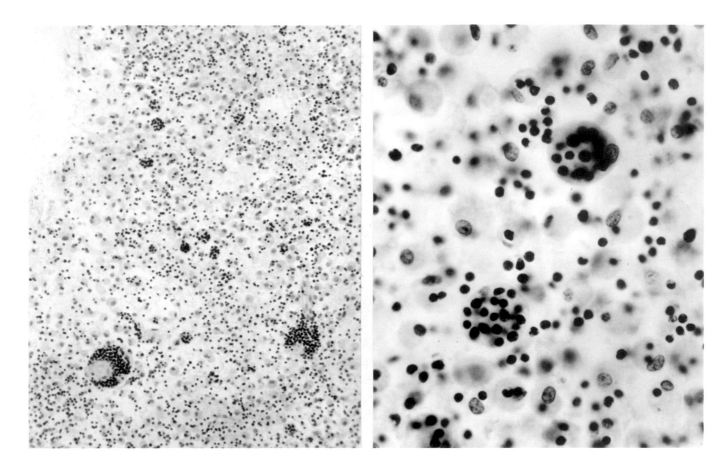

Fig. 18.13. Emperipolesis (?) *in vivo*. Uptake of intact lymphocytes by macrophages in brain lesions of familial encephalitis of unknown origin. Lesions consist of rapidly progressive and total destruction of white matter, with some accompanying gray matter damage, a tremendous outpouring of lymphocytes and larger mononuclears. The unusual phenomenon illustrated here was interpreted as ingestion of the lymphocytes by the macrophages, but it may represent an event comparable to emperipolesis.

Hematoxylin-eosin; (left) ×160, (right) ×650. Courtesy of Dr. E. P. Richardson.

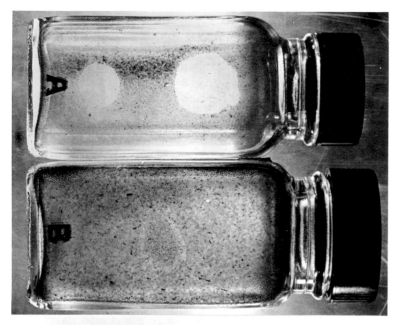

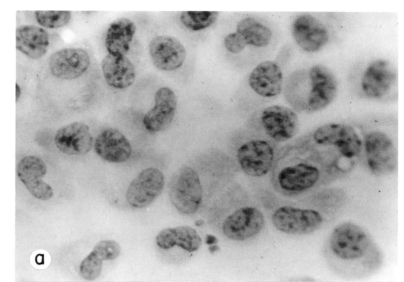

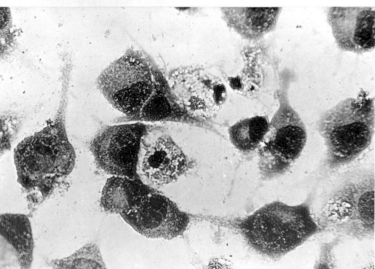

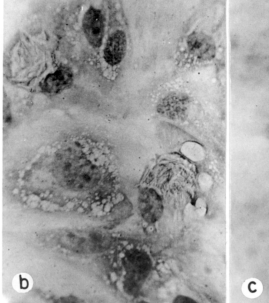

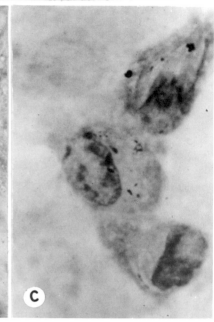

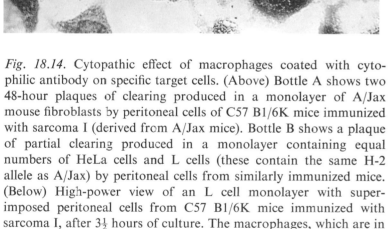

Fig. 18.14. Cytopathic effect of macrophages coated with cytophilic antibody on specific target cells. (Above) Bottle A shows two 48-hour plaques of clearing produced in a monolayer of A/Jax mouse fibroblasts by peritoneal cells of C57 Bl/6K mice immunized with sarcoma I (derived from A/Jax mice). Bottle B shows a plaque of partial clearing produced in a monolayer containing equal numbers of HeLa cells and L cells (these contain the same H-2 allele as A/Jax) by peritoneal cells from similarly immunized mice. (Below) High-power view of an L cell monolayer with superimposed peritoneal cells from C57 Bl/6K mice immunized with sarcoma I, after 3½ hours of culture. The macrophages, which are in intimate contact with the target L cells, are easily identified by numerous intracytoplasmic lipid droplets.

Stain and magnification not given. From Granger and Weiser, *Science 145*: 1427–29 (1964).

Fig. 18.15. Cellular immunity to tuberculosis. Guinea pig macrophages (5-day peritoneal exudate, elicited with glycogen), cultured in Hanks' solution and 20 per cent normal guinea pig serum and infected with tubercle bacilli in presence of streptomycin, 5 μg/ml. (a) Normal cells and BCG organisms (attenuated), 1 day after infection. A few cells contain acid-fast bacilli. (b) Same, 7 days after infection. Several cells are filled with stainable mycobacteria and there is cellular vacuolization. (c) Cells from immunized guinea pig, infected with H37Rv (virulent) organisms, 7 days. Only single organisms are seen. There is some loss of cells. Suppression of intracellular bacterial replication is due to activation of macrophages as part of usual *in vitro* delayed response.

Ziehl-Neelsen stain, modified with Tween-80, plus Giemsa. Courtesy of Dr. E. Suter

19. Homograft Rejection

Tissue or organ grafts are known as *autografts* when transplanted from one site to another of the same individual, *isografts* (isogenic or syngeneic grafts) when transplanted between genetically identical individuals, *homografts* or *allografts* (allogeneic grafts) between genetically different members of the same species, and *heterografts* or *xenografts* between members of different species. Grafted tissues such as cornea, cartilage, bone, fascia, nerve or, vessel, which provide a dead scaffolding for the host's own cells, survive indefinitely. Cellular tissues such as skin, kidney, heart, marrow, etc., heal well into place after grafting and then follow one of two courses. Autografts and syngeneic grafts survive indefinitely. Allografts and xenografts in intact adult hosts are rejected after a well-defined time interval. In the case of a *first-set graft* this interval is determined by the degree of genetic difference between donor and host, as represented by the number of antigens involved and the "strength" of those antigens, and by the dose of grafted tissue; it is usually about 10 days, when strong antigenic differences are involved (Fig. 19.1). In the case of a second graft from the same donor (or donor strain), a *second-set graft*, the interval is appreciably shortened and may be 4 or 5 days or even less. The exact figure given for the time of rejection varies with the parameter used to measure the rejection process—lymphocytic infiltration, vascular breakdown, or death of a parenchymal element such as epidermis (Figs. 19.4–9). The shortening of second-set rejection time is specific for the donor animal (or strain) and applies to all cells coming from that donor; a first-set graft of skin causes accelerated rejection of a later graft of kidney. A later graft from an unrelated donor is treated as a first-set graft.

Transplantation or *histocompatibility antigens* are genetically controlled, and some have been identified as specific lipoproteins of the cell membranes. In mice there appear to be more than 15 genetic loci controlling histocompatibility; and 15–20 different alleles, each determining a complex of several distinct antigenic factors, may be expressed at each. Yet only one locus, designated H-2, controls the expression of *strong* histocompatibility antigens. There is convincing evidence that the picture is closely similar in chickens, rats, and human subjects. In each there appears to be a single strong histocompatibility locus controlling some 15 alleles. A locus on the Y chromosome of the male determines a weak homograft antigen lacking in the female.

The immunologic basis of graft rejection may be of several types. *Cells* growing *in free suspension*, such as ascites tumor cells, are *destroyed by immune lysis* with specific antibody and complement. Marrow and lymphocyte grafts (and transplanted lymphomas) are also destroyed by antibody if the latter is passively administered within a short period before or after grafting; otherwise the cellular mechanism is operative and rejection resembles that described below for solid-tissue grafts. Even epidermal cells, if incubated with antibody and complement before grafting, are destroyed, though they become inaccessible to antibody shortly after being placed on the graft bed in the recipient (Fig. 19.1). Transfused erythrocytes, leukocytes, and platelets, if one regards the transfused cells as grafts, are "rejected" by humoral antibody. In animals with a high titer of circulating humoral antibody against the specific donor's cells (actively induced or transferred passively from animals sensitized by a powerful method such as the use of Freund's adjuvant), a skin graft may fail to take because of *antibody-mediated damage of vascular endothelium*, particularly at the site of vascular anastomosis in the base of the graft. This mechanism is of major importance *in rejection of xenografts* and may play a role in some cases of "white graft" rejection of allografts (Fig. 19.3). It rarely happens when the recipient of an allograft has been immunized only by previous grafts from the same donor.

The usual *rejection of solid, vascularized tissue allografts is* an immunologic *reaction of the cellular type*, comparable in its basic features to other delayed or cellular reactions (discussed in Sections 16, 18). Effective modes of immunization, by grafting with living cells or injection of killed tissue with adjuvant, are effective means of inducing delayed sensitization, and tests with graft antigens elicit typical delayed skin reactions in immunized animals. Immunity can be passively transferred only with living lymphoid cells. Grafts placed intraperitoneally in chambers, made of Millipore filters with pores large enough to permit the passage of antibody but too small to admit cells, survive indefinitely, even in immune animals. Finally, lymphoid cells from immune animals produce cytopathic changes in target cells of donor type in tissue culture (Figs. 18.8,9), an effect comparable to effects *in vitro* seen with other types of cellular sensitization.

The morphologic features of the rejection process also are those of cellular or delayed hypersensitivity (Figs. 19.4–9). *Vascular and perivascular infiltration of mononuclear cells* is the first change (Fig. 19.6). An *invasive–destructive lesion* is produced by the infiltrating cells in the walls of arteries and veins of the graft (Fig. 19.6) and in other parenchymal elements of the graft such as the surface and follicle epithelium (Figs. 19.6–8). The *destruction of vessels* proceeds rapidly and leads to an arrest of circulation within the graft, secondary ischemic death of its connective tissue and especially of its epidermal and vascular components, and hemorrhage (Figs. 19.7,9). The ischemia is enhanced by formation of obstructive *intravascular masses of reacting mononuclear cells* (Fig. 19.8). The relative importance of direct invasive-destruction of graft parenchyma and ischemic necrosis of the graft as a whole depends on the extent of vascularization, which is of greater importance in poorly vascularized tissues such as the flank skin of the rat. The rejection process in other organs resembles that in skin in most details. In a highly vascular organ such as the kidney, vascular damage by antibody may occur, depending on the circumstances of immunization. In general the cellular rejection mechanism is predominant here as well (Figs. 19.10–12).

The first step in immunization by a skin allograft, which is also the first step in the rejection process, has been shown by indirect experiments to occur within the graft itself. It is well seen in morphologic studies of kidney grafts. Small lymphocytes enter the graft from the blood stream within one to two days after grafting and are rapidly transformed into large basophilic (pyroninophilic) cells. This change corresponds to blast transformation in the mixed lymphocyte reaction *in vitro* (Fig. 4.2), which has been shown unequivocally to represent a primary immune response, and to the similar early appearance of large pyroninophilic cells in the cortex of lymph nodes regional to an implanted skin graft and in the splenic white pulp and lymph node cortex in systemic graft-vs.-host lesions (Section 20). It is not clear how many of the specific lymphocytes, that participate in homograft rejection are derived from these blast-like cells responding to immunization at the site and how many come via the blood stream from similar responding cells in the draining lymph nodes. The delay in skin allograft rejection when the regional nodes are removed suggests that the latter may be relatively more important.

Tumor rejection is an important special case of the general problem of allograft rejection. Experimentally transplanted tumors may differ in genetically controlled transplantation antigens from the host. Tumors produced by carcinogens frequently have characteristic *new antigens*. These differ from one tumor to the next and are not related to any specificity of the carcinogen actually used. Since many of the carcinogens are effective immunosuppressive agents, the development of a tumor in such cases frequently depends on *temporary abrogation of the immune response* and in some instances the development of *specific immunologic tolerance* to the new tumor antigen as well. In tumors produced by oncogenic viruses such as polyoma, Rous sarcoma virus, SV40, and the adenoviruses, there are neoantigens coded for by the viral genome (Section 1; Fig. 1.15). These are the same in all tumors produced by a given virus. Usually such tumors persist and grow only when viral *infection* is initiated *in early life*, when *tolerance is induced* for the neoantigens rather than transplantation immunity.

Tumors are rejected by several *different mechanisms*. Those lacking a vasculature may be rejected by immune lysis, in the rare cases where they grow freely in suspension (Figs. 10.7,8), by opsonization and actual phagocytic destruction by host macrophages, or by a similar destruction mediated by cytophilic antibody and macrophages (Fig. 18.14). Solid tumors are infiltrated by lymphocytes and destroyed by an invasive–destructive mechanism corresponding to the cytopathic action of "sensitized" lymphocytes seen *in vitro*. The role of released mediators and of the histiocytic cells, which infiltrate some tumors of this type in very large numbers (Figs. 19.13,14) as part of the immune response, remains to be evaluated. Finally, in vascularized tumors the rejection mechanism corresponds to the rejection of grafts of normal tissue such as skin, involving both vascular destruction and infarction and direct invasion and destruction of graft cells by infiltrating mononuclears. However, if the stroma is provided by the host, the tumor may be partially or completely protected against rejection (see below).

The allograft *rejection mechanism* is *inhibited* or completely lacking in animals subjected to *nonspecific depletion of* the pool of thymus-derived precursor *lymphocytes*, whether by neonatal thymectomy (Figs. 19.1,2), pyridoxine deficiency, thoracic duct drainage, antilymphocyte serum, or sufficient doses of nitrogen mustard, cyclophosphamide, steroids, or X-irradiation. It is inhibited in animals with specific immunologic *tolerance* (Fig. 19.2) or with *enhancement* resulting from the presence of circulating antibody in sufficient titer. Enhancement may result from afferent inhibition of the immunization process, when antibody combines with antigen and interferes with its dissemination to regional lymph nodes; from a central effect in the lymph node itself (Section 4); from efferent inhibition in which it combines with cells of the graft and inhibits their specific interaction with "sensitized" lymphocytes; or some combination of these events. The effect of enhancement may be much more striking with transplanted tumors, where a delay of even 2–3 days in the onset of rejection may permit sufficient tumor growth to overwhelm the rejection mechanism, than with normal tissues such as skin. There is suggestive evidence that tumors which rapidly induce a humoral antibody response may, by so doing, suppress both the cellular immune response and the efferent rejection process sufficiently to permit extensive metastasis and overwhelming of the host.

Allograft rejection is also inhibited in situations in which there is an *anatomic block to* either the *afferent* or *efferent limbs of the rejection mechanism*. Grafts of skin to the brain, which lacks draining lymphatics, fail to immunize effectively, though they are readily rejected after immunization is produced by a graft of skin from the same donor to a remote skin site. The same relationship is seen in the hamster cheek pouch. Here the absence of draining lymphatics and the presence of a mucinous connective tissue interfere with local dissemination of immunizing antigen and effectively prevent immunization by skin or tumor grafts (Fig. 19.1); these nonetheless are readily rejected after specific immunization elsewhere. With grafts which remain *in situ* a long time, specific tolerance may ultimately develop.

Conversely, grafts which are not vascularized are often not rejected even though they may induce immunization. Such cases, involving both normal and embryonic tissues and allogeneic and xenogeneic tumors, have been well studied in the anterior chamber of the eye and in Millipore diffusion chambers. The occurrence of immunization may be demonstrated by skin grafts elsewhere, but the absence of vessels prevents the cellular rejection mechanism from taking effect in the protected graft itself. This inhibition may not be effective in the case of some heterografts, where rejection by humoral antibody is important. Other anatomic barriers to the efferent limb of the response may assume great biologic importance. A surface mucopolysaccharide apparently protects trophoblast from the graft rejection mechanism, even in mothers immunized against paternal histocompatibility antigens present in the fetus. Thus rejection of the fetus and placenta is not seen, though some cases of spontaneous abortion have been attributed to this mechanism. Again, repeated pregnancies may result in a substantial degree of maternal tolerance for paternal antigen(s). Similarly, in tumors possessing a well-developed vasculature and stroma of host origin, immunization of the host against tumor antigens may fail to result in rejection of the primary tumor, which is protected from circulating "sensitized" cells by the vascular endothelium containing host antigen. Yet in the same animals, secondary implants or metastases from the primary tumor are promptly rejected (Fig. 19.14). Reports of persistent tumor allografts at subcutaneous, intratesticular, or other sites may depend on one or more of the above mechanisms.

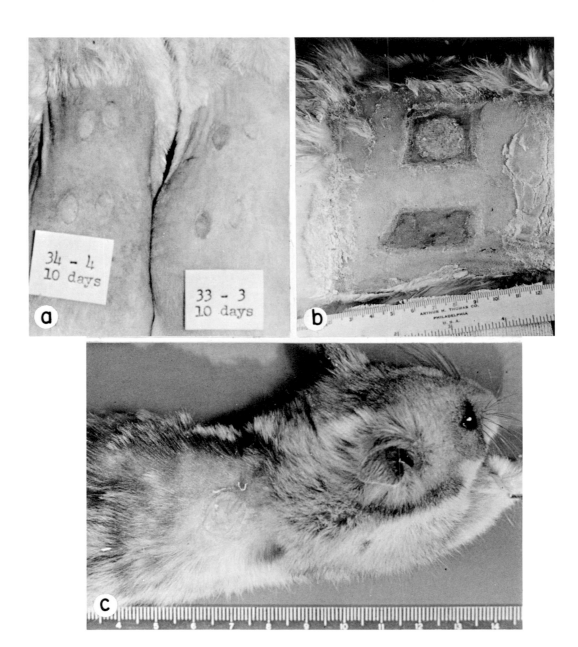

Fig. 19.1. Homograft rejection in different experimental situations. (a) Littermate Sprague-Dawley rats, thymectomized (left) and sham-operated (right) at birth and grafted at 8 weeks of age with duplicate skin homografts from Sherman strain donors on left and duplicate autografts on right. Rejection of the homografts is well advanced in the normal animal but totally lacking in the immunologically defective animal. (b) Growth of normal skin from autologous epidermal cell suspensions seeded in center of denuded areas in normal rabbit. Cells were treated before seeding with normal serum (above) and serum containing homologous antibody against the test animal's cells (below). The antibody clearly inhibited "take" of the autograft. (c) Hamster grafted with homologous cheek pouch. Graft is intact 100 days after grafting, immunization being inhibited by the mucoid ground substance and absence of lymphatics characteristic of the cheek pouch.

(a) From Arnason, Janković, Waksman, and Wennersten, *J. Exp. Med. 116*: 177–86 (1962). (b, c) Courtesy of Dr. R. E. Billingham (see Billingham, *Ann. N.Y. Acad. Sci. 64*: 799–810, 1957).

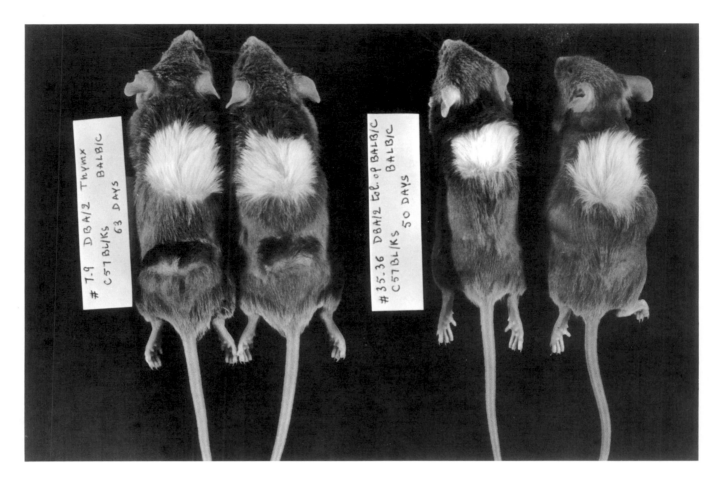

Fig. 19.2. Operational definition of tolerance as *specific* inability to respond to tolerated antigens, illustrated here for the case of tolerance to transplantation antigens and contrasted with nonspecific inability to respond after neonatal thymectomy. DBA/2 mice on left were thymectomized at birth, and those on right received an iv injection of adult BALB/c spleen cells for the induction of tolerance, also within 24 hours of birth. Both sets of mice were grafted at 5 weeks of age with skin from BALB/c and C57B1/Ks donors. The thymectomized animals show prolonged survival of both grafts. The tolerant animals have rejected the third-party C57B1/Ks grafts in a normal manner, while retaining the BALB/c skin.

Courtesy of Dr. F. T. Toullet.

Fig. 19.3. Homograft rejection in different experimental situations. Rejection of rabbit ear skin grafts after treatment locally with specific homologous antiserum. Rabbit 3301, grafted on right with skin from 3303 (test) and on left with skin from 3304 (control). At 2 days, 1.0 ml of serum from rabbit 3302, immunized with spleen cells of 3303 in Freund's adjuvant intradermally, was injected in divided doses around each graft. Test graft shows accelerated rejection by fifth day (above), while control is still intact at 7 days (below).

Courtesy of Dr. C. A. Stetson.

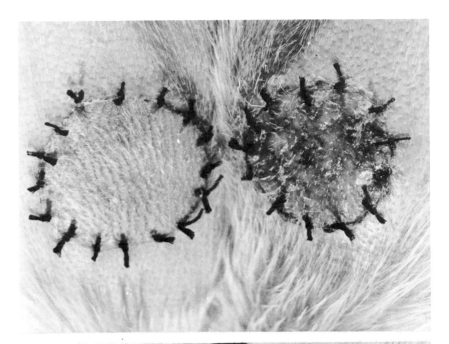

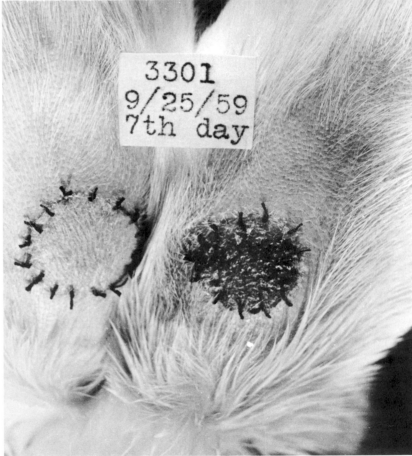

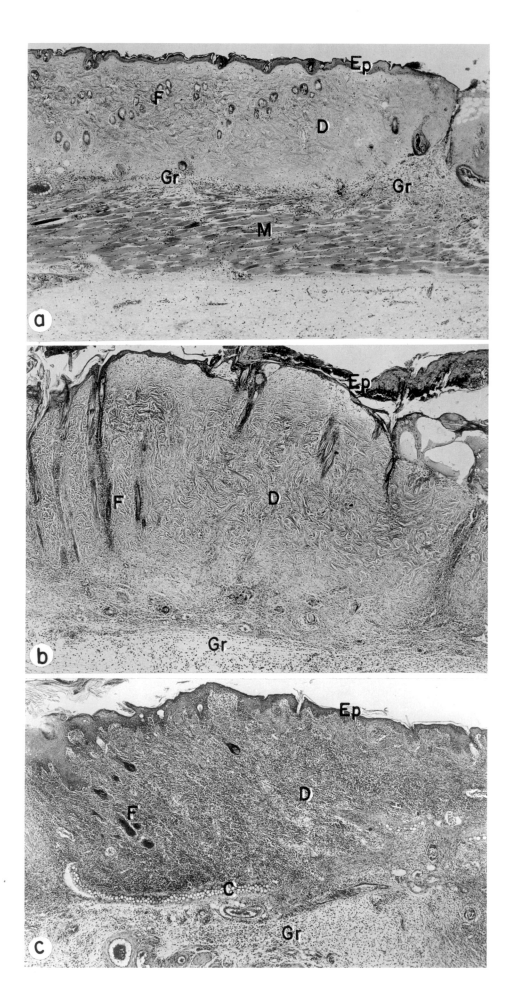

Homograft rejection in different experimental situations. Comparison of skin grafts in Sprague-Dawley rats, 7 days after grafting. Hematoxylin-eosin. From Waksman, *Lab. Invest. 12*: 46–57 (1963).

Fig. 19.4. (a) Autograft of flank skin shows normal-appearing epidermis, granulation tissue between dense dermal connective tissue and muscle, and sparse infiltration of mononuclear cells in zone of granulation. (b) Flank skin homograft shows, in addition, involvement of vessels at base of dermis and along follicles, with more intense cellular infiltrate. Edema of uppermost zone of dermis with thinning and ballooning of epidermis shows that vascular supply to graft is compromised by this infiltrative process. Dense dermal connective tissue shows little infiltration, since veins and arteries are almost entirely lacking here. (c) Similar homograft of ear skin, which is highly vascular, shows dense cellular infiltrate throughout graft (base of graft is delimited by layer of ear cartilage). Epidermis is hyperplastic and apparently undamaged, since vascular supply is still adequate. Ep, epidermis; D, dermal connective tissue; F, hair follicles; C, cartilage; Gr, granulation tissue; M, muscle; ×40.

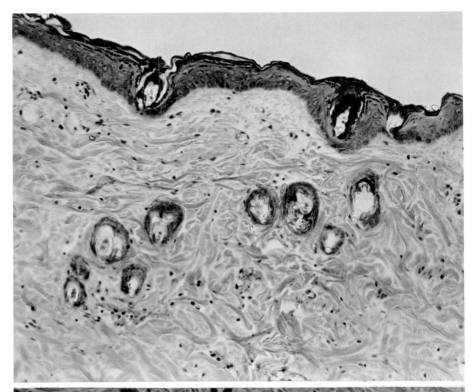

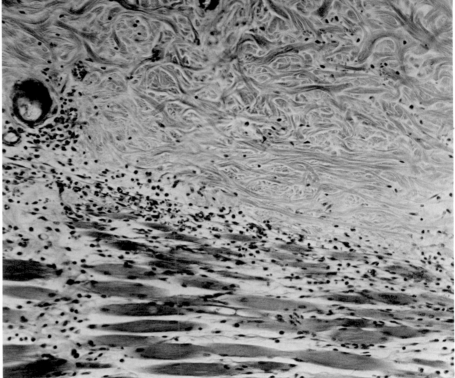

Fig. 19.5. Higher power of 19.4(a), showing normal appearance of upper dermis and epidermis, and sparse infiltrate at base of autograft and in adjacent muscle; ×120.

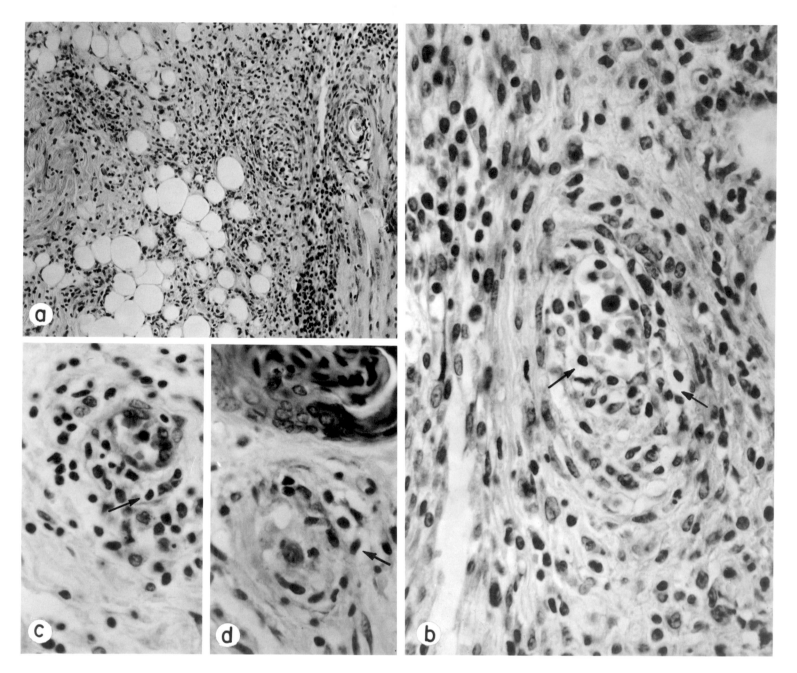

Fig. 19.6. Higher power views of grafts similar to that shown in 19.4(b). (a) Character of cellular infiltrate at base of flank skin homografts; ×120. (b) Artery from same area, showing infiltration of vessel wall by mononuclear cells and spongiosis (vacuolation, shown by arrows) of intima and media about infiltrating cells. Such vessels are rapidly obliterated and can no longer be identified in grafts taken 9 or 10 days after grafting; ×450. (c, d) Venules showing perivenous infiltration and successive stages of vessel wall destruction; ×450.

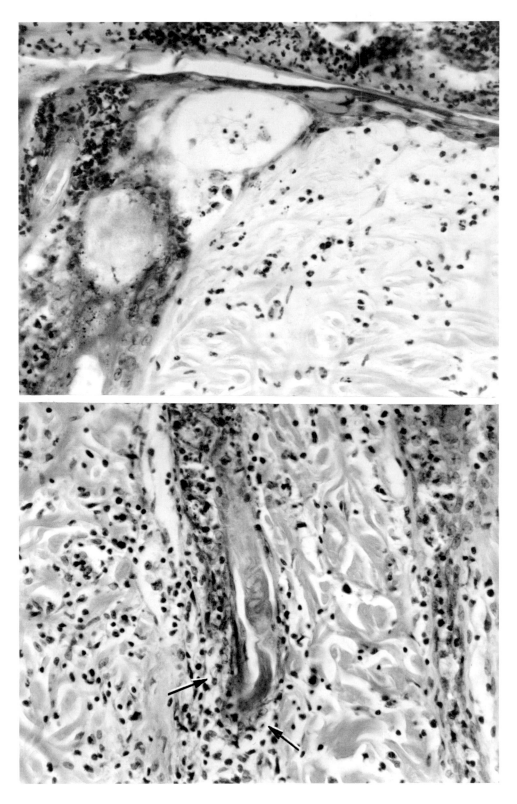

Fig. 19.7. Higher-power views of grafts shown in 19.4(b). (Above) Surface of graft, showing edema and necrosis of epidermis and upper dermis presumably consequent to ischemia. (Below) "Invasive–destructive" lesion, comparable to that in vessels (shown in Fig. 19.6), with invasion of (donor) follicles by (host) mononuclears and clear-cut destruction of follicle epithelium in invaded area (arrows); ×250.

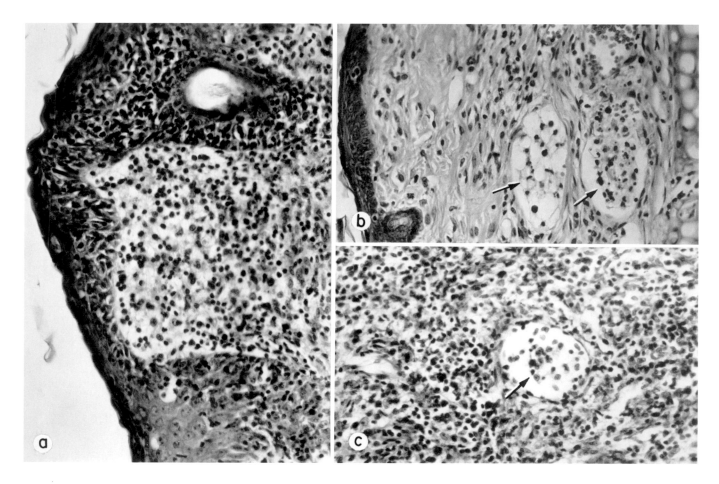

Fig. 19.8. Higher power of 19.4(c). "Invasive–destructive" lesion in ear skin homograft, with massive invasion of surface and follicle epithelium, spongiosis in zone of invasion, and hyperplasia of epithelium, in presence of adequate blood supply. (b) Thrombotic lesions (arrows), made up largely or entirely of reacting mononuclear cells within large veins at 5 days, when cellular infiltration has just begun. (c) Similar lesions at 7 days are rapidly leading to complete vascular occlusion; ×200.

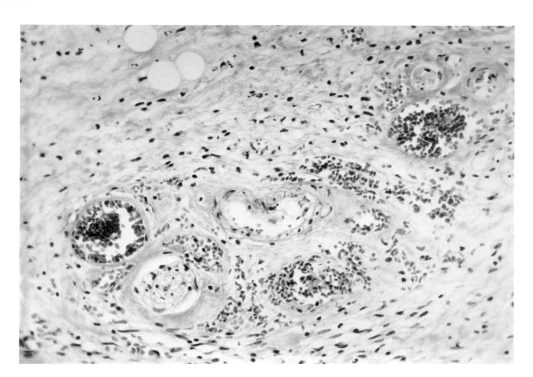

Fig. 19.9. Rat flank skin homograft at 10 days. Remaining vessels at base of graft show necrosis of vessel wall, thrombotic occlusion, or severe stasis with pooling of red cells. There is extensive hemorrhage into the surrounding connective tissue; ×200.

Fig. 19.10. Kidney homograft in dog at 12 days, showing typical features of first-set graft rejection. (a) The interstitial tissue is prominent because of the infiltration with mononuclear cells (*m*). Where tubules (*t*) are open, the epithelium is normal. In more densely cellular areas remnants of tubules can be observed, these presumably having been damaged by the infiltrating cells. Except for a slight increase in cellularity, the glomerulus (*g*) in the lower right corner appears normal. In the center of the field is an artery (*a*) which has cells infiltrating its wall. Such a cellular arteritis is common at this stage. (b) Higher magnification, showing the variety of mononuclear cells in the infiltrate. One can make out small and large lymphocytes and plasmacytes. Tubular epithelial cells appear normal in those tubules which have patent lumens. A slight increase in cellularity is the major abnormality of the glomerulus. In the lower portion of the field there is an arteriole with cells infiltrating the arteriolar wall. Here as in (a), there is a concentration of mononuclear cells around arterial structures. (c) Methyl green–pyronine stain. Cells with abundant cytoplasmic RNA stand out prominently. The dark-staining cytoplasm appears a bright red-lavender under the microscope. Nuclear detail in the infiltrating cells is also more readily visible with this stain.

(a, b) Hematoxylin-eosin; (c) methyl green–pyronine; magnifications not given. Courtesy of Dr. G. J. Dammin.

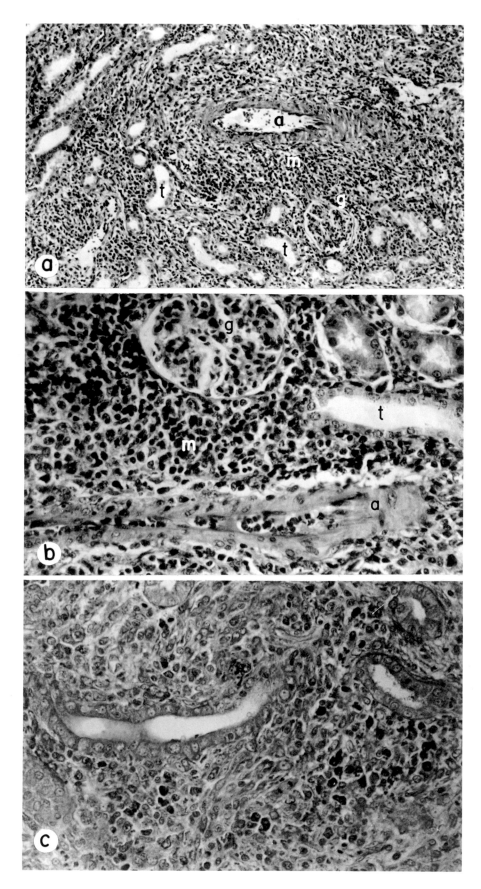

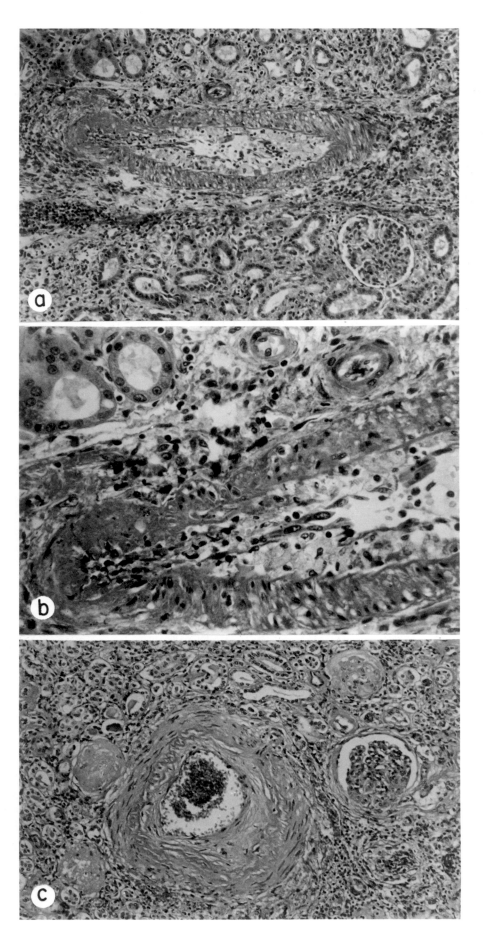

Fig. 19.11. Human kidney homograft at 28 days. (a) The prominent structure in this field is the artery which occupies the center. Its entire left extremity exhibits necrosis with fibrinoid deposition, and its lumen is narrowed by subendothelial infiltration of cells. The prominence of the interstitial tissue is due to edema, with only a slight focal increase in cellularity. The tubular epithelial cells exhibit variability in nuclear staining, and the glomerulus shows an increase in density and reduced vascularity. These manifestations have been attributed by some investigators to "humoral rejection." (b) Higher power. Necrosis and fibrinoid in the artery are better demonstrated at this magnification. Lipophages and occasional mononuclear cells are noted between the endothelial lining of the artery and the media. (c) This photomicrograph illustrates lesions in the patient's own remaining kidney, the other having been removed at the time of transplantation of the cadaver homograft. There are scattered atrophic glomeruli and tubules. The center of the field is occupied by an artery with a thickened intima. This vascular lesion of glomerulonephritis often contributes to atrophy of the grafted kidney.

Hematoxylin-eosin; magnifications not given. Courtesy of Dr. G. J. Dammin.

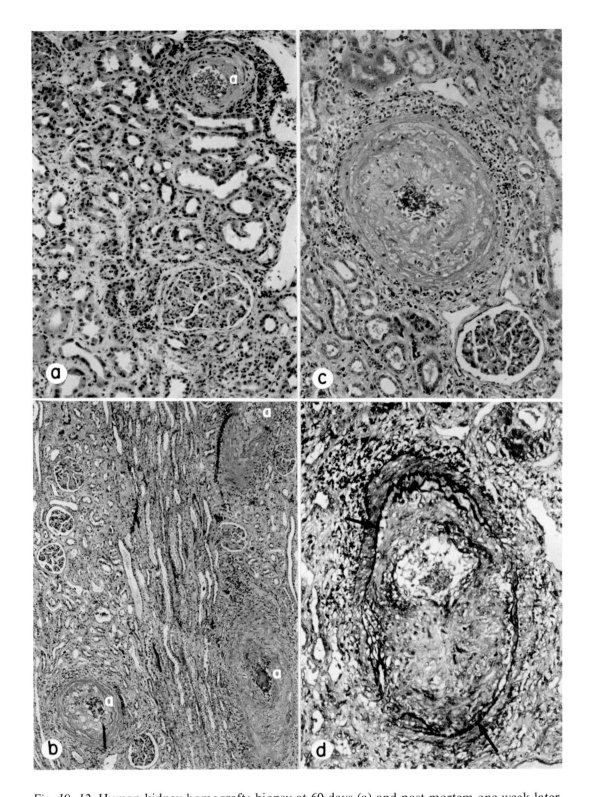

Fig. 19. 12. Human kidney homograft: biopsy at 60 days (a) and post mortem one week later (b–d). (a) The most prominent changes are interstitial edema and vascular damage suggestive of "humoral rejection." The glomerulus is dense with capillaries difficult to identify. There is irregular staining of the nuclei of tubular epithelial cells. In the upper right corner is an artery (*a*) exhibiting medial necrosis with fibrinoid, and adjacent to it a vein with infiltration of the wall and surrounding interstitial tissue. (b) At low magnification, one can recognize three arteries, all with an obliterative lesion due to intimal thickening. Prominence of the interstitial tissue is illustrated in the left half of the field. One can surmise even from this hematoxylin and eosin slide that there will be disruption of the elastica. (c) Extreme narrowing of the lumen is exhibited by the artery occupying the center of the field. Lipophages can be recognized in the thickened intima. (d) An artery similar to that shown in the previous photomicrograph illustrates well the disruption and dissolution of the elastica (arrows). The most normal portion of the wall is on the left where one can recognize the media of the artery bounded by an inner and outer elastica. Elastica is abnormal throughout the remainder of the artery. The pronounced intimal thickening is also well demonstrated.

(a–c) Hematoxylin-eosin; (d) elastic tissue stain; magnifications not given. Courtesy of Dr. G. J. Dammin.

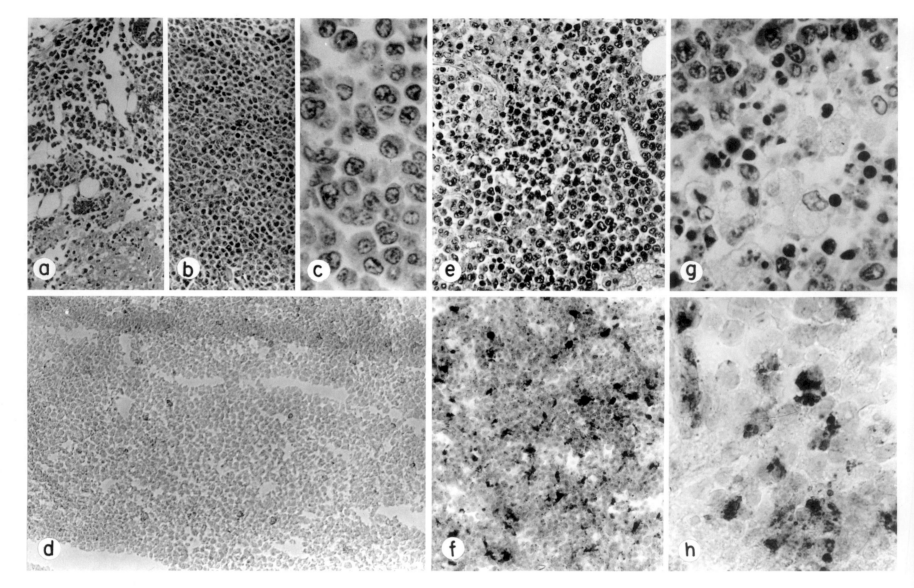

Fig. 19.13. Rejection of transplanted tumor (homograft rejection) in the absence of stroma. Nonmetastasizing lymphoma of hamster transplanted to normal (nonimmunized) animal. Sections taken at 24 hours (a), 7 days, shortly before appearance of phenomena accompanying rejection (b–d), and 14 days, when rejection is proceeding rapidly (e–h). At 24 hours, the central zone of the tumor implant is necrotic (below), but tumor cells are beginning to proliferate (above). At 7 days, tissue is replaced by a uniform sheet of tumor cells. The principal change between the 7- and 14-day specimens is the appearance of large numbers of macrophages, scattered diffusely through the graft and beginning necrosis of the tumor cells, seen especially well in the high-power photomicrograph (g). In sections stained for acid phosphatase, the 7-day specimen (d) shows absence of this enzyme from the tumor cells themselves and the almost total absence of infiltrating macrophages in the tumor. At 14 days, large amounts of acid phosphatase are seen in the numerous infiltrating macrophages (f, h). In some of these cells, enzyme-containing lyosomes are so numerous and densely packed that the particles of reaction product fuse, and individual granules become indistinguishable. Histiocytic infiltration and an apparent direct tumor cell destruction by these infiltrating cells is the characteristic mode of rejection of lymphomas and solid ascites cell tumors like that used in the present study (Gorer's type II rejection).

(a–c, e, g) Hematoxylin-eosin; (d, f, h) acid phosphatase stain. (a, b, d–f) ×94, (c, g) ×565, (h) ×375 From Gershon, Carter, and Lane, *Am. J. Path. 51*: 1111–33 (1967).

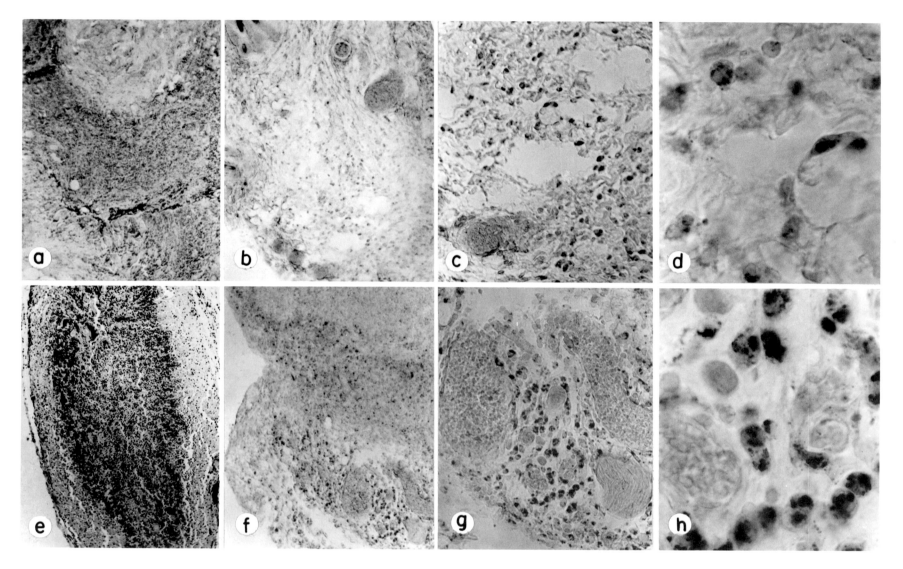

Fig. 19.14. Rejection of transplanted tumor (homograft rejection) in the absence of stroma. Same hamster lymphoma as shown in previous plate. Comparison of early macrophage infiltration within tumor in normal (unimmunized) and specifically immunized hosts. (a–d) Tumor implant at 72 hours in normal animal. (e–h) Corresponding photographs of similar implant at 24 hours in hamster immunized by earlier graft of same tumor. In the normal animal, tumor shows central ischemic necrosis (a, above) and well-defined outer zone of tumor cells beginning to in-filtrate surrounding connective tissue (below). Macrophage reaction in the connective tissue is shown in section stained for acid phosphatase (b–d). There is scattering of small cells, containing moderate complement of lysosomes, indicated by the stain. In the immunized animal, outer zone of tumor undergoes early necrosis, while central zone is preserved (e).

In section stained for acid phosphatase (f–h) it is evident that there has been rapid mobilization, in the connective tissue adjacent to the implant of large numbers of macrophages, which differ from those seen in the normal animal in number, size, number and size of lysosomes, and possibly enzyme content of the lysosomes (the darker stain in cells shown in h compared with d represents a relatively increased amount of reaction product referable to higher enzyme concentration). These macrophages are comparable to those appearing diffusely in first-set tumor implant at 8–9 days, shown in previous plate.

(a, e) Hematoxylin-eosin; other figures acid phosphatase stain. (a, b, e, f) ×38, (c, g) ×95, (d, h) ×380. From Gershon, Carter, and Lane, *Am. J. Path. 51*: 1111–33 (1967).

20. Graft-versus-Host Reactions

The injection of normal immunocompetent lymphoid cells into genetically dissimilar recipients provides the possibility that these cells will be immunized against transplantation and other antigens of the host, with a resulting production of lesions. There are two well-known examples of *local graft-vs.-host* (*GVH*) *lesions* produced in this manner. When adult chicken lymphocytes are placed on an allogeneic chick *chorioallantoic membrane* several days before hatching, the recipient does not reject the donor cells, and these give rise to local *pock-like lesions*, each reflecting the immune response of at least one donor lymphocyte (Figs. 20.16,17). Similarly, if adult mammalian lymphocytes are injected into adult allogeneic skin, they give rise over several days to erythematous, papular lesions (the *transfer reaction*) (Fig. 20.9). These reach maximum size by 5 days and regress rapidly as the host becomes immunized against the foreign cells. If the host is preimmunized against the donor's cells, no reaction occurs. Conversely if the donor is preimmunized against recipient antigen(s), the reaction occurs more rapidly and intensely, reaching a peak by 3 days but also receding after 5 days as a result of the host response. Such GVH lesions are seen only when donor and host differ at the strong histocompatibility locus and when immunocompetent cells (lymph node, spleen) are employed. A variant of the second type of lesion is seen when a mixture of lymphocytes from two dissimilar donors is injected intradermally into a heavily irradiated host, the hamster for example. This reaction is little more than a *mixed lymphocyte reaction* carried out *in vivo*, and a lesion is produced even when the cells come from a different species than the host.

The local lesion has a number of clearly defined *histological components* (Figs. 20.10–13). Some of the injected lymphocytes become large, dividing basophilic *blast-like cells*. There is rapid diapedesis throughout the site of hematogenous monocytes which rapidly give rise to *islands* (granulomas) *of dividing histiocytic cells*. These become large and pale and are variously described as histiocytes, macrophages, reticular cells, or epithelioid cells. The dermal connective tissue is replaced by the granulomas; this presumably corresponds to a conventional invasive–destructive lesion. There may be foci of ischemic necrosis and extensive areas of eosinophil infiltration (mechanism?). Labeling of donor and/or host with tritiated thymidine shows that the large cells are exclusively of host origin (Figs. 20.14,15) and presumably correspond to the bone-marrow-derived histiocytes of other delayed reactions. The extent of their proliferation is thought to depend on the continuing stimulus offered by the abundant supply of host antigen. A few of the injected lymphocytes may escape from the local site and produce systemic GVH lesions; this is especially the case in the chick with chorioallantoic lesions (Fig. 20.17).

When lymphoid cells are injected intravenously into normal allogeneic hosts, they are generally rejected as a graft of foreign tissue. However in incompetent hosts, they home in various lymphoid organs and mount a *systemic GVH response*. Such a response (runt disease, homologous disease, secondary disease) is seen in newborns given adult allogeneic cells, in neonatally thymectomized adults (Figs. 20.2–8) or adults treated with irradiation or antilymphocyte serum and similarly injected, and finally in hybrid adults given competent cells of one of the parent strains. Lesions are produced occasionally in normal adults given very large doses of allogeneic cells. The cells of lymph nodes and spleen are effective, those of marrow much less so, and those of thymus not at all. The animals, particularly if young at the time of cell injection, remain runted and show cachexia, diarrhea, dermatitis and alopecia, and other manifestations of severe illness, as well as gross splenomegaly in early phases of the disease (Fig. 20.1). The gross and histologic changes are not to be compared to the cachectic syndromes (wasting disease) which follow neonatal thymectomy or injection of steroids or antilymphocyte serum, since the latter can be shown to result from intercurrent infection in immunologically deprived animals and can be prevented by maintenance of the animals in a "germ-free" state or treatment with suitable antibiotics. However, part of the picture of runt disease may depend on such infection, since animals with systemic GVH reactions suffer a severe impairment of normal immunologic function.

The lesions of homologous disease are very similar to local GVH lesions in their pathogenesis (Figs. 20.2–8). Large, dividing, *basophilic (pyroninophilic) cells* appear in the splenic white pulp and the lymph node cortex; these have been shown to arise directly from donor lymphocytes which have settled at these sites. Secondarily, extensive *hyperplasia of large pale, reticular cells* of host origin, comparable to those in the granulomas of the local GVH response, occurs in these same organs (Fig. 20.3). Finally, reactions are seen throughout the body which resemble delayed reactions and are comparable to graft rejection or autoallergic lesions. There is massive *histiocytic infiltration* and an *invasive–destructive* lesion of parenchyma in liver (Fig. 20.2), heart (Fig. 20.5), lung (Fig. 20.7), joint synovia and skin (Fig. 20.4), and gastrointestinal tract (Fig. 20.6). These lesions too may assume a granulomatous appearance at times. There is early thymus atrophy and, at a later stage, *atrophy of all the lymphoid organs.* In one variant of the experimental procedure leading to runt disease, inbred animals made chimeric at birth with hybrid lymphoid cells, if injected with parental strain cells later in life, develop GVH lesions limited to the lymphoid organs where the hybrid cells (i.e. antigen-bearing cells) have settled.

Animals with homologous disease also develop *antibody-mediated lesions* affecting erythrocytes, leukocytes, and platelets and show large areas of hemopoietic tissue in the spleen. They frequently develop *amyloid* (Fig. 20.3) and, if the animals remain alive for long periods of time, *neoplastic lesions* affecting both *lymphoid and reticular cells* (Fig. 20.8). The latter arise as a probable consequence of the continuing immunologic deficit which these animals present and are said to resemble in some cases the lesions of Hodgkin's disease. The GVH lesions themselves, with their reticular cell granulomas, foci of necrosis, and eosinophilia, also present suggestive models for sarcoid on the one hand and such diseases as Wegener's granulomatosis and lethal midline granuloma on the other.

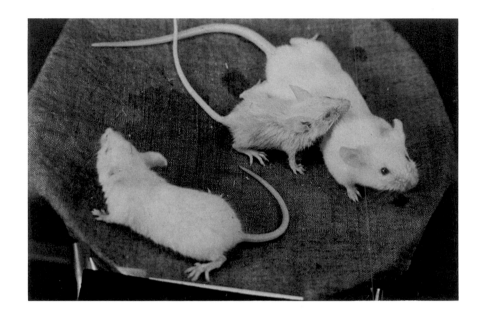

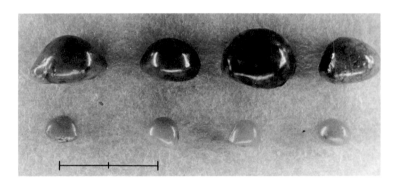

Fig. 20.1. Systemic graft-versus-host reactions. (Above) Classical runt disease, produced in A strain mice injected at birth with C3H strain adult spleen cells iv. Runted mouse is shown at 60 days of age with two normal littermates. (Below) Characteristic splenomegaly seen in runted chicks. Four spleens removed at 3 days of age from White Leghorn chicks injected at 18 days (3 days before hatching) are compared with spleens of normal chicks the same age.

(Above) From Billingham, *Ann. N.Y. Acad. 73*: 782–88 (1958). (Below) From Simonsen, (*Acta Path. Microbiol. Scand. 40*: 480–500 (1957).

Systemic graft-versus-host reactions. Lesions produced by injecting competent adult spleen cells from hooded (Long-Evans) donor rats into Sprague-Dawley recipients. Lesion shown in (a) is from an animal injected iv at 3 days of age with 0.7×10^8 cells. All others are from rats thymectomized at 3 days and injected at 9–13 weeks of age with $8-10 \times 10^8$ donor cells. Clinical disease appeared 12–14 days after injection, and animals were sacrificed at different intervals thereafter.

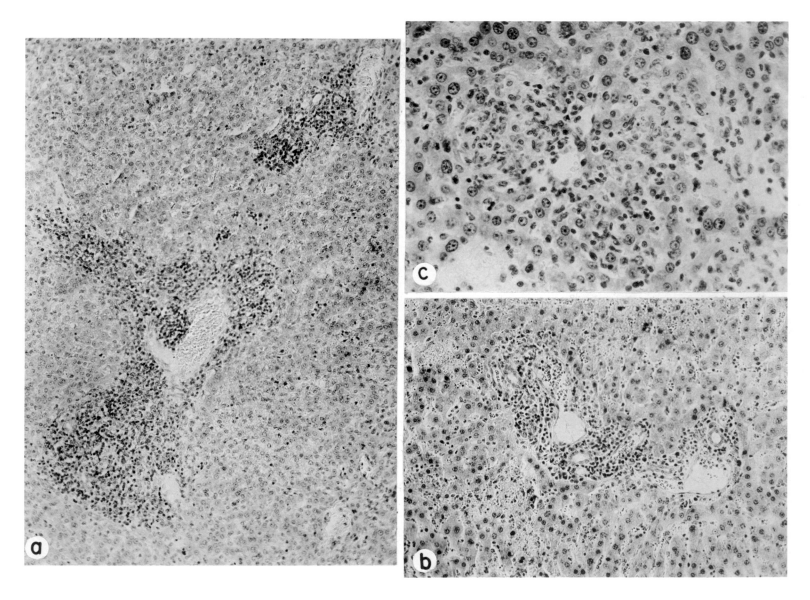

Fig. 20.2: (a, b) Liver, showing characteristic periportal cell infiltrates; ×150. (c) Higher-power view, showing mononuclear character of infiltrating cells and destruction of liver parenchyma in zone of infiltration; ×300.

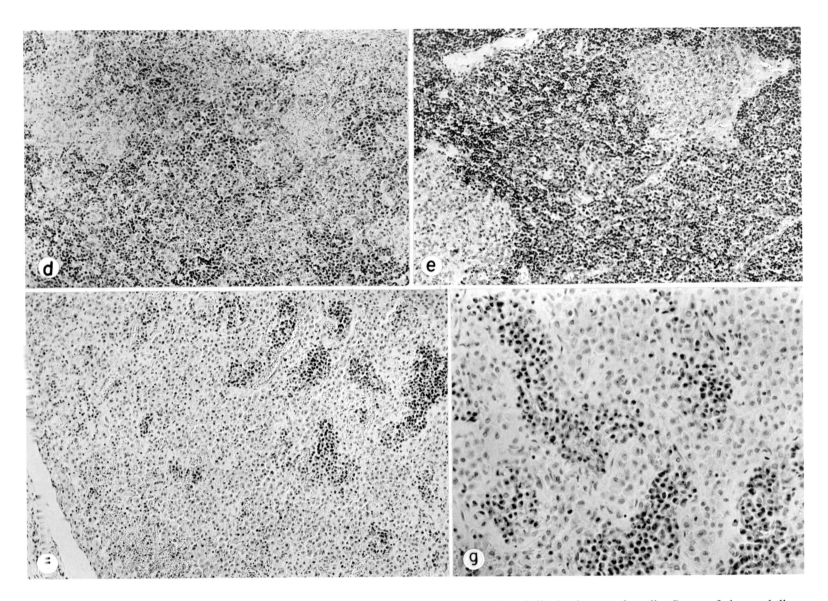

Fig. 20.3: (d) Spleen lesion: replacement of extensive areas of red pulp by large, pale reticulum cells. (e) Foci of similar pale cells developing from intermediate sinuses in lymph node cortex. (f) Maximal lymph node lesion: complete replacement of cortex and most of medulla by large pale cells. Some of the medullary cords of plasma cells are preserved. All ×130. (g) Higher power: pale cells present typical morphologic character of fully developed macrophages; ×260.

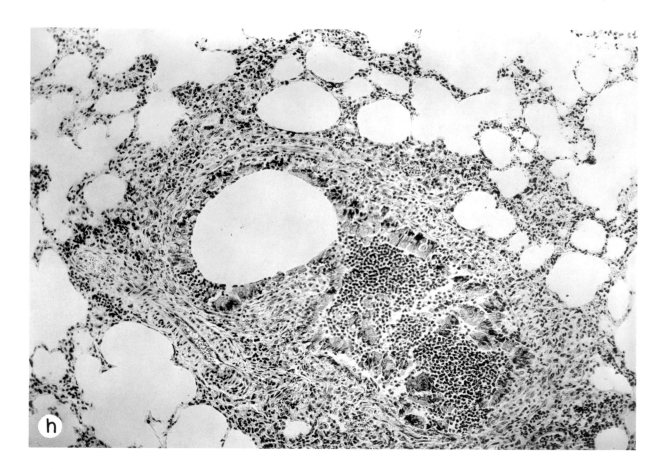

Fig. 20.4: (h) Lung: large aggregate of histiocytic cells and what appears to be invasion and destruction of bronchial epithelium. One bronchus is filled with small mononuclear cells; × 150.

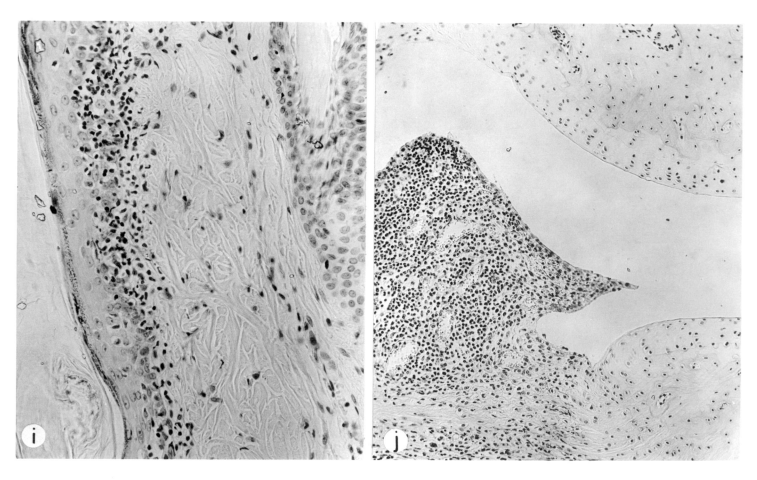

Fig 20.5: (i) Section of tail skin, showing characteristic infiltration of lymphocytes and histiocytes in upper dermis, invasion of epidermis by these cells, and formation of spongiform vesicles; × 300. (j) Wrist joint, showing synovitis without pannus formation or alteration of cartilage; × 150.

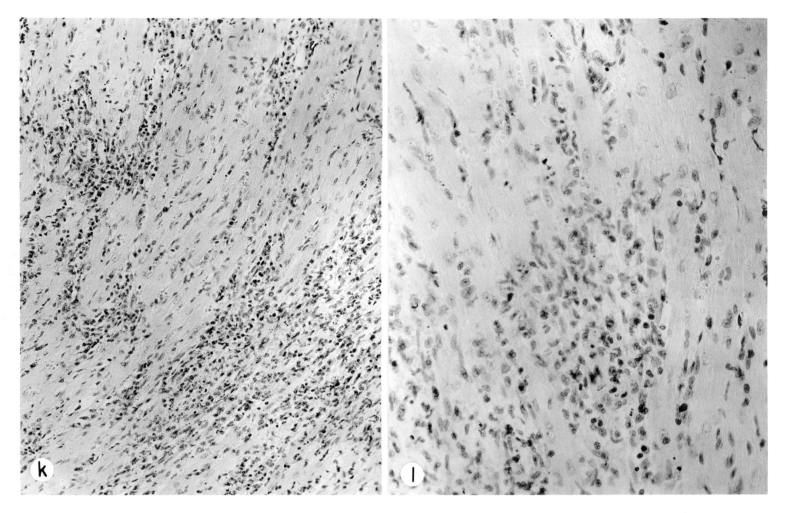

Fig. 20.6: (k) Heart, showing massive histiocytic infiltration with partial or total myofiber destruction in zone of infiltration; ×150. (l) Higher-power view of similar lesion; ×300.

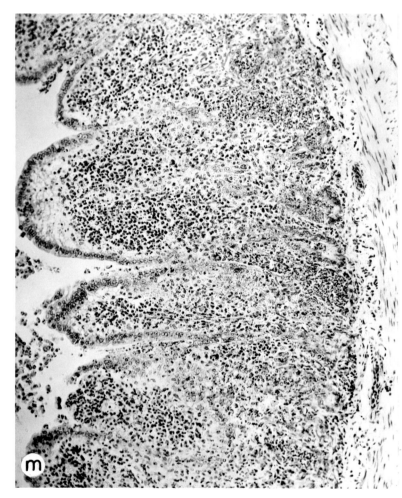

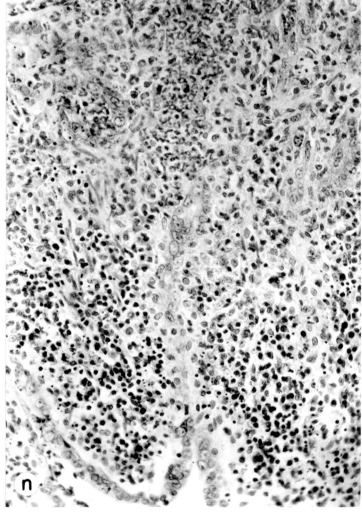

Fig. 20.7: (m) Small bowel lesion: histiocytic infiltration of lamina propria and formation of microabscesses; ×150. (n) Higher-power view shows that these are filled with polymorphonuclears; ×300.

All hematoxylin-eosin. From Aisenberg, Wilkes, and Waksman, *J. Exp. Med. 116*: 759–72 (1962).

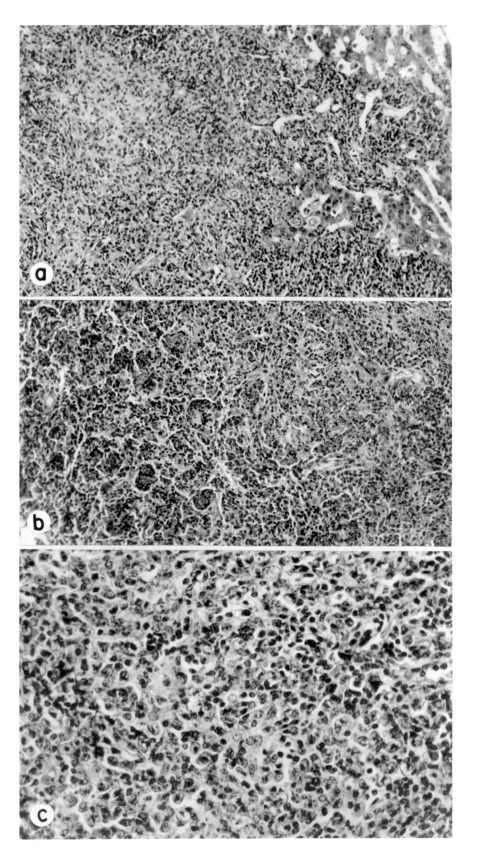

Fig. 20.8. Systemic graft-versus-host reactions. Malignant lymphomatous lesions in mice surviving for several months after production of acute runt disease. (a) Typical reticulum cell sarcoma invading liver. Residual cords of liver cells are seen to right. (b) Reticulum cell sarcoma with peculiar acinar arrangement of cells. (c) Lesion comparable to that shown in (a), under higher power. Cell infiltrate is extremely pleomorphic, containing lymphocytes, reticulum cells, blast-like cells, and multinucleate cells reminiscent of Reed-Sternberg cells.

Hematoxylin-eosin; (a, b) ×150, (c) ×450. Courtesy of Dr. R. S. Schwartz.

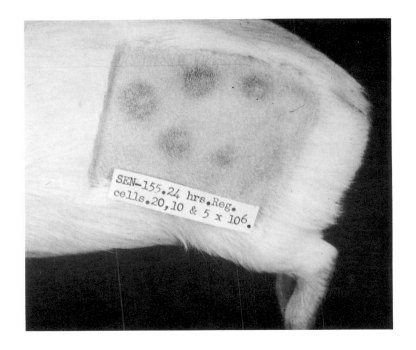

Fig. 20.9. Local graft-versus-host lesion, produced in guinea pig skin by lymph node cells from donor preimmunized against transplantation antigens of recipient; 24-hour reactions, produced by doses of 20, 10, and 5×10^6 viable cells, are seen as large, indurated, erythematous papules, grossly indistinguishable from tuberculin or other delayed skin reactions.

Courtesy of Dr. P. B. Medawar (see Brent and Medawar, *Proc. Roy. Soc. B. 165*: 281–307, 1966).

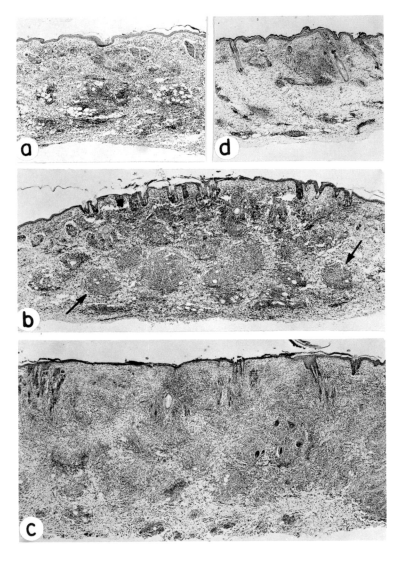

Fig. 20.10. Local graft-versus-host reactions. "Transfer reactions" produced in recipient rabbit skin (New Zealand strain) by intradermal injection of 30×10^6 popliteal lymph node cells from Dutch strain donors, sensitized 10 days previously with skin graft from the same recipient. Reactions at 1 day (a) and 3 days (b, c) contrasted with nonsensitized Dutch cells (d). Development of large islands (arrows) of uniformly staining cells is well shown in (b), and confluence of lesions in (c).

Hematoxylin-eosin; ×35. From Dvorak, Kosunen, and Waksman, *Lab. Invest. 12*: 58–68 (1963).

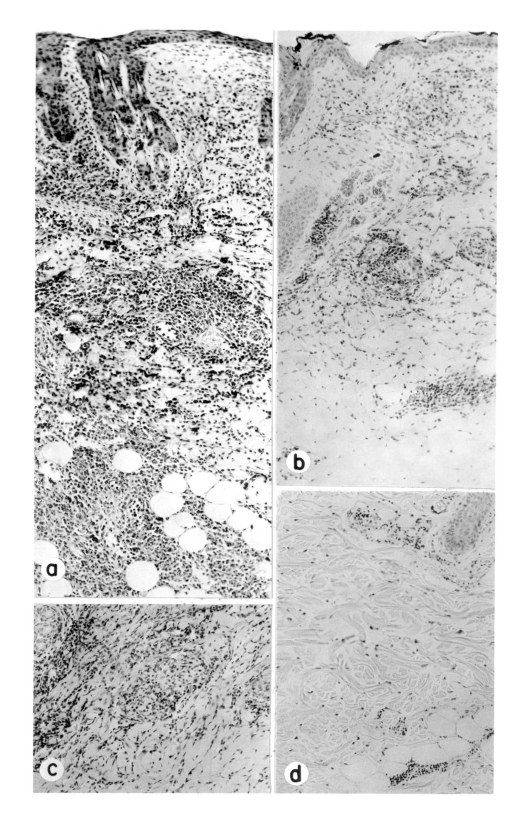

Fig. 20.11. Local graft-versus-host reactions. Character of 2-day transfer reaction produced by sensitized Dutch cells (a) is contrasted with lesions produced by nonsensitized cells (b) or sensitized cells injected into autologous (Dutch) recipients (d). Nonsensitized cells, even at 4 days (c), fail to produce lesions comparable to early specific reaction.

Hematoxylin-eosin; ×25. From Dvorak, Kosunen, and Waksman, *Lab. Invest.* *12*: 58–68 (1963).

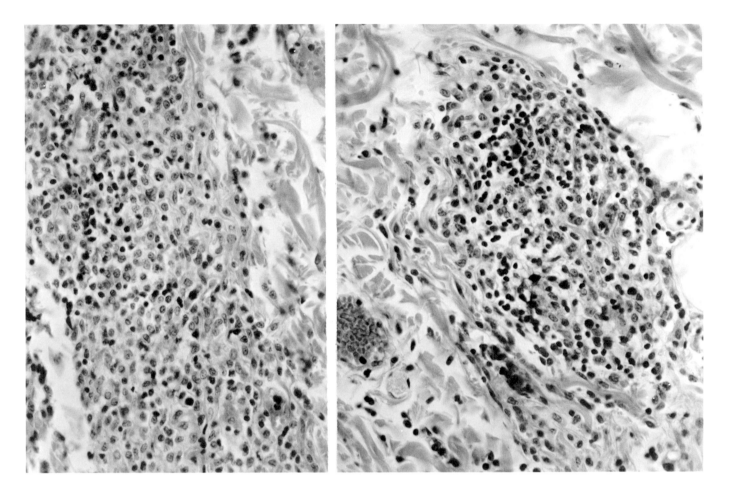

Fig. 20.12. Local graft-versus-host reactions. Two-day skin lesion (transfer reaction) produced by sensitized (left) and nonsensitized (right) homologous cells. Epithelioid character of histiocytes in island of cells characteristic of specific reaction is well shown.

Hematoxylin-eosin; ×318. From Dvorak, Kosunen, and Waksman, *Lab. Invest. 12*: 58–68 (1963).

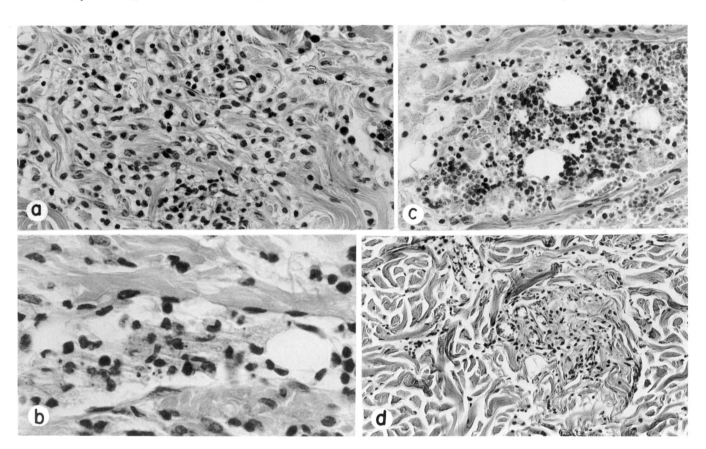

Fig. 20.13. Local graft-versus-host reactions. Resolving transfer reactions at 5 (a–c) and 8 (d) days. (a, d) Nests or islands, in which cells are decreasing progressively in number and new collagen is being formed. (b) Characteristic intravascular aggregate of mononuclear cells. (c) Focus of necrosis and hemorrhage.

Hematoxylin-eosin; (a, c) ×360, (b) ×725, (d) ×180. From Dvorak, Kosunen, and Waksman, *Lab. Invest. 12*: 58–68 (1963).

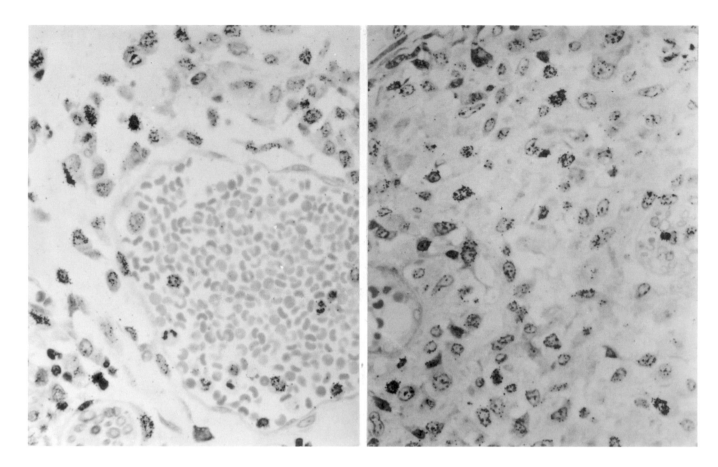

Fig. 20.14. Source of cells in local graft-versus-host reactions. Transfer reactions are shown in recipient rabbits labeled by daily iv administration of H³-thymidine, 0.75 μC/g, for 3 days prior to cell transfer from sensitized, unlabeled donors. (Left) One-day reaction, showing the exuberance with which labeled host cells (mostly medium and large "lymphocytes") are pouring out of a large venule. (Right) Three-day reaction, showing the high proportion of labeled (host) cells in a typical island. Most are pale histiocytes. Some labeled cells (lymphocytes) are seen in a venule.

Autoradiographs of thin sections, prepared with Kodak AR-10 stripping film, exposed 4 weeks, then developed and stained with May-Grünwald–Giemsa; ×650. From Kosunen and Dvorak, *Lab. Invest.* *12*: 628–37 (1963).

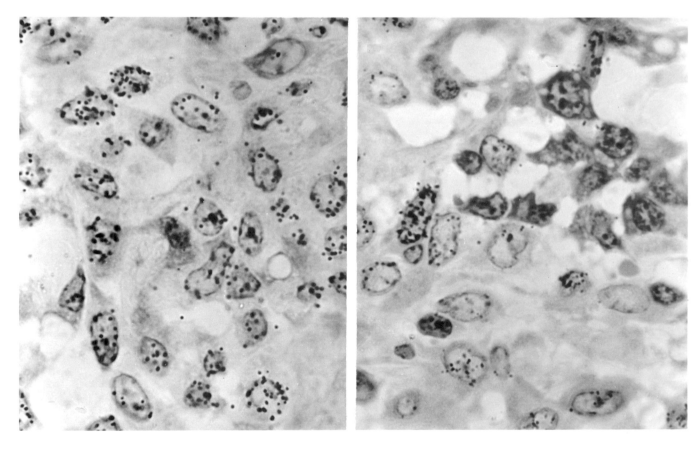

Fig. 20.15. Same as Fig. 20.14. (Left) Higher-power view of 3-day transfer reaction showing labeled (host) pale histiocytes. (Right) Five-day lesion showing prominent basophilic cells. These are a small minority (less than 6 per cent) of the cells making up the infiltrate.

Autoradiographs of thin sections, prepared with stripping film and stained with May-Grünwald–Giemsa; ×1,500. From Kosunen and Dvorak, *Lab. Invest.* *12*: 628–37 (1963).

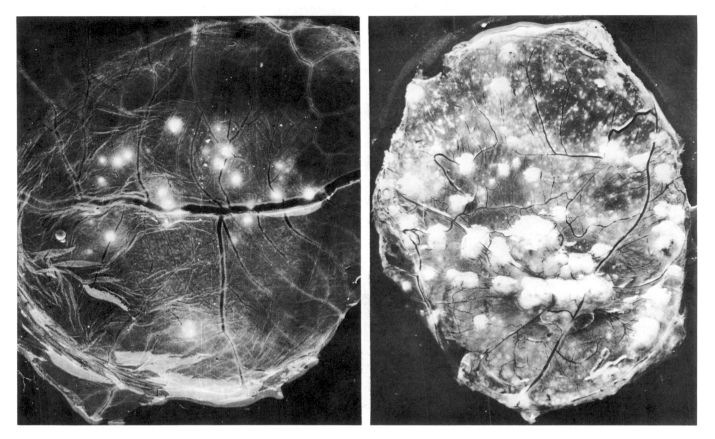

Fig. 20.16. Local graft-versus-host reactions. Pock-like lesions produced on chicken chorioallantoic membrane (CAM) by homologous blood cells. (Left) Typical 4-day lesions produced by inoculating 0.1 ml heparinized normal chicken blood on dropped CAM of a 12-day embryo. Twenty well-defined and a few smaller foci are visible. (Right) Seven days. The large lesions are hard and almost spherical, and many satellite foci are visible.

×2. Courtesy of Dr. F. M. Burnet (see Burnet and Boyer, *J. Path. Bact. 81*: 141–50, 1961).

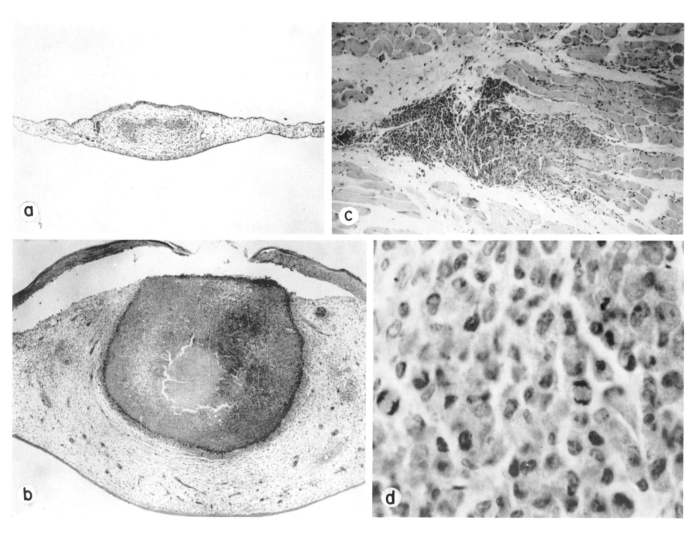

Fig. 20.17. Local graft-versus-host reactions. (a) Section of 4-day lesion on CAM. There is some thickening of chorionic epithelium, but the bulk of the lesion is made up of mesenchymal cells, mostly of host origin. (b) Section of a mature CAM lesion showing necrotic central mass sharply demarcated from surrounding tissues. (c) Lesion in occipital muscles of a chick embryo, inoculated iv with adult chicken leukocytes, shows active cell proliferation and invasion of muscle. (d) Higher-power view of same section showing mononuclear character of infiltrate and cells in mitosis.

Hematoxylin-eosin; (a–c) ×40, (d) ×615. Courtesy of Dr. F. M. Burnet (see Burnet and Boyer, *J. Path. Bact. 81*: 141–50, 1961).

21. The Experimental Autoallergies

The autoallergies are diseases produced by immunizing individuals against constituents of their own tissues. In each case, when the hypersensitive state appears, reactions are elicited wherever antigen is situated in the body and result in lesions. New experimental autoallergies have been described almost yearly over two decades. The present list of well-documented experimental diseases includes:

Organ Affected	Lesion	Figures
Central nervous system	Encephalomyelitis	21.1–7
Peripheral nervous system	Polyneuritis	21.8–10
Autonomic nervous system	Autonomic neuropathy	
Anterior pituitary	Adenohypophysitis	
Thyroid	Thyroiditis	21.14–18
Parathyroid	Parathyroiditis	
Islets of Langerhans	Insulinitis	21.20
Adrenal	Adrenalitis	21.19
Testis	Orchitis	21.21–25
Lens	Endophthalmitis	21.32
Uvea	Uveitis	21.33
Skin	Dermatosis	
Gastric mucosa	Atrophic gastritis	
Colonic mucosa	Ulcerohemorrhagic colitis	
Kidney	Glomerulonephritis	21.30,31
Heart	Carditis	21.29 (cf. 17,10)
Skeletal muscle	Myositis	
Thymus	Thymitis	

Several of the better-described cases are illustrated here. Detailed morphologic and immunologic studies thus far have been limited largely to experimental autoallergic encephalomyelitis, neuritis, thyroiditis, orchitis, and glomerulonephritis.

The *lesions* in every case are irregularly *disseminated in regions of high antigen concentration*, e.g. the white matter of the central nervous system, where there are sufficient numbers of veins or venules (Figs. 21.11–13,19,28). They are *focal perivenular inflammatory reactions* consisting of lymphocytes and histiocytes; in some instances the latter form masses of large, pale "reticular" or "epithelioid" cells, and occasional giant cells may be present (Figs. 21.1–3,8,10,16,17). Necrosis, hemorrhage, and polymorphonuclear infiltration occur only in very intense reactions and far more frequently in some species (guinea pigs) than others (rabbits, rats) (Figs. 16.21; 21.6). *Parenchymal damage* is *coextensive with* the *cellular infiltrate*: demyelination (Figs. 21.2,9,10), destruction of uveal pigment (Fig. 21.33), of testicular germinal epithelium (Fig. 21.24), of colloid in thyroid acini (Figs. 21.14, 15,17), of cells in the islets of Langerhans (Fig. 21.20), and even of connective tissue elements (Figs. 21.17,25). In lesions lasting more than a few days, plasma cells appear. Their number is apparently related to the identity of the antigen, great numbers being seen for example in autoallergic thyroiditis (Figs. 21.17; 22.1) and very few in autoallergic encephalomyelitis or polyneuritis (Fig. 21.7). In long-standing lesions typical germinal centers finally form. Late secondary parenchymal changes vary with the nature of the affected organ and may include such features as proliferation of thyroid acinar cells (Figs. 21.14,17) and aspermatogenesis (Figs. 21.26,27). The time course of the disease tends to be chronic, since it is determined by persistence of the hypersensitive state, which may wane or be boosted by renewed immunization.

54

The morphologic character of these lesions agrees with immunologic evidence that they are *mediated by the cellular type of sensitization*. Techniques of sensitization which enhance preferentially the production of such sensitization, notably the use of mycobacterial adjuvant, of repeated small intradermal doses of antigen, or of antigen–antibody precipitates, are most effective in producing experimental autoallergic disease. There is no correlation of disease with circulating antibody (Figs. 1.5,9; 22.1) or a fall in circulating complement, and lesions cannot be produced by passive transfer of antiserum from suitably immunized donors. One can demonstrate delayed skin reactivity (Fig. 16.3) with more or less highly purified antigens (e.g. thyroglobulin, encephalitogenic basic protein), and this is well correlated with the disease process. The parenchymal destruction is mimicked *in vitro* by the cytopathic effect of sensitized lymphocytes on, e.g., myelin (Figs. 18.10,11) or thyroid cells, and other *in vitro* concomitants of cellular sensitivity have been demonstrated, notably uptake of antigen by lymphocytes (Fig. 18.1), blast transformation, and the specific inhibition of macrophage migration by myelin antigen. Finally, in the better-studied cases, disease has been passively transferred with living lymphoid cells from properly immunized donors, when transfer is carried out between members of the same inbred strain of animals or when the recipient is purposely made tolerant for grafts of cells from animals of donor type. As with other categories of cellular sensitization, autoallergic disease is inhibited nonspecifically by events producing lymphopenia (such as neonatal thymectomy or the use of antilymphocyte serum) and specifically by tolerance or by the enhancement techique (active or passive introduction of sufficient humoral antibody against the same antigen.) Autoimmune disease of the kidney provides an exception to these remarks, being mediated by antibody against basement membrane antigen (Section 14) or by circulating immune complexes (Section 13).

These animal autoallergies appear to provide *models for three* distinct *classes of human disease*. Such processes as encephalomyelitis following rabies vaccination and phakogenic uveitis (phakoanaphylactic endophthalmitis) and sympathetic ophthalmia following injury to lens and uvea, respectively, almost certainly have the same mechanism, and a similar correlation of disease with delayed skin reactivity to tissue antigen can be demonstrated in each case. Post- or parainfectious processes (encephalomyelitis, polyneuritis, thyroiditis, etc.) may represent similar allergic reactions to virus, to host antigen incorporated in the viral envelope (of myxoviruses or poxviruses) or host antigens cross-reactive with viral antigens. Evidence as to mechanism is entirely lacking as yet, though the onset of postinfectious disease is closely related in time with the well-recognized delayed allergic response to the virus itself. Finally, chronic relapsing diseases like multiple sclerosis or Hashimoto's thyroiditis, the "organ-specific autoimmune diseases," may have a comparable mechanism to the autoallergies, but there is no convincing evidence of allergic reactivity either to tissue antigen(s) or to neoantigen(s) coded for by hypothetical viruses.

No simple categorization describes *antigens* responsible for the experimental autoallergies. The antigen may be: thyroglobulin in the thyroid case, a basic polypeptide of myelin in the case of encephalomyelitis, a peptide-containing carbohydrate in the testis disease, and protein in the case of the lens. In each instance, the antigen is *a constituent of a functionally specialized tissue* and is not shared with other tissues. However, one may find almost identical antigens in the same tissue of different animal species. This situation is the opposite of the homograft case, where an antigen is common to all cells of a single individual.

The question why autoimmunization is possible is related to the more general problem of tolerance. It is generally accepted that *recognition of self* is based on specific immunologic tolerance, since individuals congenitally lacking fibrinogen or other serum proteins are as readily immunized by infusions of these as if they were totally foreign materials. Therefore the induction of an immune response which permits the elicitation of lesions in a normal animal by autogenous tissue constituents implies that the tolerance mechanism has somehow been bypassed. With completely *segregated antigens*, such as those of myelin and the lens, it is probable that *tolerance never is developed*; there is no mystery involved in the fact that they can be used to induce autoimmunization. In many other instances, however, even where segregated tissue elements are concerned—thyroglobulin is a good example—antigen escapes in small amounts into the blood stream and there is *some degree of tolerance*. A comparative study of immunization against BSA, in rabbits made tolerant to BSA at birth, and against rabbit thyroglobulin in normal, intact rabbits, has shown that, in both cases, *tolerance* can be *broken* by immunization with cross-reacting antigens, i.e. the corresponding proteins from related animal species or conjugates of the homologous proteins with complex haptens. The mechanism of this "breaking" of tolerance is unclear; it may be that lymphocytes forming (or prepared to form) antibody of low combining affinity cannot react with antigen present in the circulation in low concentrations and remain available for immunization. Autoimmunization with cross-reacting antigen has been shown by the use of heterologous species' tissue (heart, kidney, GI tract) or even the use of bacteria cross-reactive with tissue antigen(s), notably streptococcal components with heart and *E. coli* with colon mucosa (Figs. 1.10; 22.3,5). Cross-reactivity between antigens of different organs in the same individual (Figs. 1.11–14) may permit elicitation of lesions at a site remote from the site of immunization.

It should be noted that autoimmunization also occurs, when cells of the *peripheral lymphocyte pool* are *replaced* experimentally *with genetically unrelated cells* not tolerant for antigen(s) of the host. Here transplantation antigens are involved; the lesion is the systemic GVH reaction, described in Section 20. Whether such reactions ever result from transplacental passage of maternal lymphoid cells is at present unknown. A more significant form of autoimmunization occurs in individuals whose lymphocytes show an *abnormality in the development of self-recognition*. The NZB mouse, which has a vertically transmitted, virus-mediated lymphoma, exhibits a marked inability to develop tolerance, accompanied by immunization against many autogenous antigens, among them even widely disseminated soluble and cellular elements of the blood (Figs. 3.7; 13.9). The same defect characterizes human subjects with systemic lupus erythematosus and partial defects of the same type appear to account for other "autoimmune" diseases of the nonorgan-specific type ("connective tissue diseases"). It has been suggested that the neoplastic lymphocytes continue to generate new specificities, a function normally limited to the thymus and other central lymphoid organs, after they enter the peripheral pool and can thus be immunized before developing tolerance to self components. In infectious mononucleosis, another viral disease of lymphocytes, autoimmunization also commonly occurs. The NZB defect can be transferred to normal recipients of the same strain by transfer of peripheral lymphocytes and to recipients of other strains by grafts of NZB thymus.

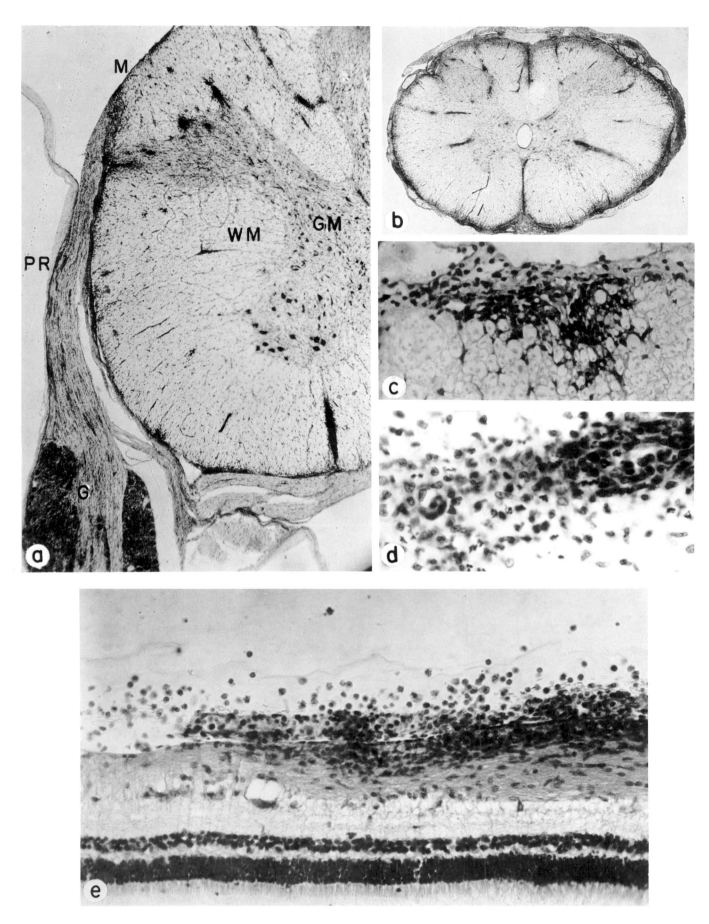

Fig. 21.1. Experimental autoallergic encephalomyelitis, the first well-studied example of the experimental autoallergies. (a) Typical picture of moderate disease in spinal cord of rabbit. Specimen shows anterior and posterior horns of gray matter (GM), the meninges (M), and the posterior (sensory) root (PR) and ganglion (G) to the left. Mild cellular infiltration of the meninges and in the subjacent cord parenchyma is seen, as well as focal perivascular infiltrates in white matter (WM) of cord and the posterior root; ×30. (b) Severe lesion of rabbit spinal cord showing much more extensive subpial invasion of parenchyma forming dark ring around entire cord; ×16. (c) Characteristic wedge-shaped subpial infiltrate of histiocytes (miroglia). Intact axis cylinders, represented by small dots in center of clear zones, are visible within the invaded area; ×160. (d) Perivascular infiltrate from cord section in (b), showing mononuclears and a few polymorphs; ×450. (e) Lesion in nerve fiber layer of the retina in the rabbit. The vitreous is shown above. Note relation of cellular infiltration to small vein on surface of the nerve fiber layer; ×250.

(a, b, d) Cresyl violet; (c, e) hematoxylin-eosin. From Waksman and Adams, *J. Exp. Med. 102*: 213–36 (1955), and *J. Neuropath. 15*: 293–333 (1956); Waksman, *Int. Arch. Allergy*, *14*, suppl.: 1–87 (1959); Bullington and Waksman, *Arch. Ophthal. 59*: 435–45 (1958).

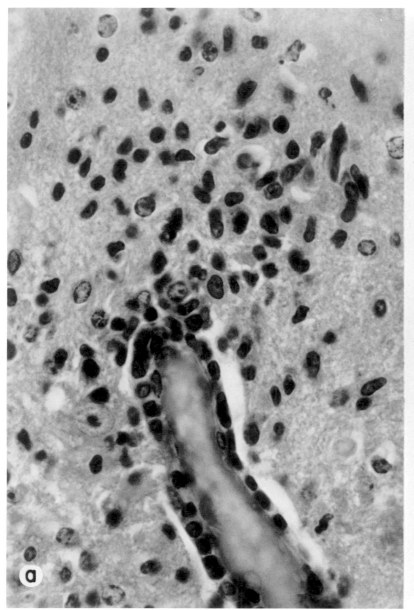 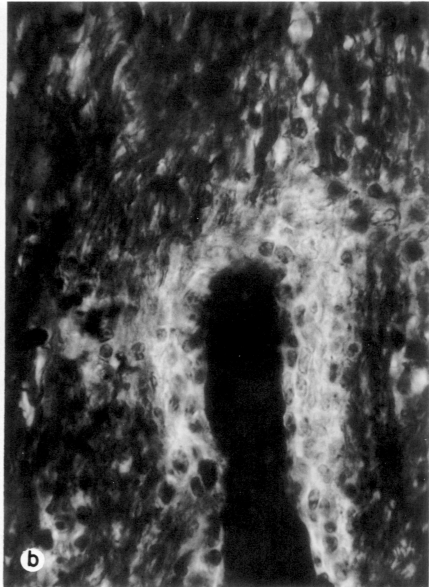

Fig. 21.2. Experimental autoallergic encephalomyelitis. Early lesions in guinea pigs, 8 days after inoculation with nervous tissue and adjuvant. (a) Most of the cells infiltrating the white matter appear intermediate in character between lymphocytes and histiocytes. (b) Myelin destruction in infiltrated zone extends well beyond the pia–glia membrane. Nuclei of infiltrating cells are seen at and just beyond the advancing edge of the zone of demyelination. It is clear from other data that these lesions are less than 48 hours old and perhaps no more than 24.

(a) Hematoxylin-eosin; (b) Loyez stain for myelin; ×680. From Waksman and Adams, *Am. J. Path. 41*: 135–62 (1962).

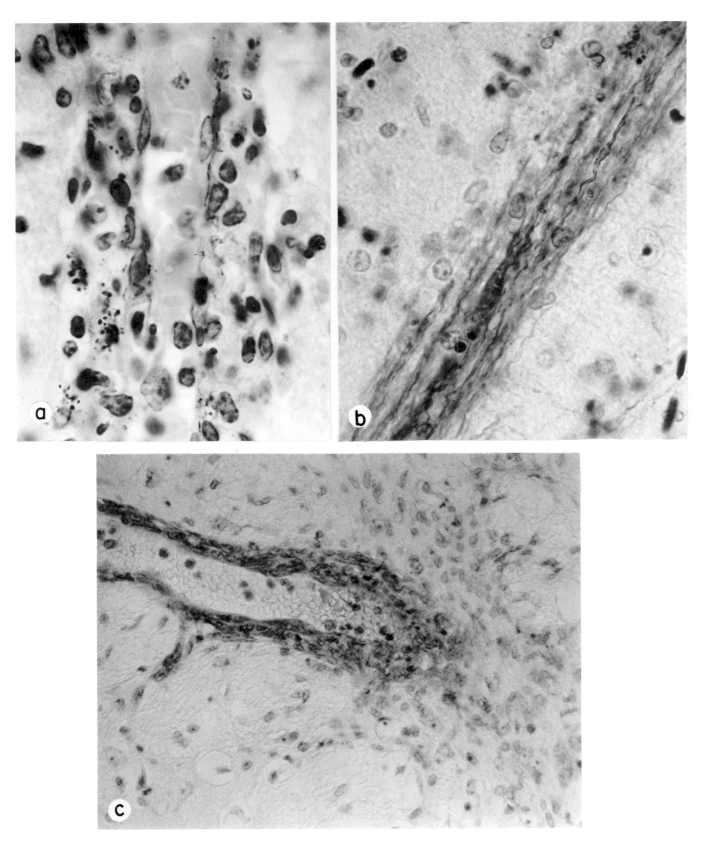

Fig. 21.3. Experimental autoallergic encephalomyelitis. Character of the cells in early guinea pig lesions and their relation to the demyelinative event. (a) Guinea pig injected iv with colloidal carbon at onset of clinical neurological signs and sacrificed 24 hours later. Carbon is present in almost half the infiltrating cells and some is also seen trapped beneath the endothelium. Thus these cells are clearly phagocytic. (b) A small fascicle of myelinated nerve fibers crossing the field is interrupted by mononuclear cells coming from a vessel to the left (outside the field). Destruction of fibers in close proximity to the invading cells is clearly shown. (c) In a methyl green–pyronine stain it is clear that there are no cells of the plasma cell series (which are dark red with this stain) in perivascular infiltrate. All are histiocytic in character; (b, c) are comparable lesions from a guinea pig sacrificed 8 days after inoculation, before onset of clinical disease.

(a) Hematoxylin-eosin; ×1,050. (b) Loyez myelin stain; ×655. (c) Methyl green–pyronine; ×435. From Waksman and Adams, *Am. J. Path. 41*: 135–62 (1962), and unpublished.

Experimental autoallergic encephalomyelitis. Use of labeling with tritiated thymidine (H³T) to identify source of infiltrating cells and occurence of cell division in lesions.

Stripping-film autoradiographs, stained with Giemsa; 21.4 (b) ×1100; all others ×500. From Kosunen, Waksman, and Samuelsson, *J. Neuropath. 22:* 367–80 (1963).

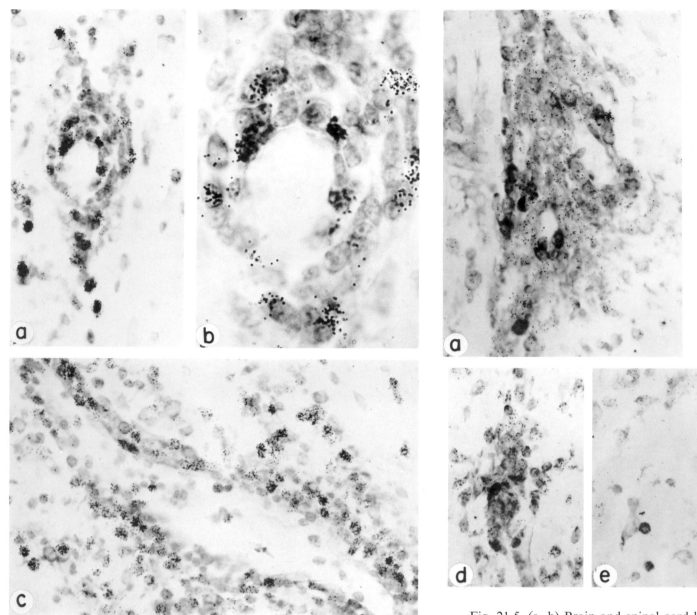

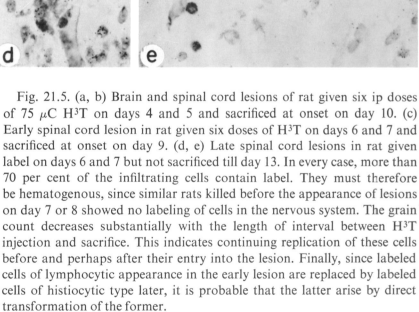

Fig. 21.4. (a, b) Cerebellar lesion in rat sacrificed at onset of clinical disease, 9 days after inoculation and 4 hours after iv injection of H³T (1 μC/g). (c) Similar lesion in rat given H³T at onset on day 10 and sacrificed 24 hours later. Early labeling of mononuclear cells indicates that they divide in lesion. Rapid increase in labeled cells over a 24-hour period implies both cell division and emigration from the blood.

Fig. 21.5. (a, b) Brain and spinal cord lesions of rat given six ip doses of 75 μC H³T on days 4 and 5 and sacrificed at onset on day 10. (c) Early spinal cord lesion in rat given six doses of H³T on days 6 and 7 and sacrificed at onset on day 9. (d, e) Late spinal cord lesions in rat given label on days 6 and 7 but not sacrificed till day 13. In every case, more than 70 per cent of the infiltrating cells contain label. They must therefore be hematogenous, since similar rats killed before the appearance of lesions on day 7 or 8 showed no labeling of cells in the nervous system. The grain count decreases substantially with the length of interval between H³T injection and sacrifice. This indicates continuing replication of these cells before and perhaps after their entry into the lesion. Finally, since labeled cells of lymphocytic appearance in the early lesion are replaced by labeled cells of histiocytic type later, it is probable that the latter arise by direct transformation of the former.

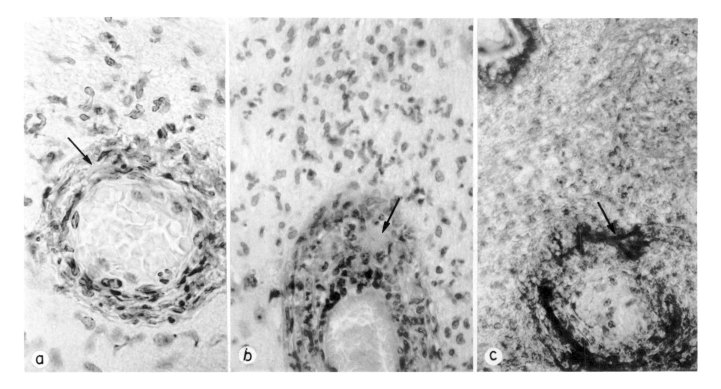

Fig. 21.6. Experimental autollergic encephalomyelitis. Evolution of vascular necrosis in unusually intense lesions. Lesions found 7 days (a) or 8 days (b, c) after inoculation in guinea pig brain, before onset of clinical abnormality. All show the characteristic mononuclear infiltration. Picture is dominated, however, by impregnation of vessel wall with serum protein (arrows), seen in (a) and (b) as grayish homogeneous material, and by massive diapedesis of polymorphonuclear leukocytes, which is just beginning in the very early lesion (a) but is extensive 24 hours later (b). The phosphotungstic acid stain (c) shows presence of "fibrin" in the exudate and confirms the impression that the primary event here involves leakage of plasma proteins.

(a, b) Hematoxylin-eosin, (c) phosphotungstic acid–hematoxylin; (a) ×505, (b, c) ×335. From Waksman and Adams, *Am. J. Path. 41*: 135–62 (1962).

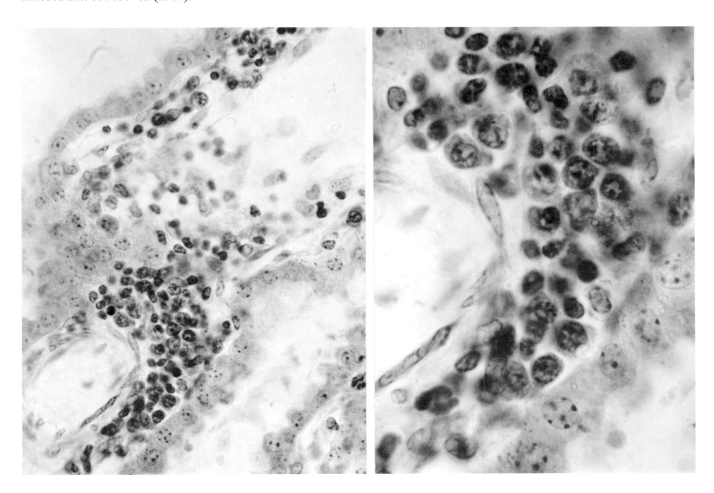

Fig. 21.7. Experimental autoallergic encephalomyelitis. Plasma cells in choroid plexus of guinea pig with disease of several days' duration. These cells are not near the white matter, which contains the antigen to which the animal has been sensitized, nor are they seen in the early phases of lesion formation, illustrated in Figs, 21.2 and 21.3. They are interpreted as representing a local antibody-formation reaction to antigen released into the cerebrospinal fluid, comparable to that seen in the eye (Fig. 5.22, 23).

Methyl green–pyronine; ×400, ×795. Waksman, unpublished.

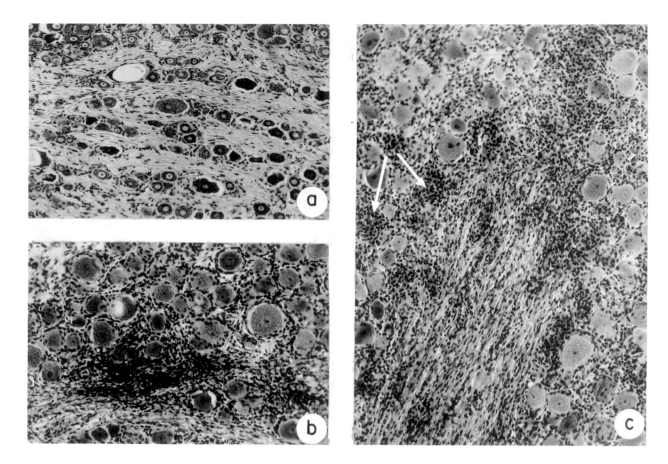

Fig. 21.8. Experimental autoallergic neuritis lesions, produced in rabbit by inoculation with rabbit sciatic nerve and adjuvant. (a) Normal sensory ganglion, showing nerve cells with pale nuclei and prominent nucleoli and myelinated fibers which pass through the ganglion. Schwann cell and fibroblast nuclei appear as dots among the fibers. (b) Focal infiltration of mononuclear cells, mainly lymphocytic in character. (c) Multiple coalescing foci of histiocytic infiltration between myelinated fibers, apparently replacing some of the ganglion cells (arrows).

  (a) Cresyl violet; ×110. (b, c) Hematoxylin-eosin; ×165. From Waksman and Adams, *J. Exp. Med. 102*: 213–36 (1955).

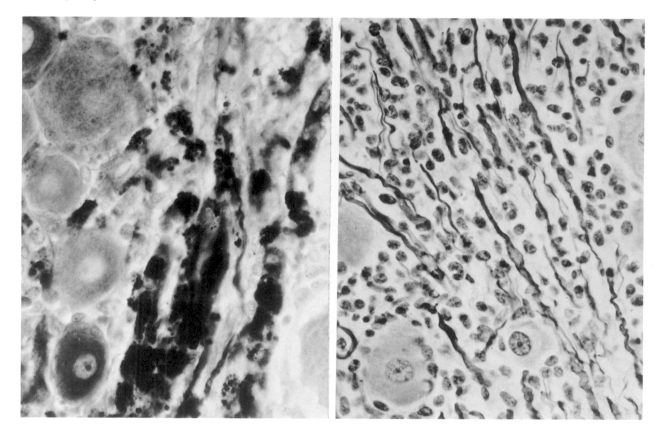

Fig. 21.9. Experimental autoallergic neuritis in rabbit. Involved area of ganglion comparable to that shown in Fig. 21.8(c). (Left) In appropriately stained sections there is extensive breakdown of myelin, with loss of normal tubular structure and appearance of droplets of lipid within macrophages, seen here as clusters or masses of dark-staining material. (Right) Axis cylinders are well preserved, appearing as wavy lines among cellular infiltrates. A few tortuous or dilated segments are seen and may represent degenerating fibers.

  (a) Swank-Davenport stain for myelin and degenerating myelin; ×420. (b) Bodian axis cylinder stain; ×395. From Waksman and Adams, *J. Neuropath. 15*: 293–333 (1956), and *J. Exp. Med. 102*: 213–36 (1955).

Fig. 21.10. Experimental autoallergic neuritis. Severe sciatic nerve lesions in three different experimental species. (a) Rabbit; large, dense lymphohistiocytic infiltrate in center of nerve, accompanied by small lesions above and moderate-sized infiltrate below to the left. In cell stain, myelin damage is not shown, but absence of distortion of fibers above and below major lesion suggests that parenchyma is largely destroyed in region of infiltration. (b) Guinea pig; with this stain, normal myelin (to right) is well shown, and disappearance of myelinated fibers in zone of infiltration is apparent. (c) Rat; again, with myelin stain, destruction of parenchyma and its replacement by granular material within cytoplasm of histiocytes, above and below, is clear. Only a few normal fibers are seen, and most of these possess clearly abnormal segments.

(a) Van Gieson–hematoxylin; ×150. (b) Oil-red-O-hematoxylin; ×250. (c) Weigert's myelin stain; ×250. From Waksman and Adams, *J. Exp. Med. 102*: 213–36 (1955), *J. Neuropath. 15*: 293–333 (1956), and unpublished.

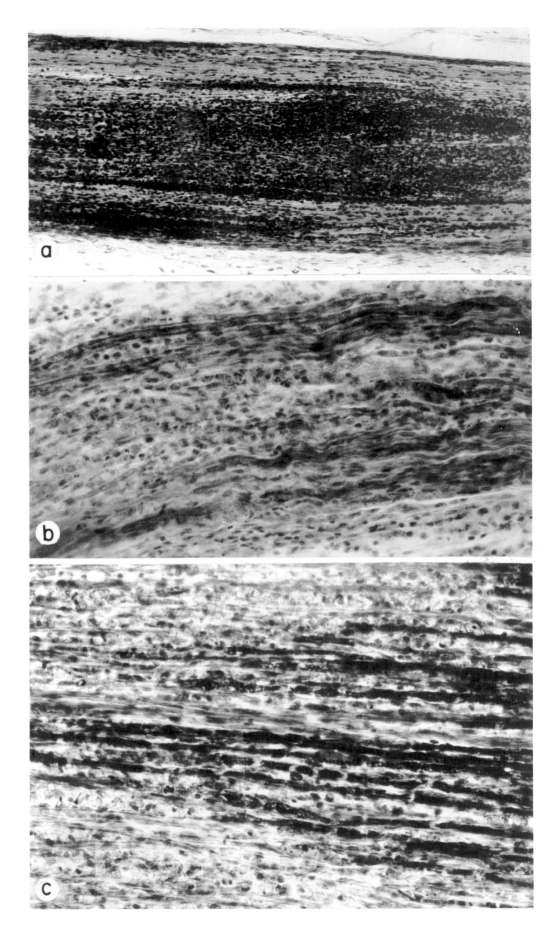

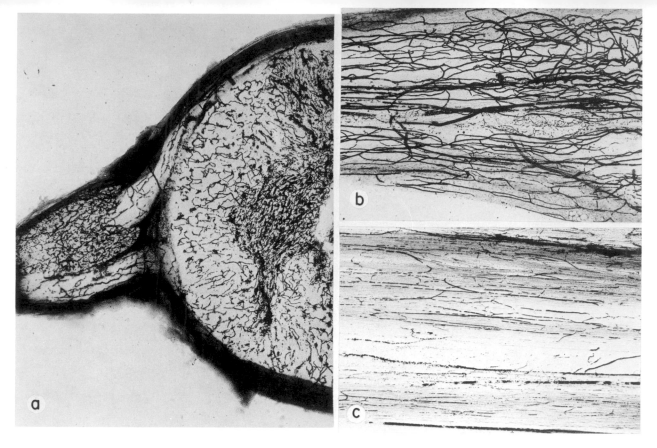

Fig. 21.11. Normal vasculature of nervous system in guinea pig and rabbit. (a) Thoracic spinal cord of guinea pig, with sensory and motor roots (left and right, above) and sensory ganglion. Note dense vascularization of gray matter in cord and of ganglion, areas which are primarily cellular. Most vessels shown are capillaries. A few larger veins are seen at edge of the gray matter and in meninges on surface of the cord, regions where autoallergic encephalomyelitis lesions occur predominantly. (b) Guinea pig sciatic nerve, showing extensive network of veins and venules. Lesions of autoallergic neuritis in this species are diffuse and may occupy entire nerve parenchyma. (c) Rabbit sciatic nerve, showing poorly filled network of capillaries and occasional larger vessel of venous type. Lesions of autoallergic neuritis in rabbit nerve, which are necessarily perivenous, are found accordingly to consist of isolated inflammatory foci.

250μ frozen sections. Pickworth benzidine stain; $\times 28$. From Waksman, *J. Neuropath. Exp. Neurol. 20*: 35–77 (1961).

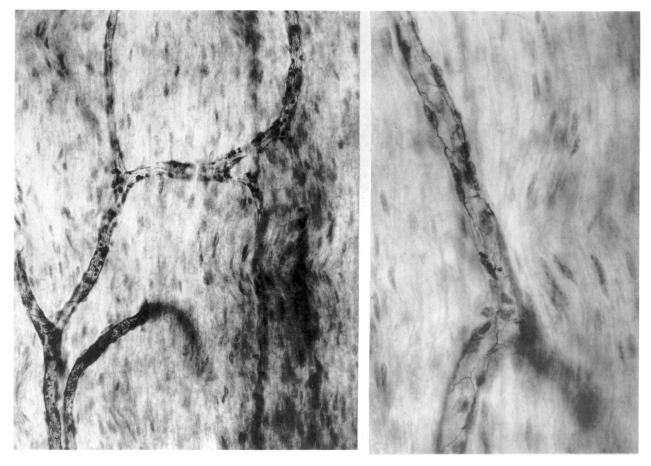

Fig. 21.12. Normal vasculature of guinea pig sciatic nerve. (Left) There is an extensive network of vessels of venous caliber unlike the network in rabbit nerve, which consists largely of capillaries; $\times 200$. (Right) One of the veins under higher power. Irregular junctions between endothelial cells are well shown; $\times 375$.

80μ paraffin sections treated with ammonium sulfide after venous perfusion with lead sulfamate and fixation in Carnoy's fluid; hematoxylin counterstain. From Waksman, *J. Neuropath. Exp. Neurol. 20*: 35–77 (1961).

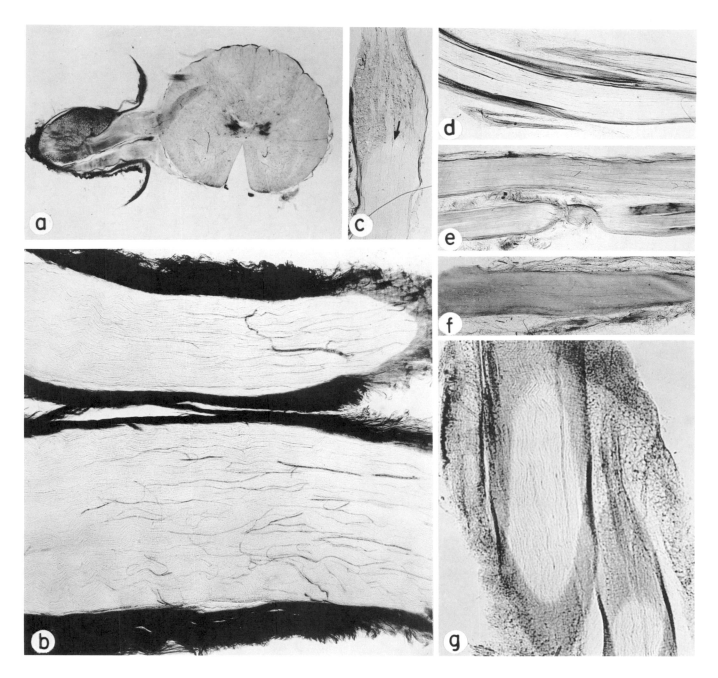

Fig. 21.13. Diffusion of macromolecular acid dyes into parenchyma as index to presence of venous network which favors development of autoallergic lesions. (a) Spinal cord, sensory, and motor spinal nerve roots, and sensory ganglion of monkey injected subcutaneously with Niagara sky blue 6B 5 hours before sacrifice. Slight staining is seen in gray matter and moderate to intense staining in distal portion of roots and in ganglion itself. (b) Sciatic nerve of the same monkey, showing intense staining of peri- and epineurial connective tissue, unstained parenchyma of nerve, and dye-filled capillary plexus. (c) Rabbit sensory ganglion, 1 hour after iv dose of trypan blue. There is sharp demarcation (arrow) between ganglion (above), in which dye has diffused extensively from vessels, and distal portion of sensory root (below), which resembles peripheral nerve and in which no diffusion has occurred. (d) Sciatic nerve of rabbit, 24 hours after trypan blue. Perineurium is deeply stained, but parenchyma of nerve remains free of dye. (e) Sciatic nerve of guinea pig, 1 hour after iv Niagara sky blue 6B, shows moderate to intense staining throughout nerve. (f) Rabbit sciatic, 1 hour after neutral red, shows diffuse staining. (g) Hamster sciatic, 18 hours after Niagara sky blue 6B, shows staining of perineurium but not of nerve parenchyma. Distribution of trypan blue and Niagara sky blue in each case corresponds to distribution of lesions of autoallergic neuritis. Neutral red stains tissue indiscriminately and does not provide a suitable index to location of veins or to lesion distribution.

All sections except (f) were formalin-fixed, 200μ frozen sections, photographed with yellow filter. (f) Fresh tissue, 80μ frozen section, photographed with green filter; (a) ×6.4, (b, g) ×36, remaining photographs ×10.5. From Waksman, *J. Neuropath. Exp. Neurol. 20*: 35–77 (1961).

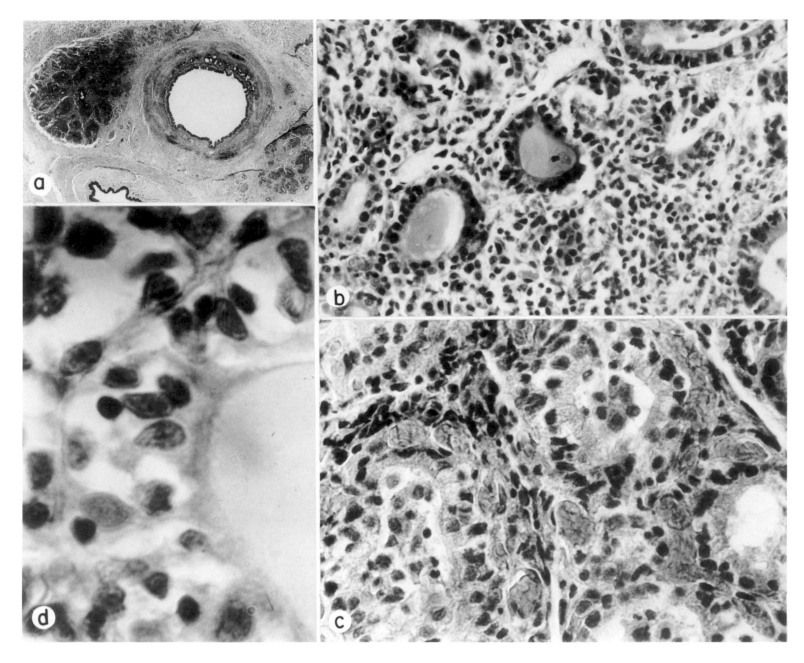

Fig. 21.14. Experimental autoallergic thyroiditis in the rat. (a) Extremely severe disease of one thyroid lobe, in rat given 2 mg rat thyroglobulin, boosted at 3 weeks, and autopsied 1 week later. Thyroid shows massive cell infiltration and disappearance of follicular architecture, under low power; ×13.5. (b) Early, moderately intense lesion, with extensive lymphohistiocytic infiltrate and beginning invasion of follicular epithelium by cells of the infiltrate, in rat immunized with sheep thyroglobulin 13 days earlier; ×350. (c) Later lesion, with many intrafollicular cells, mainly of mature macrophage type, loss of colloid, increased height of follicular epithelium, and dilation of perifollicular vascular plexus; ×675. (d) Detail, showing invasion of follicle epithelium by cells resembling lymphocytes or histiocytes and spongiosis of the epithelium in their immediate vicinity, i.e. formation of fluid-filled spaces between epithelial cells; ×980.

Hematoxylin-eosin. From Jones and Roitt, *Brit. J. Exp. Path.* *42*: 546–57 (1961).

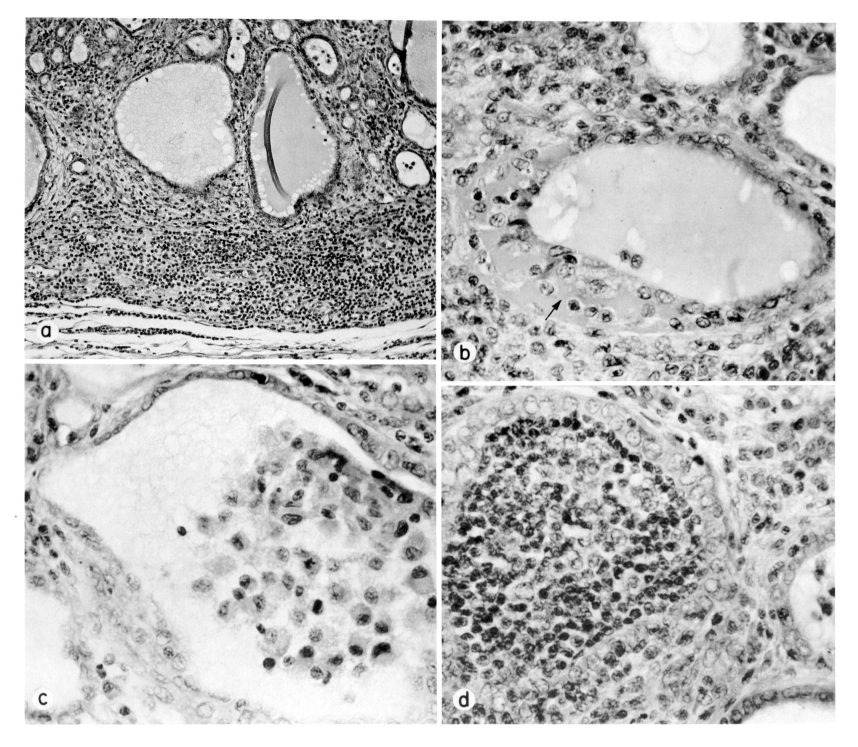

Fig. 21.15. Autoallergic thyroiditis in the rabbit. (a) Inflammation and fibrosis in severely damaged thyroid. Many follicles show resorption of colloid. (ɔ) Leakage of colloid (arrow) from damaged follicle. (c) Invasion of follicle by histiocytes, with formation of mature macrophages and what may be phagocytosis of colloid. (d) Lympho-cyte–histiocyte mass in follicle, probably the end stage of the process shown in (c).

Hematoxylin-eosin; (a) ×76, (b-d) ×430. Material of Drs. Witebsky, Rose, and Terplan; from Waksman, *Int. Arch. Allergy, 14*, suppl.: 1–87 (1959).

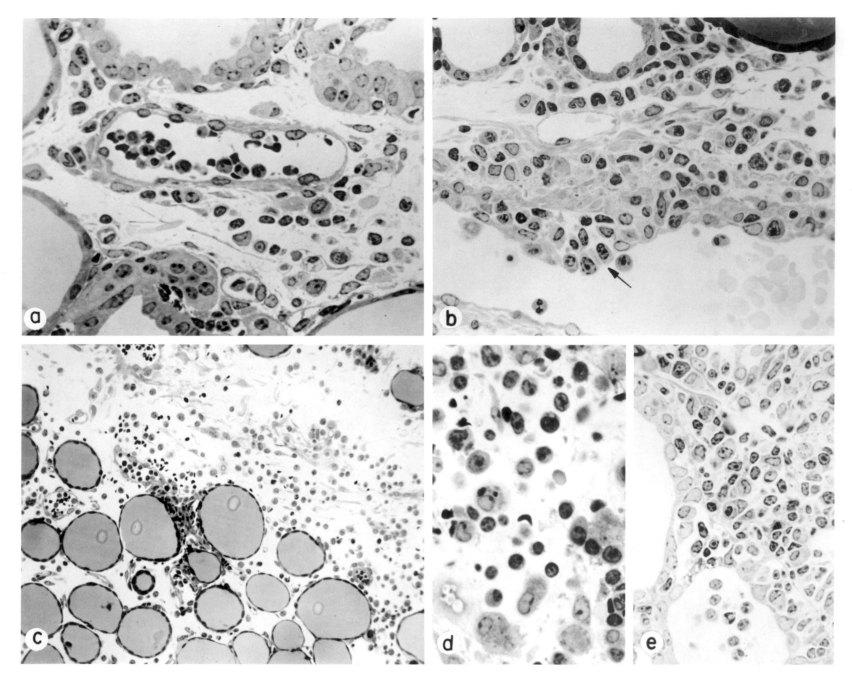

Fig. 21.16. Experimental autoallergic thyroiditis in guinea pigs sensitized with whole guinea pig thyroid extract (1 mg in Freund adjuvant) in footpads. Early evolution of lesions. (a) Four days after inoculation: minimal focal infiltrate of lymphoid mononuclear cells and histiocytes in interstitial tissue adjacent to small vein; ×660. (b) Eight days: similar lesion involving the wall of a vein and producing focal disruption of the normal continuity of endothelial cells (arrow); ×515. (c) Eight days: diffuse interstitial infiltration and edema with no alteration of acini (follicles); ×190. (d) Eight days: cells in the infiltrate are lymphocytic or histiocytic in appearance, and polys are completely lacking. Several histiocytes contain phagocytized material; ×670. (e) Ten days: cell infiltrate has not changed in character, but there is now early invasion of acini by mononuclears. Invading cells within wall of follicle appear to have disrupted attachment of acinar epithelial cells to basement membrane but themselves remain extracellular. Several mononuclears are seen within the lumen of one follicle; ×515.

Methacrylate embedding; thin sections stained with Giemsa. From Flax, *Lab. Invest. 12*: 199–213 (1963).

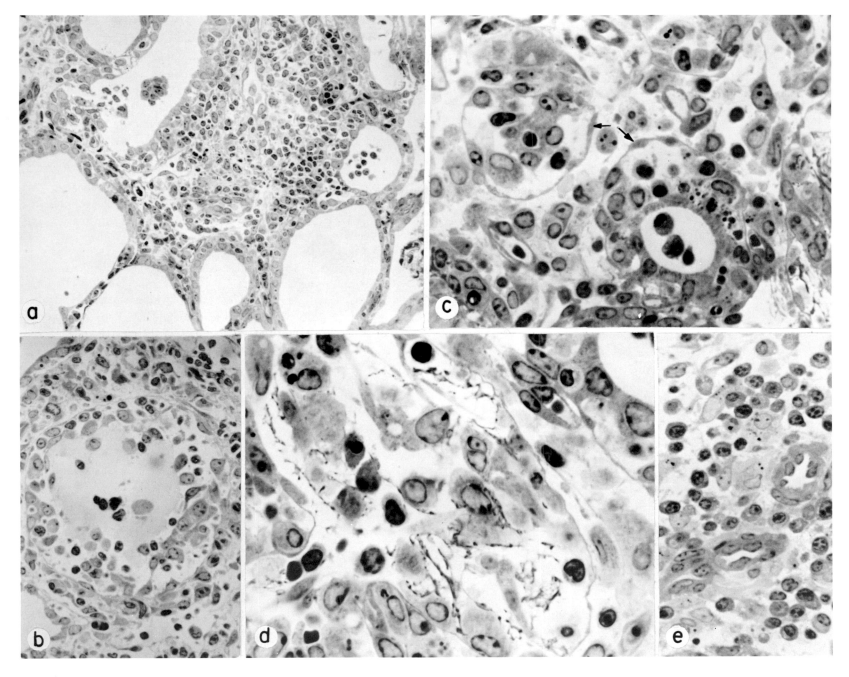

Fig. 21.17. Experimental autoallergic thyroiditis in guinea pigs sensitized with homologous thyroid extract (as in Fig. 21.16). Secondary evolution of lesions. (a) 12 days: cellular infiltrate is more extensive than at 8 days, and almost all acini in field show invasion by mononuclear cells; ×270. (b) Later stage in disruption of follicle by invading cells. Most of the epithelial cells are displaced from the basement membrane and from their neighbors; ×670. (c) Similar changes in several acini, with persistence (and thickening?) of basement membrane (arrows). Many of the invading cells are now typical histiocytes and contain phagocytized material. Similar material

is seen free in acinar wall. The increase in extracellular space (unstained) may represent fluid. This change closely resembles spongiosis of epidermis in lesion of contact allergy (Fig. 16.18); ×465. (d) Still more advanced lesion, in adjacent section, with focal disruption of basement membrane. Enough basement membrane remains to show outline of former follicle. The remaining epithelial cells are mixed with mononuclears; ×975. (e) At 21 days: many typical plasma cells are now present in lesion; ×720.

Methacrylate embedding; thin sections stained with Giemsa. From Flax, *Lab. Invest. 12*: 199–213 (1963).

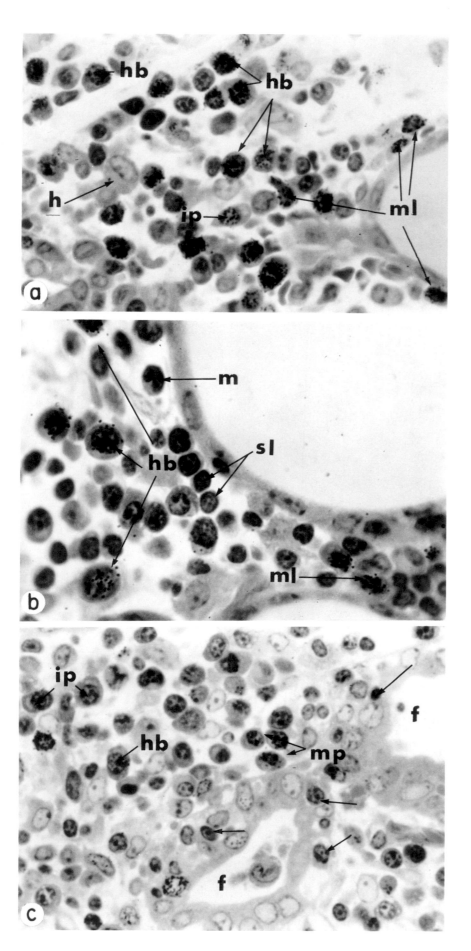

Fig. 21.18. Experimental autoallergic thyroiditis in guinea pig. Analysis of cell infiltrates by use of H³-thymidine and autoradiography. (a) Infiltrate 12 days after sensitization; 1 μC/g of tritiated thymidine was injected iv 1 hour prior to biopsy. Note the high proportion of labeled cells, predominantly medium-large lymphocytes and "hemocytoblasts"; ×900. (b) Infiltrate 20 days after sensitization. One μc/g of tritiated thymidine was injected 1 hour prior to biopsy. Contrast the labeling of "hemocytoblasts" and immature plasma cells with the lack of label in small lymphocytes and mature plasma cells; ×1,280. (c) Mononuclear infiltrate 35 days after sensitization; 1 μc/g of tritiated thymidine was injected 48 hours prior to sacrifice. Mature plasma cells and small lymphocytes are labeled, while "hemocytoblasts" are less heavily labeled than at 1 hour after thymidine administration. Invasion of several follicles, f, by lymphoid cells is indicated by arrows; ×900. h, Histiocyte; m, monocyte; sl, small lymphocyte; ml, medium-large lymphocyte; hb, "hemocytoblast"; ip, immature plasma cell; mp, mature plasma cell.

Thin sections; stripping-film autoradiographs, stained with Giemsa. From Kosunen and Flax, *Lab. Invest. 15*: 606–16 (1966).

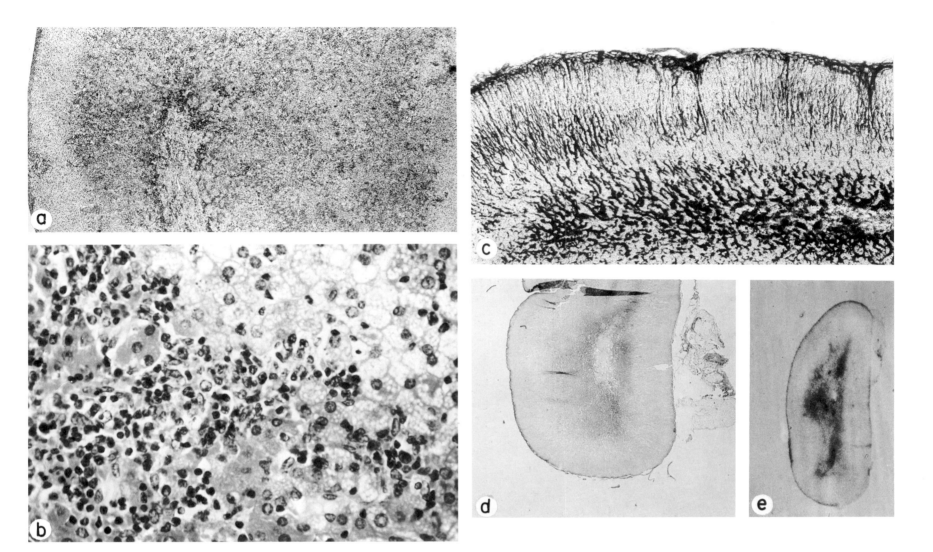

Fig. 21.19. Experimental autoallergic adrenalitis in the guinea pig and its relation to vascular network in this organ. (a) Massive cellular infiltration of zona reticularis and scattered inflammatory foci in much of the remainder of cortex and in medulla. (b) Infiltrating cells are almost entirely pleomorphic lymphocytes and histiocytes. In invaded zone, parenchymal elements of adrenal cortex have been destroyed (note lack of compression by infiltrate). (c) Vessels of the normal guinea pig adrenal. Veins are largely limited to the zona reticularis and inner portion of the zona fasciculata. This distribution corresponds to the distribution in which the lesions, illustrated in (a) and (b), develop. (d) Staining of same region (inner zone of cortex), 20 minutes after iv injection of Niagara sky blue 6B. (e) Penetration of I^{131}-labeled human serum albumin into the same zone, 18 hours after its injection iv.

(a, b) Hematoxylin-eosin; $\times 31$, $\times 400$. (c) Frozen section, 250 μ; Pickworth benzidine stain; $\times 32$. (d) Carnoy's fixative, paraffin section, 16μ; $\times 10.5$. (e) Stripping-film autoradiograph, $\times 5.5$. (a, b) Preparation of Dr. J. Colover. From Waksman, *Int. Arch. Allergy*, *14*, suppl.: 1–87 (1959). (c–e) From Waksman, *Am. J. Path. 37*: 673–93 (1960).

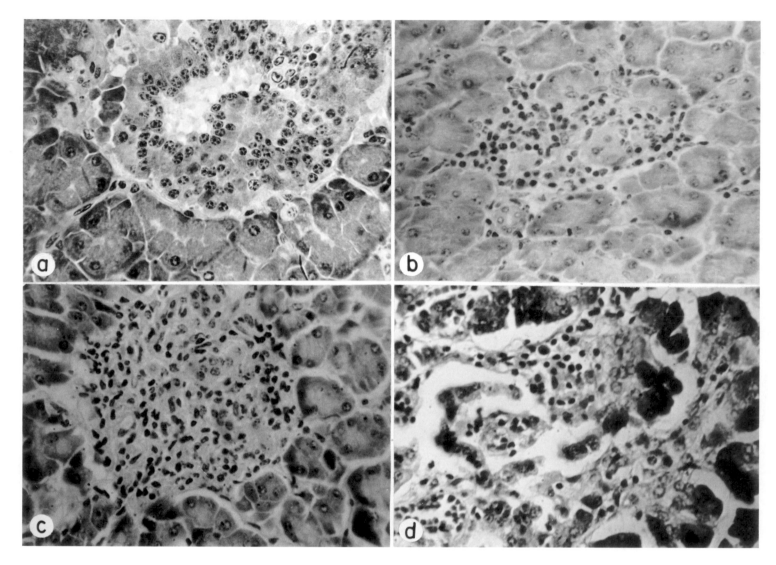

Fig. 21.20. Inflammatory lesions of pancreatic islets of Langerhans produced by immunization of heifers with isologous or heterologous insulin. (a) Normal islet showing ellipsoidal shape, regular, closely packed nuclei of B cells, and open space in center, all characteristics of bovine islets. (b) Abnormal islet in pancreas of heifer injected repeatedly for almost 2 years with bovine insulin in adjuvant. The outstanding change is lymphocytic infiltration, and almost every islet shows this in some degree. There is clear-cut loss of B cells in area of infiltration. The exocrine tissue about the islet appears normal. (c) More advanced islet lesion, showing lymphocytic in-filtration, extensive destruction of islet cells, and fibrosis, in pancreas of cow receiving seven injections of pork insulin followed by seven injections of beef insulin, both in adjuvant. Again, exocrine tissue is normal. (d) Islet lesion ("insulitis") from human subject (17-year, male), dying in coma after showing diabetic symptoms for 2 weeks. There is lymphocytic infiltrate, and most of the islet has been destroyed.

All hematoxylin-eosin, at same magnification. From Le-Compte, Steinke, Soeldner, and Renold, *Diabetes 15*: 586–96 (1966).

Autoallergic orchitis produced in adult (500-g) Hartley guinea pigs by single subcutaneous or intradermal injection of guinea pig testis homogenate plus Freund's complete adjuvant.

Figure 21.22 is from Waksman, in *CIBA Foundation Symposium on Cellular Aspects of Immunity*, G. E. W. Wolstenholme and M. O'Connor, eds., Churchill, London, 1960, pp. 280–322. Other plates are from Waksman, *J. Exp. Med. 109*: 311–24 (1959).

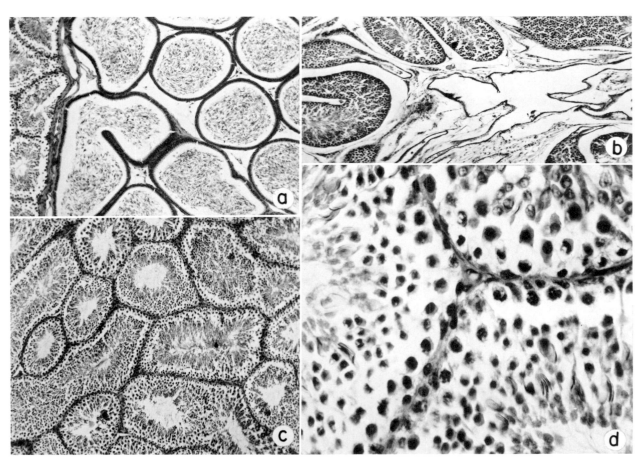

Fig. 21.21. Control testis, from animal given adjuvant alone intradermally and sacrificed at 26 days, showing normal appearance of epididymis (a), filled with mature spermatozoa; rete testis (b); and seminiferous tubules (c, d), containing all stages of maturation of the germinal epithelium from spermatogonia to spermatozoa.
Hematoxylin-eosin; (a–c) × 72, (d) × 410.

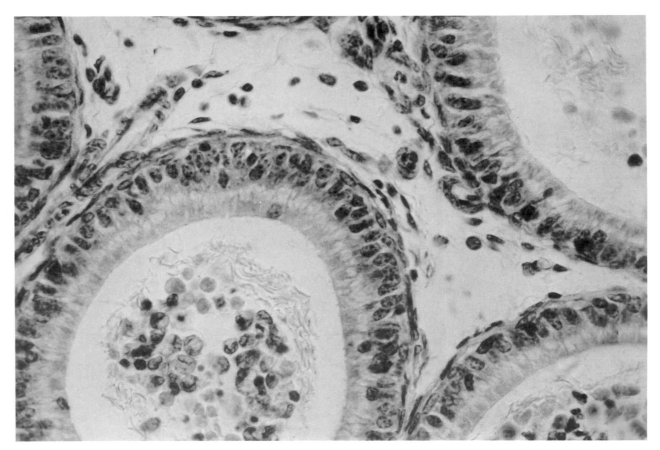

Fig. 21.22. Early epididymitis, 12 days after intradermal inoculation of testis plus adjuvant. A few lymphocytes and histiocytes have appeared in mesenchyme between tubules, and many histiocytes are seen within the tubules. There are no pyroninophilic cells at either locus.
Methyl green–pyronine; × 360.

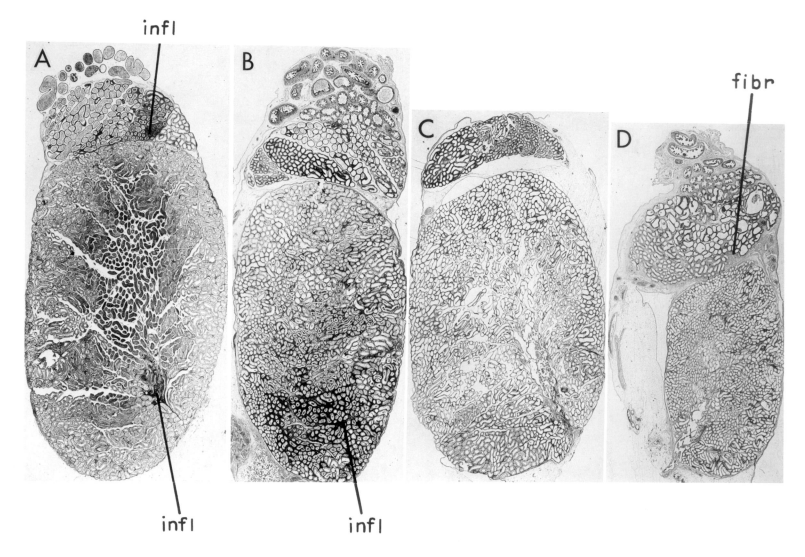

Fig. 21.23. Successive stages of orchitis and aspermatogenesis in animals given testis plus adjuvant intradermally and sacrificed at 12, 19, 26, and 36 days. Higher-power views are given in succeeding plates.

Hematoxylin-eosin; ×6.0.

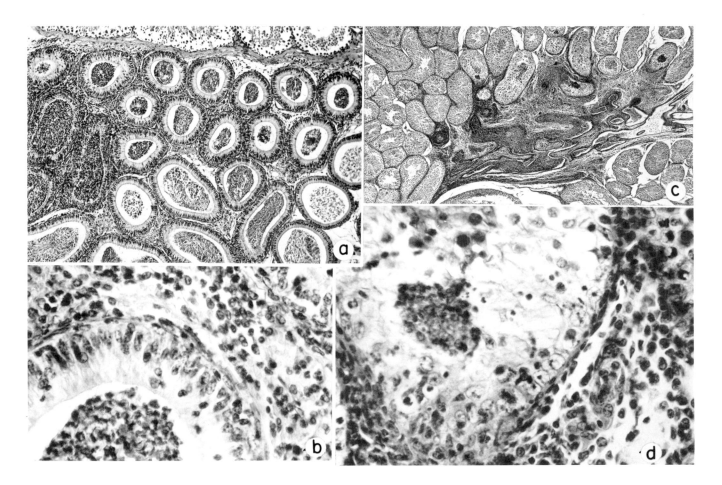

Fig. 21.24. Inflammatory lesions of epidymis (a, b) and rete testis (c, d) from testis shown in Fig. 21.23(a). There is massive interstitial infiltrate of lymphocytes and histiocytes, with invasion of tubules and destruction of tubular contents (spermatozoa in epididymal tubules, germinal epithelium in seminiferous tubules near rete). There are many polymorphonuclears in the inflammatory mass within tubules. Note completely normal tubules adjacent to involved area.

Hematoxylin-eosin; (a) ×66, (c) ×31, (b, d) ×375.

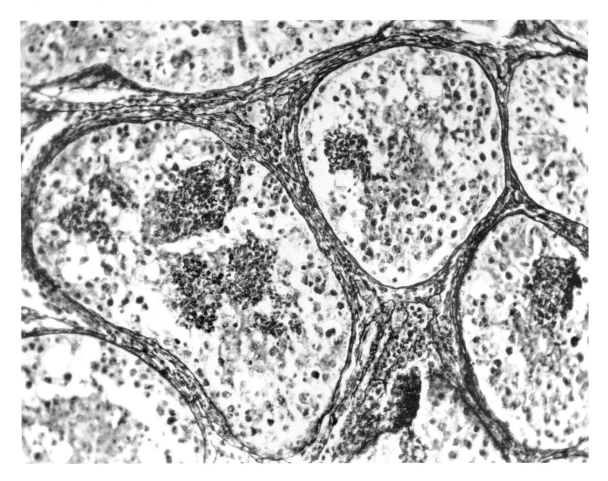

Fig. 21.25. Formation of masses of inflammatory cells within seminiferous tubules with preservation of tubular architecture. Except at one point, basement membrane of tubules appears intact.

Sweet's reticulum stain; ×225.

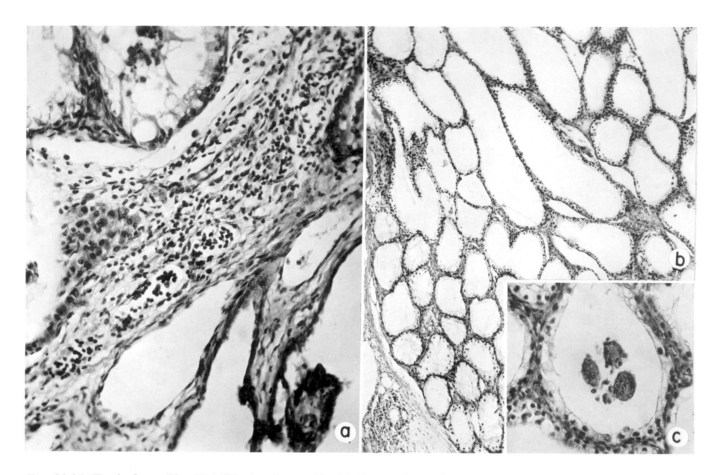

Fig. 21.26. Testis from Fig. 21.23(c) showing residual inflammation adjacent to rete tubules (a), advanced general aspermatogenesis (b), and histiocytic giant cells remaining in empty seminiferous tubule (c). Inflammation has largely resolved.

Hematoxylin-eosin; (a, c) ×200, (b) ×72.

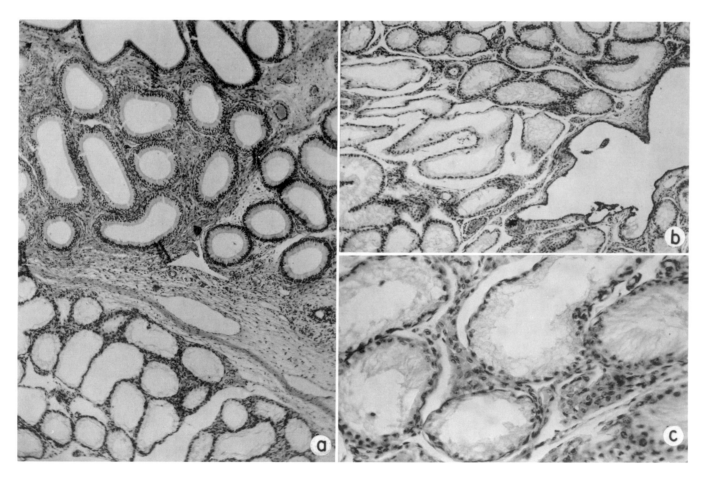

Fig. 21.27. Testis from Fig. 21.23(d). (a) Empty epididymal tubules and fibrosis, interpreted as secondary to the inflammation seen in earlier specimens. (b, c) Rete and seminiferous tubules, showing complete aspermatogenesis, proliferation of Sertoli cells, and hypertrophy of Leydig cell masses between tubules.

Hematoxylin-eosin. (a, b) ×70, (c) ×200.

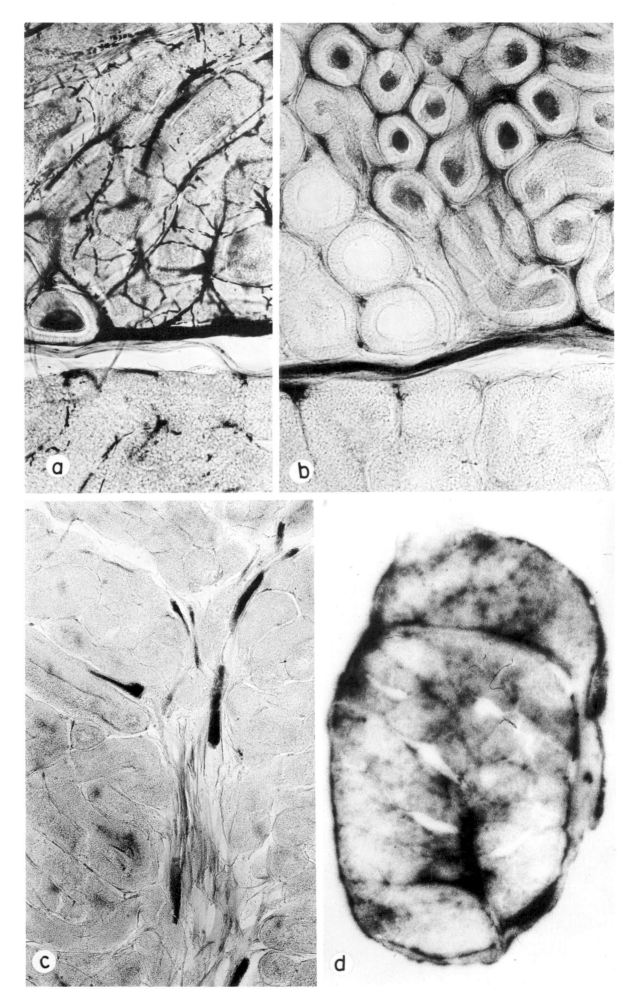

Fig. 21.28. (a) Character of vessels in guinea pig epididymis and testis and their relation to distribution of lesions in experimental autoallergic orchitis. Many veins and venules are seen in epididymis (above) while almost no vessels larger than capillaries are present among seminiferous tubules (below). (b) Injected dye, Niagara sky blue 6B given iv 20 minutes earlier, impregnates the epididymis but does not leave the vascular compartment in the zone of tissue lacking veins. (c) Rete testis in same guinea pig, showing dye within large veins and *in vivo* staining of adjacent tubules. (d) Leakage from vessels of I[131]-HSA, injected iv 18 hours earlier. Accumulation of label is most apparent in subcapsular distribution and in area of rete testis; lesser amounts are seen in epididymis and in central part of testis along branches of rete veins.

   (a) Frozen section, 250 μ; Pickworth benzidine stain; ×80. (b, c) Frozen sections, 200 μ; ×80 and ×37, photographed through orange filter. (d) Stripping-film autoradiograph; ×6.5. From Waksman, *Am. J. Path.* 37: 673–93 (1960).

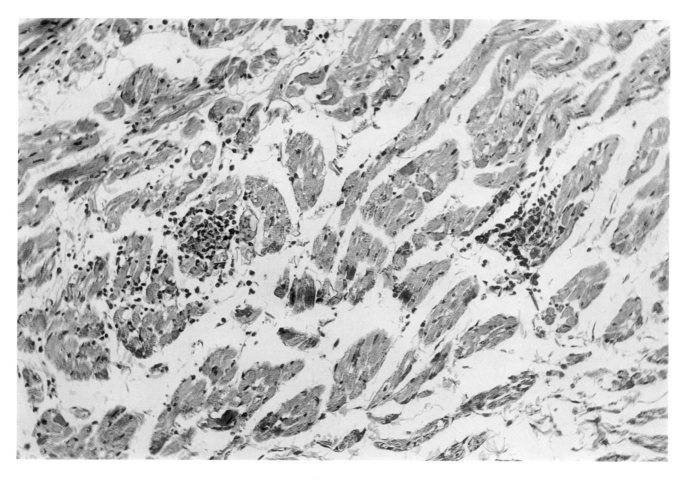

Fig. 21.29. Autoallergic lesions of ventricular myocardium in rabbit immunized with beef heart muscle homogenate, injected subcutaneously in aluminum hydroxide gel at weekly intervals for approximately 2 months. There are focal infiltrates of poly- and mononuclear cells and vacuolization and necrosis of myofibers in zone of infiltration.

Hematoxylin-eosin; × 240. From Kaplan and Craig, *J. Immunol. 90*: 725–33 (1963).

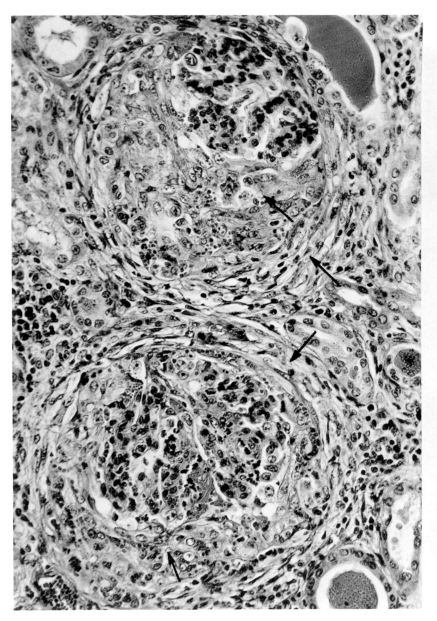 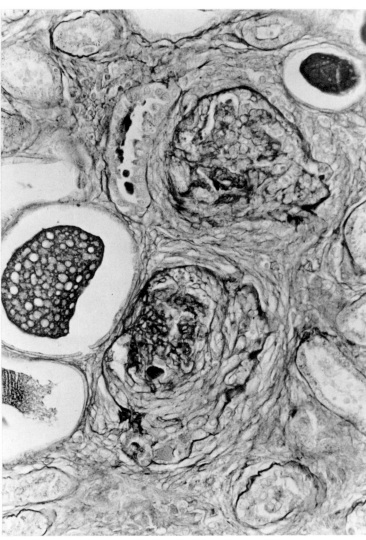

Fig. 21.30. Autoallergic renal lesion from sheep, injected repeatedly with human glomerular basement membrane in complete Freund adjuvant (total dose 912 mg) and sacrificed at 50 days (blood urea nitrogen 300). (Left) Typical subacute glomerulonephritis, with marked fibroepithelial proliferation of Bowman's capsule (cresent formation; arrows) and compression of glomerular tufts, which are hypercellular and show both areas of necrosis and poly-morphonuclear infiltration. Blood and casts are present in the tubules, and the interstitial spaces show mononuclear cell infiltration and some increase of connective tissue. (Right) Two obsolescent glomeruli are shown with disruption of the original Bowman's capsule and extensive fibrosis inside and outside the glomerulus.

(Left) Hematoxylin-eosin; ×320. (Right) Periodic acid-Schiff; ×350. From Steblay, *J. Exp. Med. 116*: 253–72 (1962).

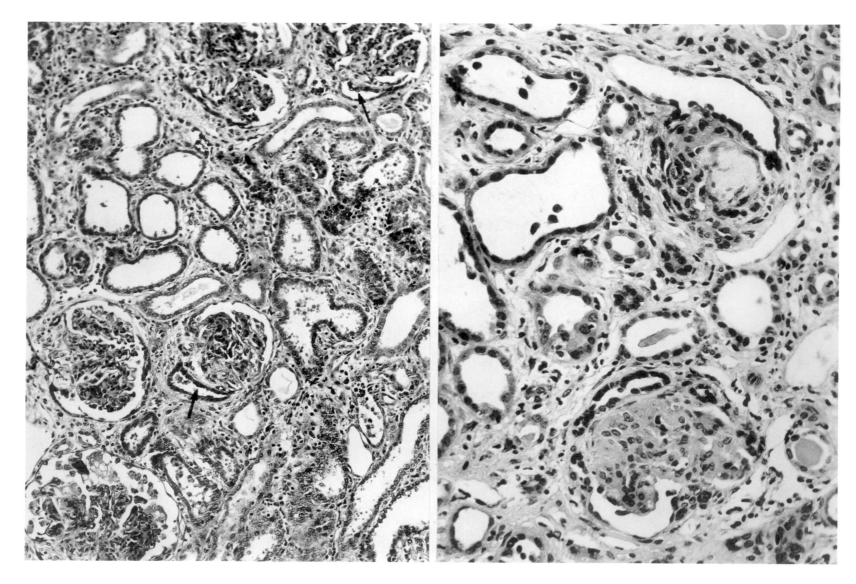

Fig. 21.31. Autoallergic renal lesion in the monkey. (Left) Animal immunized repeatedly by multiple portals with human glomerular basement membrane and adjuvant (total dose 250 mg) and sacrificed at 102 days. There is cellular proliferation and distortion of glomerular tufts, with adhesions and formation of pseudotubles (arrows) whose cuboidal epithelium is derived from parietal epithelium of Bowman's capsule and visceral epithelium of the glomerulus. Marked interstitial infiltration of mononuclear cells and fibrosis are present, as well as tubular dilatation and atrophy. Small, darkly stained mononuclears surrounded by a clear halo resemble closely the infiltrating cells seen in other autoallergies and other reactions of cellular sensitivity; × 155. (Right) Similar lesion in a monkey given 400 mg of dog glomerular basement membrane and adjuvant and biopsied at 161 days. Glomeruli show advanced degree of scarring; × 355.

Hematoxylin-eosin. From Steblay, in *Thirteenth Annual Nephrotic Conference*, J. Metcoff, ed., Northwestern Univ. Press, Evanston, Ill., 1962, pp. 105–16; and unpublished.

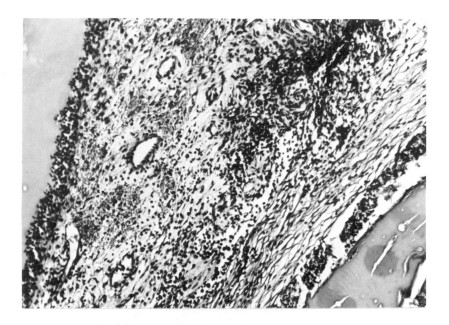

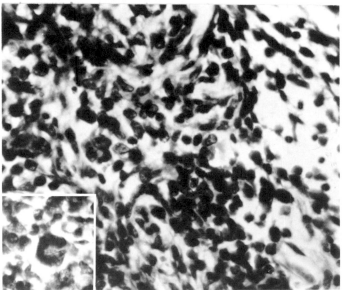

Fig. 21.32. Autoallergic uveitis in response to lens antigen in the rabbit. (Above) Ten-day lesion in eye shows massive iris inflammation. There is a band of necrotic tissue between the iris and the traumatized lens (right), and numerous macrophages and polymorphonuclears have accumulated on anterior surface of the iris (left); ×125. (Below) Higher-power view of iris lesion shows that the principal infiltrating cell is histiocytic. Insert shows a histiocytic giant cell from another part of the same lesion; ×450.

Hematoxylin-eosin. Courtesy of Drs. A. M. Silverstein and L. Zimmerman, unpublished studies, 1958.

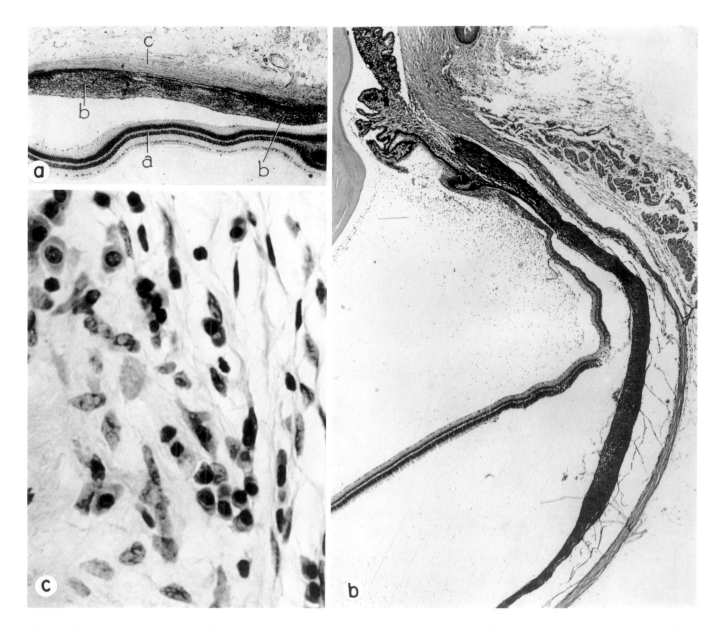

Fig. 21.33. Experimental autoallergic uveitis in guinea pigs immunized repeatedly with homologous uvea (iris, ciliary body, and choroid) plus Freund adjuvant. Both (a) and (b) show severe chronic choroiditis, with massive diffuse infiltrations of mononuclear cells and formation of large nodular aggregates of these cells. There is mild involvement of the ciliary body and iris (b, above), and the retina is undamaged. The letters a, b, and c in (a) designate the retina; nodules of lymphocytes, histiocytes, and plasma cells; and the sclera, respectively. (c) Mild ciliary body lesion with predominantly plasma cellular reaction.

Hematoxylin-eosin; (a) ×19, (b) ×9.5, (c) ×380. (a) From Collins, *Am. J. Ophthal. 32*: 1687–99 (1949), and *36*, part II: 150–62 (1953). (b, c) From Aronson, Hogan, and Zweigart, *Arch Ophthal. 69*: 208–19 (1963); and Aronson, *Ann. N.Y. Acad. Sci. 124*: 365–76 (1965).

22. Autoantibodies in Human Disease

Circulating autoantibodies have been demonstrated, accompanying a number of human diseases and experimental animal lesions, by the use of sensitive serological methods. Among these are gel diffusion, passive hemagglutination and agglutination of other particles (such as collodion, latex, and bentonite), the Coombs method, antiglobulin consumption, and immunofluorescence. Several examples are shown here and in Section 1 (Figs. 1.3–5,9,10,12–14; 22.1,3,5,6). Pathologic effects which are produced by autoantibody depend entirely on the location and nature of the antigen. These are described earlier and listed here merely for convenience. Antibody against biologically active materials, present in body fluids in low concentration (Fig. 9.1), may neutralize their activity (Section 9). Antibody against serum proteins or other body constituents present in higher concentration in the circulation may produce immune complex disease (Fig. 13.10) with renal, joint, or other lesions (Section 13). Antibody against intercellular substances (Fig. 22.4) may produce cell separation and bullous lesions (Section 10). Antibody against basement membrane (and other connective tissue antigens?) (Fig. 1.17) may produce immune complex disease limited to the glomerular basement membrane, the lung, or other discrete organ sites (Section 14). Antibody against cells in suspension (Figs. 1.4,5; 10.2) or monolayer may produce disease of cellular elements of the blood (Figs. 10.12–15), vascular endothelium, and possibly other endothelial or mesothelial tissues (Section 10). Finally, antibody against cellular antigens of solid tissues may produce little pathologic effect.

The production of autoantibody is essentially unrelated to the autoallergy problem, except that most modes of immunization which induce cellular sensitization also give rise to antibody formation against the same (auto)-antigen. In many of the cellular lesions affecting organs like the thyroid (both animal and human), antibody-forming cells appear in the lesion itself (Figs. 6.11,12; 22.1); in such cases its presence may be used as an index for the presence of lesions. The antibodies that have been described, however, play no apparent role in the pathogenesis of the corresponding lesions. Yet it is widely thought that they may modify the alterations produced by the cellular mechanism. In such instances as the aspermatogenesis that accompanies autoallergic orchitis (Figs. 21.21–27) antibody may play a pathogenetic role, but it remains to be demonstrated by convincing passive transfer experiments. In autoimmune renal disease, humoral antibody is the effective mediator, as noted earlier.

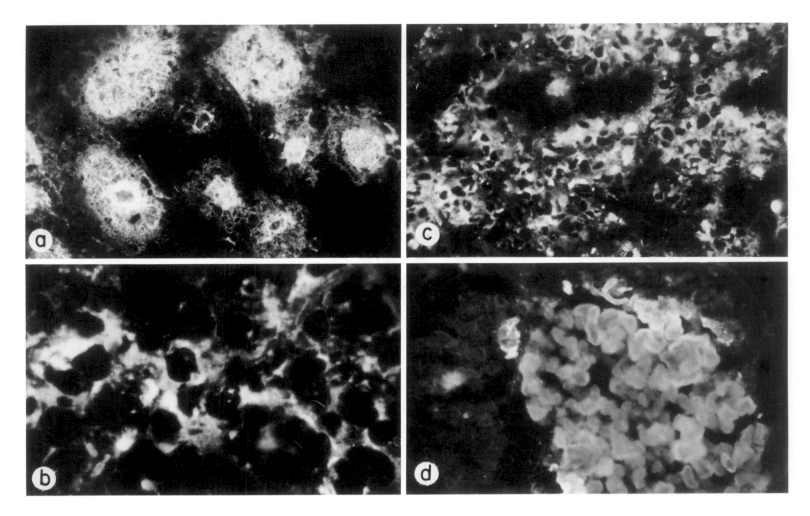

Fig. 22.1. Immunohistochemistry of chronic nonspecific thyroiditis in man. (a) Thyroglobulin, stained with fluorescent rabbit antibody to human thyroglobulin, shows lacelike distribution within small, colloid-containing follicles (bright areas); ×265. (b) Thyroglobulin distributed outside of thyroid follicles, between. and possibly within cells of the dense plasma cell and lymphoid infiltrate; ×1,330. (c) Cells containing, and apparently forming, antibody to thyroglobulin are plasma cells of immature and mature types distributed in the dense mononuclear cell infiltrate surrounding and replacing the follicular epithelium and colloid. Stained with fluorescent human thyroglobulin; ×490. (d) Follicular thyroglobulin intimately associated with human 7S γ-globulin and having a globular or lobulated appearance. Stained with fluorescent rabbit antibody to human 7S γ-globulin; ×390.

From Mellors, Brzosko, and Sonkin, *Am. J. Path. 41*: 425–37 (1962).

Fig. 22.2. Homogeneous nuclear staining by antinuclear antibody. (Left) Specific fluorescence of leukocytes in a positive lupus erythematosus preparation (normal human white cells plus serum from a patient with systemic lupus erythematosus). γ-Globulin localization in the nuclei of leukocytes which are undergoing transformation prior to phagocytosis and formation of LE cells. Unfixed LE preparation treated with acetone for 10 minutes and stained with fluorescent antibody for human γ-globulin. (Right) Total absence of specific fluorescence in nuclei (arrows) of leukocytes in a negative LE preparation.

Both ×500. From Mellors, Ortega, and Holman, *J. Exp. Med. 106*: 191–202 (1957).

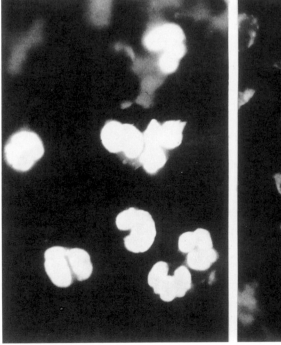
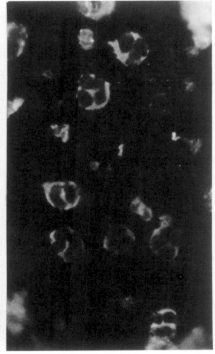

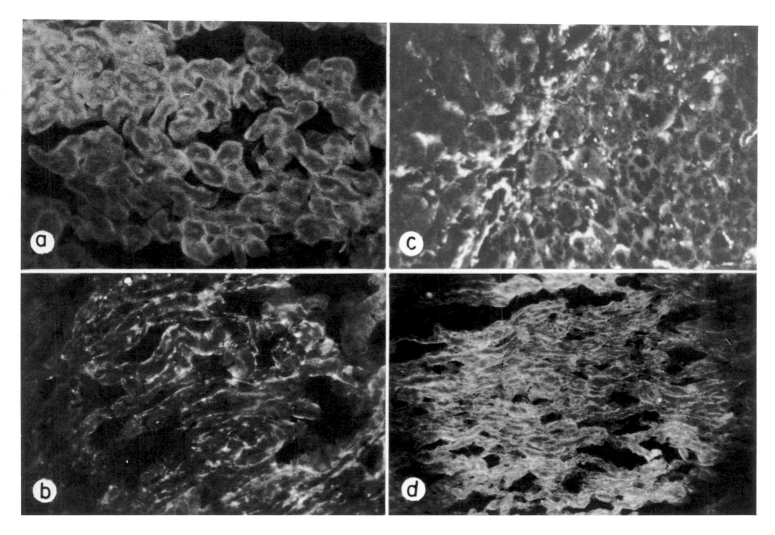

Fig. 22.3. Immunohistochemistry of rheumatic fever. (a, b) Cross-reaction, shown by fluorescence staining, of rabbit antiserum against group A streptococcal cell walls (strain Tripp, type 5) with normal human heart. Reactive site localized to sarcolemma of cardiac myofibers; ×300. (a) Unfixed, frozen section, (b) is alcohol-fixed. Staining reaction is enhanced in (b). (c) "Bound" γ-globulin in auricular appendage of patient with rheumatic heart disease, demonstrated by fluorescence technique. Staining is seen in interstitial connective tissue, apparently fused with segments of sarcolemma, and extends into subsarcolemmal sarcoplasm; ×200.

(d) Localization of β_{1c}-globulin, identified as part of the C′3 component of human complement, in sarcolemma of myofibers in left ventricle of 5-year-old boy dying of rheumatic fever; ×125.

Indirect fluorescence technique. (a, b) Courtesy of Dr. M. Kaplan (see Kaplan, *J. Immunol.* *90*: 595–606, 1963). (c) From Kaplan and Dallenbach *J. Exp. Med.* *113*: 1–16 (1961). (d) From Kaplan, Bolande, Rokita, and Blair, *New Engl. J. Med.* *271:* 637–45 (1964), reproduced with permission of *The New England Journal of Medicine.*

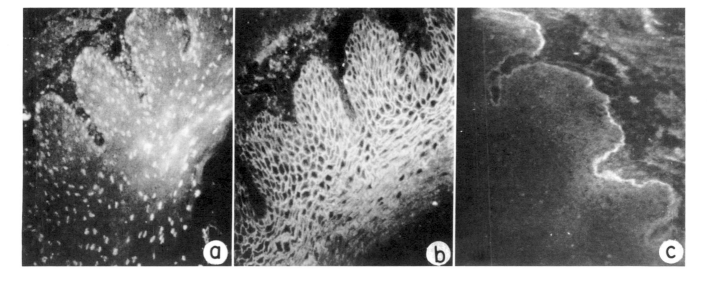

Fig. 22.4. Indirect immunofluorescence staining reactions of human sera with the epithelium of unfixed sections of monkey esophagus; a conjugate of a rabbit antiserum to chromatographically pure human γG was used. (a) Reaction of nuclear antibodies. Section treated with a 1:10 dilution of serum from patient with a "collagen disease." Lumen of esophagus is at lower right. Only nuclei are stained. (b) Section treated with 1:10 serum from a fatal case of pemphigus vulgaris shows intercellular staining pattern characteristically produced by pemphigus serum. Lumen of esophagus lower right. (c) Staining of basement membrane by antibodies in serum of a patient with active bullous pemphigoid (bullous dermatitis herpetiformis). Lumen of esophagus lower left.

    All ×120. From Beutner, *Derm. Digest* *6*: 55–63 (1967).

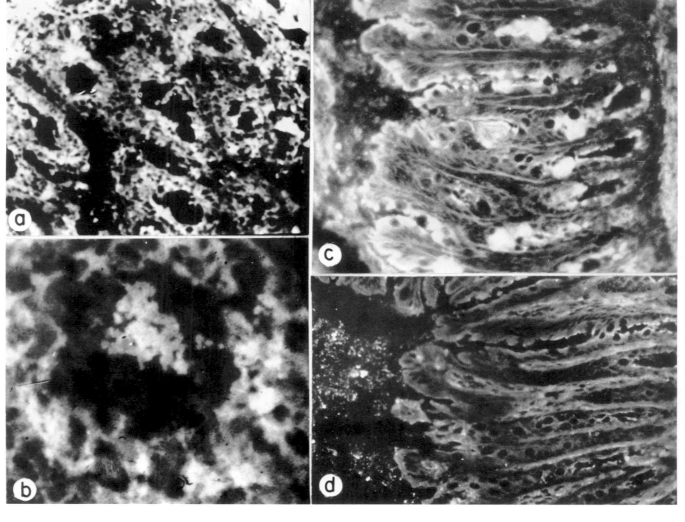

Fig. 22.5. Immunohistochemistry of chronic ulcerative colitis. (a) Human colonic mucosa stained by fluorescein-labeled serum from human patient with the disease. Specific antibody in serum stains epithelial cells, nuclei remaining unstained; ×290. (b) Cross section of colonic crypt, similarly treated, shows staining of epithelial cells and central secretory mass; ×485. (c, d) Sections of rat colon, stained by the indirect technique with ulcerative colitis serum and normal human serum respectively. The goblet cells in particular contain an organ-specific antigen and show specific staining; ×405.

From Broberger and Perlmann, *J. Exp. Med. 115*: 13–26 (1962), and unpublished; and Lagercrantz, Hammarström, Perlmann, and Gustafsson, *Clin. Exp. Immunol. 1*: 263–76 (1966).

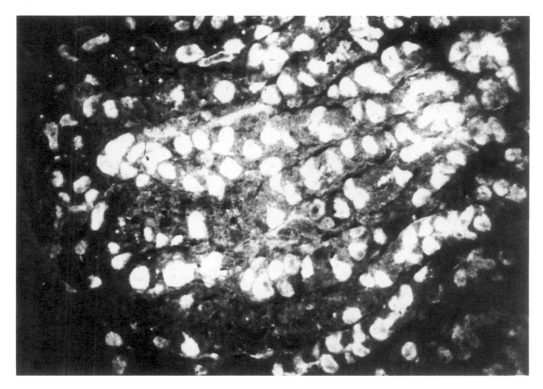

Fig. 22.6. Immunohistochemistry of pernicious anemia. Diffuse cytoplasmic staining of the parietal cells in unfixed section of human gastric mucosa treated with serum from a patient with pernicious anemia. The pepsin-producing (chief) cells are not stained. Parietal cell antibodies are complement fixing and react with the microsomal fraction of gastric mucosal homogenates. In these respects, they resemble complement-fixing antibodies found in sera of patients with chronic thyroiditis, and a considerable overlap is found between the two diseases. Sixty per cent of pernicious anemia sera also contain intrinsic factor antibodies, but these cannot be detected by immunofluorescence.

Immunofluorescence technique; ×420. Courtesy of Drs. I. Roitt and D. Doniach.

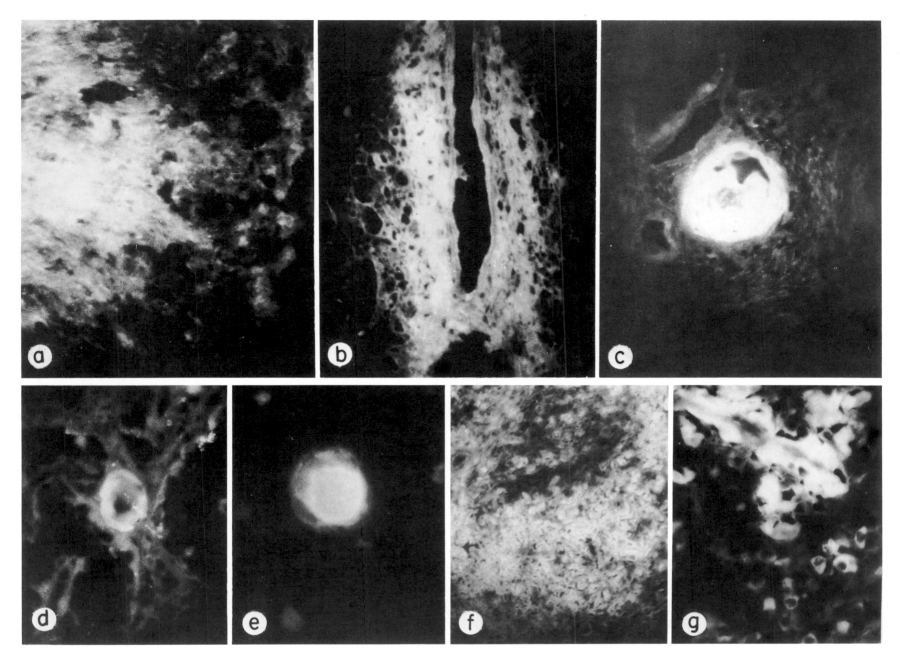

Fig. 22.7. Immunohistochemistry of human diseases of unknown origin. (a) Rheumatoid arthritis. Subcutaneous nodule, stained with fluorescent anti-HGG, shows specific localization of γ-globulin in areas of fibrinoid. (b) Rheumatic fever. Myocardium, similarly stained, shows localization of γ-globulin in altered perivascular connective tissue in area containing many Aschoff bodies. (c) Thrombotic thrombocytopenic purpura. Section stained for human fibrinogen shows localization of fibrinogen in fibrinoid in an arteriole with fibrinoid change. (d) Systemic lupus erythematosus. Kidney, stained with fluorescent anti-HGG. Arteriole with fibrinoid change in wall shows specific fluorescence indicating localization of γ-globulin in fibrinoid; all ×48. (e) Systemic lupus erythematosus. LE cell, stained similarly, shows γ-globulin localization in altered nucleus which has been phagocytized; ×420. (f, g) Experimental RNA amyloid in rabbit. Spleen, stained for rabbit γ-globulin, shows localization both in the cytoplasm of plasma cells and in amyloid deposits; ×34, ×150.

From Vazquez and Dixon, (a, d, e) *Lab. Invest. 6*: 205–17 (1957). (b, c) *Arch. Path. 66*: 504–17 (1958). (f, g) Unpublished (see Vazquez and Dixon, *J. Exp. Med. 104*: 727–36, 1956).

23. Nonimmunologic Lesions: Primary Tissue Damage

In general, nonimmunologic lesions do not resemble those produced by the immunologic mechanisms illustrated in this volume. Lysis of single cells by a toxin or surface-active material, for example, is quite distinct at the ultrastructural level from specific immune (complement-mediated) lysis (Fig. 10.11).

Nonimmunologic events which have been confused with immunologic lesions result from primary tissue damage by any of a variety of agents. Examples are illustrated here of lesions produced by toxins; necrotizing agents such as trauma, burn, croton oil, and turpentine; and infectious agents, notably viruses. *Toxins* such as streptolysin O (Figs. 10.11; 23.1) and diphtheria toxin (Fig. 23.2) may produce primary cell damage, with breakdown of such specialized cellular elements as the red cell, the myofiber, or myelin. A polymorphonuclear response occurs in very acute lesions and a mild mononuclear response (infiltration of hematogenous monocytes and activation of local resting histiocytes) in more chronic lesions. Regenerative changes are usually seen in lesions lasting more than a few hours or days, e.g. proliferation of myocardial cells, Schwann cells, etc. In no case does the degree of cellular response equal that seen in an Arthus reaction (polys) or delayed hypersensitivity reaction (mononuclears).

With *necrotizing agents* (Fig. 23.7) there may be extensive tissue destruction but the cellular response, as in the toxin case, is relatively mild. Irritants, applied to the skin, may kill large areas of epidermis without eliciting a cellular response which approaches that of a delayed reaction in intensity (Figs. 16.16,17). Agents that produce primary vascular damage, burn or ultraviolet irradiation for example, lead to capillary leakage with a prolonged time course, quite distinct from the transient venular leakage characteristic of anaphylactic phenomena. The changes produced by so-called histamine-releasers do, however, mimic anaphylactic reactions (Section 11). Primary tissue necrosis may lead to characteristic products, such as the C_x-reactive protein (Fig. 23.7), which are not in any way pathognomic of immunologic processes.

Finally, infectious agents, notably *viruses*, produce changes in infected host cells which may be manifested by actual cell breakdown (see cellular debris in Fig. 23.4), breakdown of specialized cellular elements such as myelin (Figs. 23.4,5), formation of syncytial giant cells and development of characteristic inclusion bodies (Figs. 23.4,5), etc. Again the response to tissue damage is a mild poly or mononuclear response (Fig. 23.4), which cannot be mistaken for an immunologic reaction.

Lesions produced by infectious agents may be expected to show, in addition to tissue damage directly attributable to toxin or to unrestrained growth of the organism and the mild nonspecific reaction described above, specific immunologic changes (see Postscript). These depend on the host's immune response and may present anaphylactic, Arthus, or delayed components. Similarly, constituents of common organisms, such as the endotoxin of enteric bacteria, may elicit reactions which depend in part on the presence of pre-existing antibody (Fig. 15.1). In prolonged viral or other infection, perivascular lymphocyte or plasma cell cuffs appear, which may represent a local immune response comparable to the "progressive immunization reaction" (Section 5). There are as yet few cases where toxic, nonspecific, and immunologic components have been sorted out. Such an analysis is made possible by observations in subjects with specific immunologic deficiencies (Fig. 23.5). The occurrence of measles infection without a rash in certain lymphoma patients suggèsts that the rash is indeed partly determined by the immunologic response. The same principle is demonstrated in mice rendered tolerant to lymphocytic choriomeningitis virus by intracerebral injection at birth. These animals, when they become adult, present no neural lesions, though their nervous system contains large amounts of virus. If normal mouse lymph nodes are transferred to such mice, they develop typical disease after the usual immunologic latent period. Therefore the brain lesions must be largely immunologic.

It may be noted finally, that lesions resulting from other common pathogenetic mechanisms—congenital anomalies, degenerative and deficiency diseases, metabolic diseases, and neoplastic states—show few features in common with lesions produced by antibody or sensitized cells. The thyroid acted on by long-acting thyroid stimulator, a γG-autoantibody to a microsomal component of the acinar epithelium, behaves much like the thyroid acted on by TSH. Neoplasms of lymphoid cells and organs may resemble lesions of cellular hypersensitivity and, in cases where the neoplastic cells retain immunologic reactivity, this resemblance may not be fortuitous (Sections 8,16). Here there remains insufficient evidence in many interesting cases—Hodgkin's disease is a striking example.

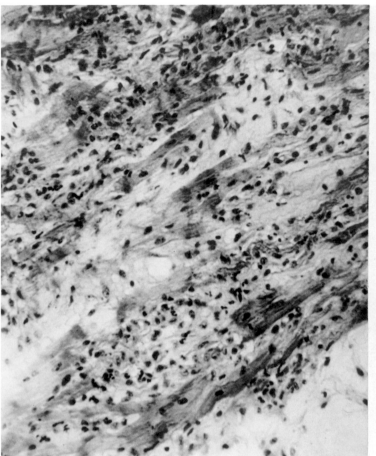 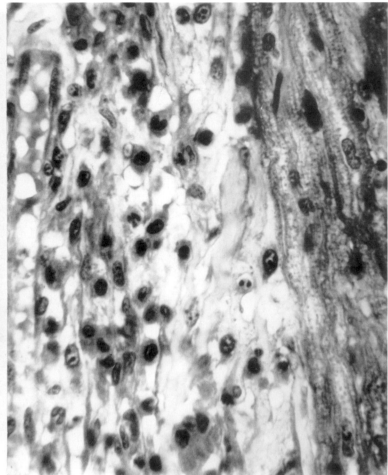

Fig. 23.1. Primary toxic lesion produced in rabbit heart by streptolysin O. At 24 hours, damage of myofibrils and a mild reaction of polymorphonuclear leukocytes are the main findings. Later, some infiltration of "round cells" is also seen. Lesions shown here illustrate changes in right ventricle of two different rabbits 48 hours after iv toxin. In field at left, few intact muscle fibers remain. In field at right, some normal fibers are seen at the right. The rest of the field is filled with sarcolemmal nuclei, and there are no normal myofibers. (Left) Hematoxylin-eosin; ×190. (Right) Masson-trichrome; ×385. From Halbert, Bircher, and Dahle, *J. Exp. Med. 113*: 759–84 (1961).

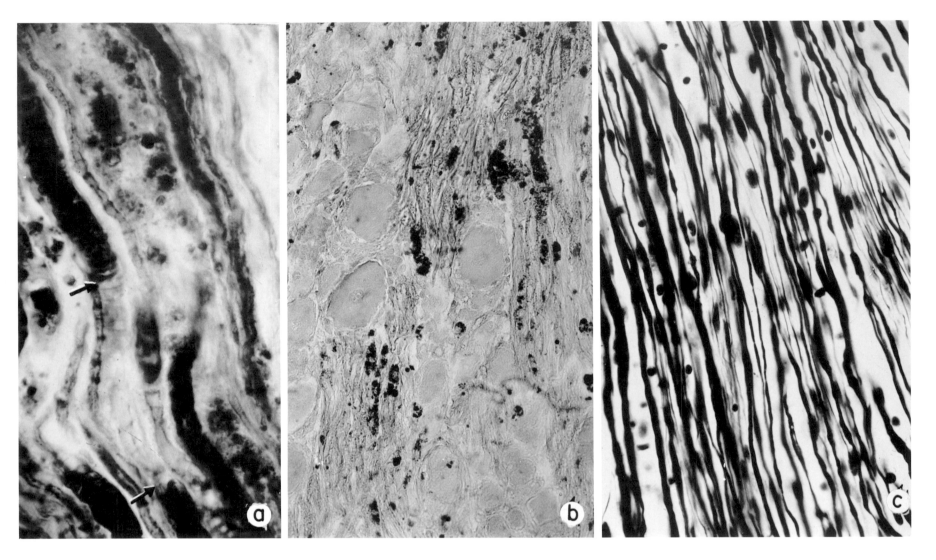

Fig. 23.2. Primary toxic lesion produced by diphtheria toxin in rabbit posterior root and ganglion. Moderately severe disease of several weeks' duration. This lesion, like that seen in guinea pig nerve, is a destructive event affecting myelin, with minimal effect on other tissue elements and little or no inflammation. (a) Segments of the myelin sheaths of several fibers have either disappeared or disintegrated into amorphous granular masses. In fiber marked by arrows, a bare segment of neurilemma and axon is faintly visible. (b) Ganglion, showing degenerating myelin in the form of granular masses of black material. Normal myelin is unstained. (c) Axis cylinder stain, show-

ing integrity of the majority of axons in severely diseased area of the root. They appear as fine or coarse lines of uneven caliber. This lesion should be compared with autoallergic lesion affecting myelin (Figs. 21.8, 10), in which marked infiltration of mononuclear cells is the main feature, preceding demyelination.

(a) Myelin stain (osmic acid); ×417. (b) Marchi stain for degenerating myelin; ×238. (c) Glees silver stain; ×428. From Waksman, Adams, and Mansmann, *J. Exp. Med. 105*: 591–614 (1957).

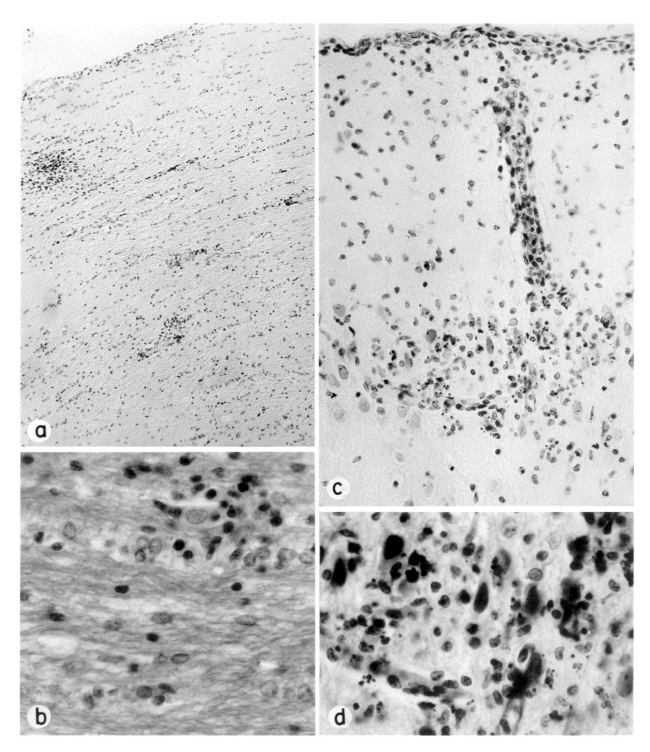

Fig. 23.3. Primary viral lesion affecting nerve cells, glia, and myelin. Acute lesion produced in rabbit by injecting *Herpes simplex* virus intracisternally. (a) White matter of brain stem at 10 days shows minimal focal aggregates of cells; ×80. (b) Similar lesion at 7 days, in white matter of cortex entorrhinalis, shows inclusion bodies in glia, proliferation of glia, and a few lymphocytes; ×450. (c, d) Cortex entorrhinalis at 7 days. Many nerve cells and glia show homogenization of nuclei or intranuclear inclusions, and there is some nuclear debris. A few polys are seen and a scattering of lymphocytes and histiocytes; ×250, ×450.

Hematoxylin-eosin. From Waksman and Adams, *J. Neuropath. 21*: 491–518 (1962).

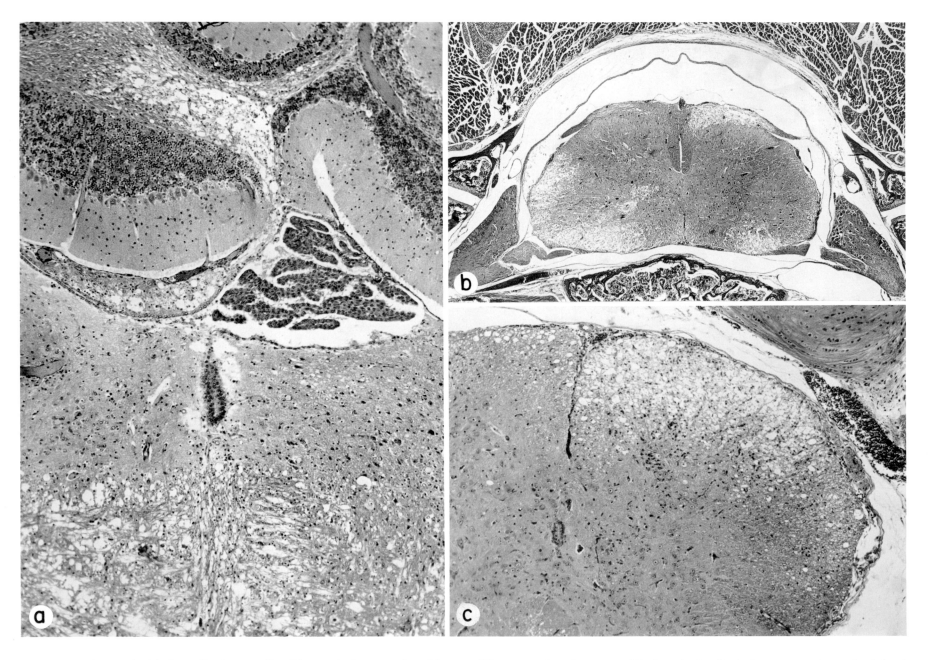

Fig. 23.4. Primary viral lesion affecting myelin. Chronic lesions produced by *JHM* virus in the mouse. (a) Cerebellum (above) and medulla (below); × 80. Patchy, vacuolating lesion of white matter with minimal inflammatory reaction. (b, c) Spinal cord showing extensive myelin destruction. Note diffuse, patchy character of lesion, lack of relation to vessels, and minimal meningeal inflammation; × 37, × 80.

Hematoxylin-eosin. From Waksman and Adams, *J. Neuropath. 21*: 491–518 (1962).

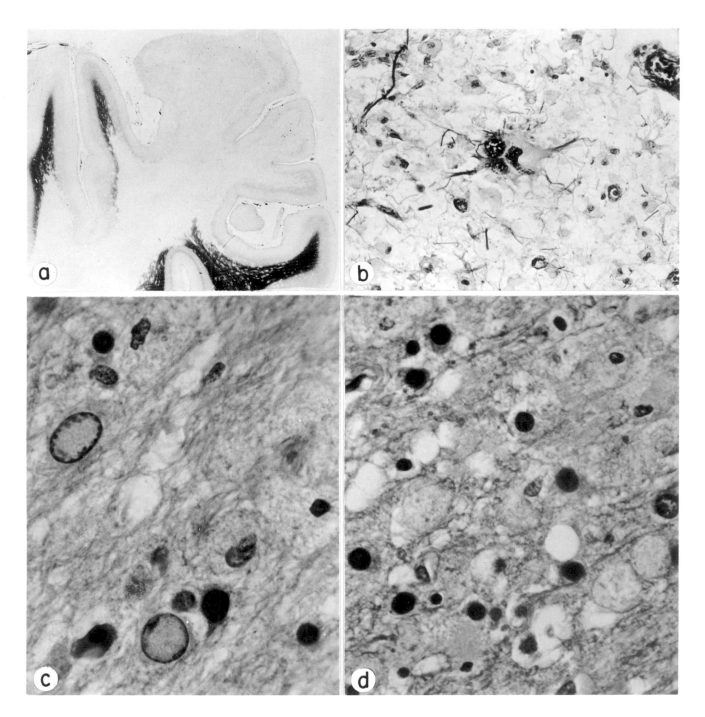

Fig. 23.5. Effects of viral disease in the absence of normal immune responses. Progressive multifocal leukoencephalo-pathy occurring in subjects with Hodgkin's disease or other processes which interfere with immune responses of the cellular type. (a) Cerebral hemisphere showing patchy demyelination and extensive zone of complete demyelination; ×1. (b) Multinucleated astrocyte; ×200. (c) Two enlarged oligodendroglia with eosinophilic inclusions; ×900. (d) Several enlarged, densely basophilic oligodendroglia nuclei, showing loss of nuclear detail. The small round nuclei are normal oligos ×450. These glial abnormalities suggest viral infection, and typical papova virus has been demonstrated in the lesions by electron microscopy; yet there is no perivascular lymphocyte cuffing.

(a) Loyez myelin stain. (b) Holzer method for glial fibrils. (c, d) Hematoxylin-eosin. From Richardson (a) in *Remote Effects of Cancer*, Brain and Norris, eds., Grune and Stratton, 1965, p. 8; (b–d) *New Engl. J. Med. 265*: 815–23 (1961), reproduced with permission of *The New England Journal of Medicine*.

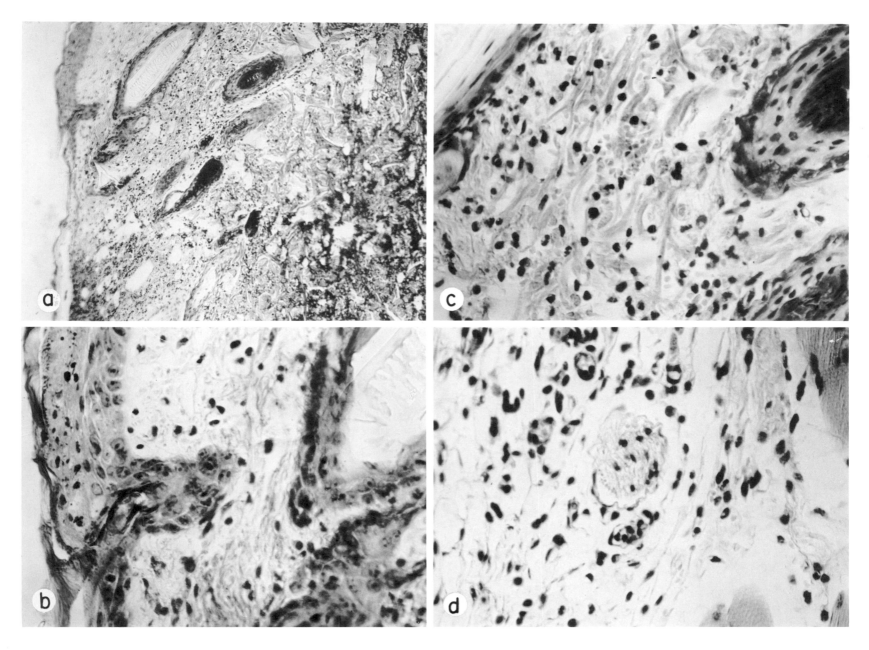

Fig. 23.6. Cell response to nonspecific tissue damage. Reaction produced in guinea pig skin by intradermal injection of 0.05 ml turpentine, diluted 1:5 in olive oil. (a) Lesion (24-hour) consists of massive necrosis of dermal connective tissue (right) and of overlying epidermis (left), with mild cellular reaction; ×120. (b–d) Fields near edge of epidermal damage, the adjacent hair follicles, and the underlying muscle show minimal response of mononuclear cells and slight infiltration of polymorphonuclears. Necrotic zone (not illustrated) contains cell debris, many polys, and almost no mononuclear cells; ×400.

Hematoxylin-eosin. Waksman, unpublished.

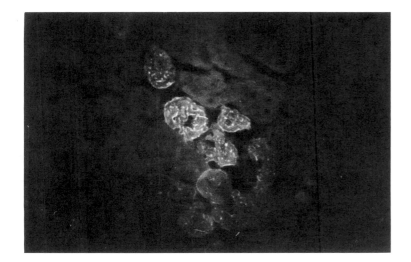

Fig. 23.7. Formation of C_x–reactive protein in area of local inflammation and necrotic change, produced in rabbit muscle by intramuscular injection of typhoid vaccine.

Fluorescence technique; ×250 From Kushner and Kaplan, *J. Exp. Med. 114*: 961–74 (1961).

Postscript: Immunity and Host–Parasite Relationships

There is a broad spectrum of host–parasite relationships. At one extreme are organisms like *E. coli*, which are present as commensals or parasites throughout the life of the host, causing disease only when host resistance is lowered by some means. At the other are organisms like the smallpox virus, which always cause disease. Many microbes of course fall between these extremes.

The *pathogenicity* of an organism is related to its possession of "pathogenic factors" or "virulence" factors, which enable it to establish or extend an established infection. In general, for the class of obligate, extracellular parasites such as the pneumococcus or streptococcus, these are properties that inhibit phagocytosis, kill host tissue, or break the mechanical barriers to spread of the organism in infected tissue. For facultative intracellular parasites, i.e. organisms which can survive and multiply inside phagocytic cells such as the tubercle bacillus or brucella, most fungi, and many protozoan parasites, and obligate intracellular parasites such as the leprosy bacillus and many viruses, the properties that make intracellular survival possible constitute the major virulence factors. The degree of pathogenicity, the *virulence*, depends on the amount of virulence factor produced and is given quantitative expression in such terms as minimum lethal dose, 50 percent lethal dose, 50 per cent infective dose (MLD, LD_{50}, ID_{50}) etc.

The best-understood virulence factors are *toxins*, substances that kill host tissue or derange its function. So-called exotoxins are extracellular proteins, usually heat-labile and fair to good antigens. Well-known examples are the toxins of the tetanus and diphtheria organisms; of *Clostridium botulinum*, *Shigella dysenteriae*, and *Pasteurella pestis*; and streptolysin O and the *Staphylococcus aureus* α toxin. These produce highly specific pharmacologic effects, e.g. on synapses in the central nervous system, on the myoneural junction, on red cells, white cells, or heart muscle, on smooth muscle or renal tubular epithelium, or on protein synthesis or mitochondrial function in all cells. They are extremely potent. No more than 2×10^7 molecules of tetanus or botulinus toxin may suffice to kill a mouse. "Endotoxins" in contrast are lipopolysaccharide–polypeptide complexes forming part of the cell wall of many Gram-negative organisms and corresponding to their "O" (somatic) antigens. These are stable at 100°C and are poorly antigenic. They produce fever, vascular damage, and a number of other relatively nonspecific effects (Section 15). They are much less potent than the exotoxins. Many bacterial products are intermediate in their properties between classical exo- and endotoxins. Protein toxins are altered by heat or aging or by agents, such as formaldehyde, iodine, and ketene, which act on free amino groups, to form *toxoids* which have lost their toxicity while retaining antigenicity. Antibody, whether formed in response to natural infection, induced by active immunization with toxin or toxoid, or passively transferred to the infected subject, can neutralize toxin and thereby inhibit its biological action. Endotoxins are less effectively neutralized by specific antibody than are exotoxins.

Toxins which kill leukocytes are of course effective in preventing phagocytosis. However, some pathogens have nontoxic *surface materials which prevent phagocytosis*. The pneumococcal capsular polysaccharide and streptococcal cell wall M protein are prototypes of this class of product. These are antigenic, and specific antibody by combining with them can render the organism in each case susceptible to phagocytosis. On the other hand, the capsular hyaluronic acid of highly virulent group A streptococci is nonantigenic, and its efficacy as a virulence factor is thereby greatly enhanced.

Various microbial products are *enzymes*, which by their action on cells and connective tissue components favor the spread of infection. These include such substances as streptokinase, streptodornase, staphylococcal coagulase *Clostridium welchii* lecithinase, collagenase, hyaluronidase, etc. Antibody against any of these appears to play at best a limited role in protection.

60

Finally, certain *cell wall materials protect* phagocytized *organisms* from destruction *within the phagocytic cell.* Their presence thus distinguishes virulent from avirulent strains. One may mention as an example the "cord factor" (trehalose 6, 6'-dimycolate) of virulent tubercle bacilli. Antibody against such cellular constituents has no effect *in vitro* and can be expected to have little protective action in the intact animal.

The mechanisms described here allow us to distinguish *toxemic disease,* produced largely or entirely by toxin (e.g. tetanus or botulism), from *invasive disease,* produced by the survival and multiplication of the pathogen in the tissues (e.g. pneumococcal pneumonia). Again a spectrum exists of intermediate forms of disease.

The host's defenses include *nonspecific humoral factors* such as lysozyme, certain basic proteins and polyamines, several imperfectly characterized substances released from leukocytes and platelets (β-lysins, leukins, and plakins), and bactericidal or virus-neutralizing substances in serum, milk, and colostrum (properdin, lactenin). The last are frequently difficult to distinguish from *natural antibodies* formed in response to antigens of organisms in the gastrointestinal and other normal flora. Interferon release from cells infected by virus is an important adaptive but nonspecific mechanism of antiviral defense. Perhaps the most important mechanism of defense, however, is the *phagocytic uptake* of microbial pathogens or their products by polymorphonuclear leukocytes (Figs. 2.8,17), eosinophils (Fig. 2.18), and reticuloendothelial cells (Figs. 2.16; 6.4) and their destruction within the phagocytes by lysosomal hydrolases discharged into phagocytic vacuoles (Figs. 2.17,19) (see discussion in Section 2). These defense mechanisms are markedly strengthened by the specific immune responses which follow infection or purposeful immunization.

The role of specific immunologic mediators in defense includes two major elements. *Humoral antibody* (Fig. 1.1) neutralizes exotoxins and, to a limited extent, endotoxins. With obligate extracellular parasites (bacterial), i.e. organisms which are destroyed once they are phagocytized, antibody's major role is to promote phagocytosis by opsonizing (coating) the target organism. It is particularly effective when it is directed against cell surface components such as pneumococcal capsular polysaccharide or streptococcal M protein, which inhibit phagocytosis. Phagocytosis is also promoted by cytophilic antibody (Fig. 10.4) and by the immune adherence mechanism (Fig. 10.5). Antibody sensitizes a small number of Gram-negative organisms to complement-mediated lysis. By agglutinating organisms, it may tend to localize them at their point of entry into the tissues. Antibody neutralizes some viruses while they are extracellular, i.e. at a mucosal surface or during hematogenous or local dissemination. It has no effect on facultative or obligate intracellular parasites, bacterial, viral, or other, nor does its presence affect the rate of intracellular destruction of opsonized organisms after they have been phagocytized.

In the *cellular (delayed) type of hypersensitivity,* organisms possessing antigens to which the host is sensitized elicit a reaction which consists of a rapid and intense local accumulation of highly phagocytic reticuloendothelial cells (histiocytes, macrophages) (Figs. 16.7–9). These cells, activated as a result of the specific reaction, can suppress intracellular replication of even highly virulent organisms of the facultative and obligate intracellular class (Fig. 18.15). This mechanism has been shown to apply to a number of bacteria (tubercle bacillus, brucella), fungi (histoplasma), protozoa (toxoplasma), and several viruses. The activated macrophages produce interferon as well.

Finally, *immunologic memory* itself plays a major role in specific defense, leading as it does to an intense and rapid synthesis of antibody and/or production of sensitized cells.

The relative roles *in vivo* of these different immunologic mediators may be inferred from experiments *in vitro* but are proved convincingly only by *passive transfer* experiments with serum or cells. Thus passive antibody can protect against exotoxin if it is given in sufficient amount before toxin becomes fixed in its target tissue. It can cure as well as protect against infection with pyogenic bacteria like the pneumococcus. It gives limited protection against enteric bacteria and virtually none against the tubercle bacillus, various fungi, and other agents of chronic infection. It prevents hematogenous dissemination of many viruses, but does not prevent or cure intracellular infection. With sensitized cells, on the other hand, protection against viral and chronic bacterial, fungal, or protozoal infection is readily transferred.

Strong supporting evidence as to mechanisms of defense is provided by study of *immunologic deficiency syndromes* (Section 8). Subjects with hypogammaglobulinemia or agammaglobulinemia are highly susceptible to various pyogenic bacteria but resist almost normally infection with most viruses and chronic bacterial and mycotic agents. Conversely, patients with Hodgkin's disease or sarcoid, lacking the cellular type of immune response, show loss of immunity to mycobacteria, fungi, and some viruses. Hecht's giant cell pneumonia is produced by measles virus infection in leukemic subjects. Progressive multifocal leukoencephalopathy (Fig. 23.5) is due to infection with a virus of the papova group in subjects with the same type of deficiency.

An interesting group of problems arises, on the one hand, from the *mimetic relationships* which may exist *between* antigen(s) of *the parasite and the host* and, on the other, from the induction of *tolerance* or partial tolerance *to parasite antigen(s)*. Hyaluronic acid in the capsule of virulent group A streptococci is enough like hyaluronic acid in mammalian connective tissue to inhibit antibody formation against this antiphagocytic virulence factor. This is an adaptation of the organism favoring its pathogenicity. With some antigens showing a comparable degree of similarity to host antigen, immunization when it occurs effectively breaks tolerance to the host material and leads to autoimmunization and lesion formation. A clear-cut example is the response against heart resulting from immunization with group A streptococcal cell wall antigens (Fig. 1.10) and the resulting production of lesions (Fig. 21.29). Another interesting type of case involves chronic immune complex disease, resulting from long-standing viral infection (lymphocytic choriomeningitis, adenovirus, rubella) in hosts with partial tolerance which fail to develop the cellular type of hypersensitivity but produce antibody. Antibody does not terminate the intracellular infection but forms immune complexes with circulating virus (Section 13). In the LCM case, which has been thoroughly investigated, tolerance may be produced by neonatal infection, by infection of the adult with overwhelming amounts of virus, or finally by infection in the presence of immunosuppressive treatment. A more acute type of lesion is seen in dengue-hemorrhagic fever, where the anamnestic production of antibody following reinfection with a strain of dengue different from that which induced priming leads to severe disease, probably of the immune complex type. A similar disease is seen with measles reinfection following inactivated virus vaccination by a sufficient interval.

With intracellular parasites growing within reticuloendothelial cells, a series of conditions is observed whose form is determined by either mimetic relationships or the balance between immunization and tolerance. The tubercle bacillus possesses antigens which tend to induce both cellular sensitization and antibody formation readily. The closely related leprosy bacillus may do the same—in this case the lesions are tuberculoid and the infection is well controlled. On the other hand, this organism frequently induces specific immunologic tolerance. In the tolerant subject, the organism proliferates freely inside macrophages, there is little inflammatory response, and the disease is poorly controlled (lepromatous leprosy). With fungi such as blastomyces, coccidioides, and histoplasma, the usual response is cellular sensitization and control of infection. The occasional development of an anergic state, though accompanied by antibody formation, permits uncontrolled growth of the organism. The proliferation of *Histoplasma capsulatum* in reticuloendothelial cells in this situation deserves comparison with lepromatous leprosy. Similarly, cutaneous leishmaniasis is usually tuberculoid in character, but some strains of leishmania tend to give rise to anergy (tolerance?) and produce a typical lepromatous lesion. Kala azar is a visceral lesion of the same type. Here sensitization is not usually seen, and there may be a mimetic relationship with host antigen(s) rather than tolerance.

It should finally be remarked that the usual *antithesis between "immunity" and "hypersensitivity"* results from the artificial view of immune reactions imposed by laboratory experimentation. The amount of antigen entering the body with a bacterial, viral, or other infection is the equivalent of a very tiny dose compared with what is injected in the laboratory. Antibody has, in relation to invading organisms, the defensive properties noted: localization, lysis, and opsonization. Opsonization is, of course, an effect on the host. The anaphylactic mechanism, expressed in histamine release for example, can result at this low dose level in nothing more than slight vasodilatation and slightly increased vascular permeability, both effects interpreted in classical pathology as aiding defense. The inflammatory effect of antigen–antibody aggregates (the Arthus mechanism), resulting in stickiness of leukocytes, platelets, and endothelium and increased local permeability, are effects promoting defense by promoting localization and diapedesis of granulocytes. At the dose level of a usual infection, this is not an effect harmful to the host. Finally the cellular or tuberculin type of reaction, at this dose level, results largely or entirely in local mobilization of phagocytic and possibly antibody-forming cells.

Phenomena such as anaphylactic shock and the wheal and flare, the Arthus reaction, tuberculin shock, serum disease, transfusion reactions, and graft rejection result from the abnormal doses of antigen employed in the laboratory and in medical practice or from the use of unphysiological routes of entry (intravenous injection). With frequent ingestion or contact with drugs and other chemicals, one gets other "unnatural" diseases— hemolytic anemia, agranulocytosis, thrombocytopenia, contact dermatitis, and other "drug allergies." Naturally occurring diseases include erythroblastosis and neonatal thrombocytopenic purpura, acquired hemolytic anemias, leukopenias, and purpuras, atopy, polyarteritis nodosa (rare), contact dermatitis, and the various "autoimmune" diseases. In these, infectious agents are not involved, and it may properly be said that the immunologic apparatus is being used for the wrong purpose or there is an actual abnormality of the immune apparatus, as in some of the autoimmune conditions.

In infection, the necrosis associated with cellular hypersensitivity is clearly harmful to the host. Yet prominent necrosis occurs in only a few infectious diseases, such as tuberculosis. In others, hypersensitivity appears to be a highly effective mechanism of defense.

Bibliography

Within each subsection, references to books and major reviews are listed in chronological order. These are followed, in each case, by a few references to illustrative articles grouped by subject matter and not necessarily in chronological sequence.

Introduction: The Immune Response

General

F. M. Burnet and F. Fenner: *The Production of Antibodies*. Macmillan, Melbourne, 1949.

A. M. Pappenheimer, Jr. (ed.): *The Nature and Significance of the Antibody Response*. Columbia Univ. Press, New York, 1953.

J. H. Humphrey and R. G. White: *Immunology for Students of Medicine*, 2d ed. Little, Brown, Boston, 1964.

W. C. Boyd: *Fundamentals of Immunology*, 4th ed. Wiley, New York, 1966.

J. W. Uhr: The heterogeneity of the immune response. *Science 145*: 457–64 (1964).

J. L. Fahey: Antibodies and immunoglobulins. I. Structure and function. II. Normal development and changes in disease. *J. Am. Med. Ass. 194*: 71–74, 255–58 (1965).

S. V. Boyden: Natural antibodies and the immune response. *Adv. Immunol. 5*: 1–28 (1966).

T. A. Waldmann and W. Strober: Metabolism of immunoglobulins. *Progr. Allergy 13*: 1–110 (1969).

T. B. Tomasi, Jr., and J. Bienenstock: Secretory immunoglobulins. *Adv. Immunol. 9*: 2–96 (1968).

Antibody Structure and Function

E. A. Kabat and M. M. Mayer: *Experimental Immunochemistry*, 2d ed. Thomas, Springfield, Ill., 1961.

H. Fudenberg: The immune globulins. *Ann. Rev. Microbiol. 19*: 301–38 (1965).

D. Gitlin: Current aspects of the structure, function, and genetics of the immunoglobulins. *Ann. Rev. Med. 17*: 1–175 (1966).

S. Cohen and C. Milstein: Structure and biological properties of immunoglobulins. *Adv. Immunol. 7*: 1–89 (1967).

A. S. Kelus and P. G. H. Gell: Immunoglobulin allotypes of experimental animals. *Progr. Allergy 11*: 141–84 (1967).

D. Pressman and A. L. Grossberg: *The Structural Basis of Antibody Specificity*. Benjamin, New York and Amsterdam, 1968.

Antibody Formation and Memory

Symposium: *Mechanisms of Antibody Formation*. Czechoslovak Acad. Sci., Prague, 1960.

CIBA Foundation Symposium: *Cellular Aspects of Immunity*. Churchill, London, 1960.

L. A. Steiner and H. N. Eisen: Variations in the immune response to a simple determinant. *Bact. Rev. 30*: 383–96 (1966).

J. W. Uhr and M. S. Finkelstein: The kinetics of antibody formation. *Progr. Allergy 10*: 37–83 (1967).

G. J. V. Nossal: Mechanisms of antibody production. *Ann. Rev. Med. 18*: 81–96 (1967).

G. Edsall, H. J. Banton, and R. E. Wheeler: The antigenicity of single graded doses of purified diphtheria toxoid in man. *Am. J. Hyg. 53*: 283–95 (1951).

W. H. Taliaferro and L. G. Taliaferro: The dynamics of hemolysin formation in intact and splenectomized rabbits. *J. Infect. Dis. 87*: 37–62 (1950).

F. J. Dixon, P. H. Maurer, and M. P. Deichmiller: Primary and specific anamnestic antibody responses of rabbits to heterologous serum protein antigens. *J. Immunol. 72*: 179–86 (1954).

M. Heidelberger et al.: Persistence of antibodies in human subjects injected with pneumococcal polysaccharide. *J. Immunol. 65*: 535–41 (1950).

J. W. Uhr and M. S. Finkelstein: Antibody formation. IV. Formation of rapidly and slowly sedimenting antibodies and immunological memory to bacteriophage ϕX174. *J. Exp. Med. 117*: 457–77 (1963).

A. I. Fecsik, W. T. Butler, and A. H. Coons: Studies on antibody production. XI. Variation in the secondary response as a function of the length of the interval between two antigenic stimuli. *J. Exp. Med. 120*: 1041–49 (1964).

64

G. J. V. Nossal, C. M. Austin, and G. L. Ada: Antigens in immunity. VII. Analysis of immunological memory. *Immunology 9*: 333–48 (1965).

S. Fazekas de St. Groth and R. G. Webster: Disquisitions on original antigenic sin. *J. Exp. Med. 124*: 331–45, 347–61 (1966).

COMPETITION OF ANTIGENS

F. L. Adler: Competition of antigens. In *Mechanisms of Hypersensitivity* (J. H. Shaffer et al., eds.). Little, Brown, Boston, 1959, p. 539.

F. L. Adler: Competition of antigens. *Progr. Allergy 8*: 41–57 (1964).

A. A. Amkraut, J. S. Garvey, and D. H. Campbell: Competition of haptens. *J. Exp. Med. 124*: 293–306 (1966).

TOLERANCE

Symposium: *Mechanisms of Immunological Tolerance*. Czechoslovak Acad. Sci., Prague, 1962.

A. L. de Weck and J. R. Frey: Immunotolerance to simple chemicals. *Monogr. Allergy 1*: 1–142 (1966).

S. Leskowitz: Tolerance. *Ann. Rev. Microbiol. 21*: 157–80 (1967).

W. O. Weigle: *Natural and Acquired Immunologic Unresponsiveness*. World Publ. Co., Cleveland, 1967.

D. W. Dresser and N. A. Mitchison: The mechanism of immunological paralysis. *Adv. Immunol. 8*: 129–81 (1968).

R. E. Billingham, L. Brent, and P. B. Medawar: Quantitative studies on tissue transplantation. III. Actively acquired tolerance. *Phil. Trans. Roy. Soc. B. 239*: 357–414 (1956).

E. E. Sercarz and A. H. Coons: The absence of antibody-producing cells during unresponsiveness to BSA in the mouse. *J. Immunol. 90*: 478–91 (1963).

N. A. Mitchison: Induction of immunological paralysis in two zones of dosage. *Proc. Roy. Soc. B. 161*: 275–92 (1964).

M. M. Dorner and J. W. Uhr: Immunologic tolerance after specific immunization. *J. Exp. Med. 120*: 435–57 (1964).

P. C. Frei, B. Benacerraf, and J. G. Thorbecke: Phagocytosis of the antigen, a crucial step in the induction of the primary response. *Proc. Nat. Acad. Sci. 53*: 20–23 (1965).

P. J. Staples, I. Gery, and B. H. Waksman: Role of the thymus in tolerance. III. Tolerance to bovine gamma globulin after direct injection of antigen into the shielded thymus of irradiated rats. *J. Exp. Med. 124*: 127–39 (1966).

D. A. Follett, J. R. Battisto, and B. R. Bloom: Tolerance to a defined chemical hapten produced in adult guinea pigs after thymectomy. *Immunology 11*: 73–76 (1966).

N. A. Mitchison: The dosage requirements for immunological paralysis by soluble proteins. *Immunology, 15*: 509–30 (1968).

HOMEOSTATIC EFFECT OF ANTIBODY

J. W. Uhr and G. Möller: Regulatory effect of antibody on the immune response. *Adv. Immunol. 8*: 81–127 (1968).

N. Kaliss: Immunological enhancement of tumor homografts in mice. *Cancer Res. 18*: 992–1003 (1958).

M. S. Finkelstein and J. W. Uhr: Specific inhibition of antibody formation by passively administered 19S and 7S antibody. *Science 146*: 67–69 (1964).

G. Möller: Regulation of cellular antibody synthesis. Cellular 7S production and longevity of 7S antigen-sensitive cells in the absence of antibody feedback. *J. Exp. Med. 127*: 291–306 (1968).

GENETIC BASIS OF IMMUNE RESPONSE

F. Haurowitz: The mechanism of the immunological response. *Biol. Rev. 27*: 247–80 (1952).

R. S. Schweet and R. D. Owen: Concepts of protein synthesis in relation to antibody formation. *J. Cell. Comp. Physiol. 50*, Suppl. 1: 199–228 (1957).

F. M. Burnet: *The Clonal Selection Theory of Acquired Immunity*. Vanderbilt Univ. Press, Nashville, Tenn., 1959.

G. J. V. Nossal: Cellular genetics of immune responses. *Adv. Immunol. 2*: 163–204 (1962).

L. Mårtensson: Genes and immunoglobulins. *Vox Sang. 11*: 521–45 (1966).

M. Potter and R. Lieberman: Genetics of immunoglobulins in the mouse. *Adv. Immunol. 7*: 91–145 (1967).

E. S. Lennox and M. Cohn: Immunoglobulins. *Ann. Rev. Biochem. 36*: 364–406 (1967).

T. J. Greenwalt: *Advances in Immunogenetics*. Lippincott, Philadelphia and Toronto, 1967.

J. Cairns (ed.): Cold Spring Harbor Symposium: *The Structure and Synthesis of Antibodies*. Cold Spring Harbor Symposia on Quantitative Biology, 1968.

65

BIBLIOGRAPHY

J. Lederberg: Genes and antibodies. Do antigens bear instructions for antibody specificity or do they select cell lines that arise by mutation? *Science 129*: 1649–53 (1959).

L. Szilard: The molecular basis of antibody formation. *Proc. Nat. Acad. Sci. 46*: 293–302 (1960).

G. M. Edelman and B. Benacerraf: On structural and functional relations between antibodies and proteins of the gamma-system. *Proc. Nat. Acad. Sci. 48*: 1035–42 (1962).

I. Green, W. E. Paul, and B. Benacerraf: Hapten carrier relationships in the DNP-PLL-foreign albumin complex system: Induction of tolerance and stimulation of cells in vitro. *J. Exp. Med. 127*: 43–53 (1968).

IMMUNOPATHOLOGY

C. F. von Pirquet: Allergy. *Arch. Intern. Med. 7*: 259–88, 383–436 (1911).

B. N. Halpern and B. Benacerraf: Allergy. *Ann. Rev. Med. 5*: 167–82 (1954).

H. S. Lawrence (ed.): *Cellular and Humoral Aspects of the Hypersensitive States*. Hoeber, New York, 1959.

J. H. Shaffer et al. (eds.): Henry Ford Hospital Symposium: *Mechanisms of Hypersensitivity*. Little, Brown, Boston, 1959.

P. G. H. Gell and R. R. A. Coombs (eds.): *Clinical Aspects of Immunology*, 2d ed. Blackwell, Oxford, 1968.

L. Thomas, J. Uhr, and L. Grant (eds.): International Symposium: *Injury, Inflammation, and Immunity*. Williams and Wilkins, Baltimore, 1964.

J. D. Feldman: Ultrastructure of immunologic processes. *Adv. Immunol. 4*: 175–248 (1964).

M. Samter and H. L. Alexander (eds.): *Immunological Diseases*. Little, Brown, Boston, 1965.

P. A. Miescher and H. J. Müller-Eberhard (eds.): *Textbook of Immunopathology*. Grune and Stratton, New York, 1968.

1. ANTIGENS

GENERAL

K. Landsteiner: *The Specificity of Serological Reactions*. Harvard Univ. Press, Cambridge, Mass., 1947.

H. N. Eisen and J. H. Pearce: The nature of antibodies and antigens. *Ann. Rev. Microbiol. 16*: 101–26 (1962).

D. A. L. Davies: Antigens. In *Modern Trends in Immunobiology* (R. Cruickshank, ed.). Butterworth, Washington, 1963, pp. 1–24.

B. Cinader (ed.): Antibody to enzymes. A three-component system. *Ann. N.Y. Acad. Sci. 103*: 493–1154 (1963).

E. Zuckerkandl: The evolution of hemoglobin. *Sci. Am. 212*: 110–18 (1965).

FOREIGNNESS AND RECOGNITION

S. Boyden: Cellular recognition of foreign matter. *Int. Rev. Exp. Path. 2*: 311–56 (1963).

G. J. V. Nossal: Self-recognition. *Ann. N.Y. Acad. Sci. 124*: 37–49 (1965).

SPECIFICITY AND STRUCTURE

M. Heidelberger: Chemical constitution and immunological specificity. *Ann. Rev. Biochem. 25*: 641–58 (1956).

E. Haber, J. C. Bennett, and J. A. Mills: The relationship of the three dimensional conformation of proteins to their antigenic specificity. *Medicine 43*: 305–14 (1964).

E. A. Kabat: The nature of an antigenic determinant. *J. Immunol. 97*: 1–11 (1966).

M. Sela: Immunological studies with synthetic polypeptides. *Adv. Immunol. 5*: 29–129 (1966).

P. G. H. Gell and B. Benacerraf: Delayed hypersensitivity to simple protein antigens. *Adv. Immunol. 1*: 319–43 (1961).

EXOGENOUS ANTIGENS

J. F. Wilkinson: The extracellular polysaccharides of bacteria. *Bact. Rev. 22*: 46–73 (1958).

G. H. Beale and J. F. Wilkinson: Antigenic variation in unicellular organisms. *Ann. Rev. Microbiol. 15*: 263–96 (1961).

M. McCarty and S. I. Morse: Cell wall antigens of gram-positive bacteria. *Adv. Immunol. 4*: 249–86 (1964).

O. Lüderitz, A. M. Staub, and O. Westphal: Immunochemistry of O and R antigens of *Salmonella* and related *Enterobacteriaceae*. *Bact. Rev. 30*: 192–255 (1966).

TISSUE ANTIGENS

W. M. Watkins: Blood group substances. *Science 152*: 172–81 (1966).

M. M. Rapport and L. Graf: Immunochemical reactions of lipids. *Progr. Allergy 13*: 273–331 (1969).

O. J Plescia and W. Braun: Nucleic acids as antigens. *Adv. Immunol. 6*: 231–52 (1967).

D. C. Dumonde: Tissue-specific antigens *Adv. Immunol. 5*: 245–412 (1966).

R. A. Flickinger: Embryological development of antigens. *Adv. Immunol. 2*: 310–66 (1962).

D. A. L. Davies: The purification and chemical composition of a mouse histocompatibility antigen. *Ann. N.Y. Acad. Sci. 101*: 114–20 (1962).

B. D. Kahan and R. A. Reisfeld: Transplantation antigens. *Science 164*: 514–21 (1969).

F. H. Bach and D. B. Amos: Hu-l: Major histocompatibility locus in man. *Science 156*: 1506–8 (1967).

D. Franks: Antigens as markers on cultured mammalian cells. *Biol. Rev. 43*: 17–50 (1968).

TUMOR ANTIGENS

L. J. Old and E. A. Boyse: Antigens of tumors and leukemias induced by viruses. *Fed. Proc. 24*: 1009–17 (1962).

L. J. Old, E. A. Boyse, D. A. Clarke, and E. A. Carswell: Antigenic properties of chemically induced tumors. *Ann. N.Y. Acad. Sci., 101*: 80–106 (1962).

G. I. Abelev: Antigenic structure of chemically-induced hepatomas. *Progr. Exp. Tumor Res. 7*: 104–57 (1965).

R. J. C. Harris (ed.): Symposium: *Specific Tumor Antigens*. Med. Exam. Publ. Co., New York, 1967.

C. M. Southam: Evidence for cancer-specific antigens in man. *Progr. Exp. Tumor Res. 9*: 2–39 (1967).

J. J. Trentin (ed.): Conference on *Cross Reacting Antigens and Neoantigens*. Williams and Wilkins, Baltimore, 1967.

B. Hattler, Jr., and B. Amos: The immunobiology of cancer: Tumor antigens and the responsiveness of the host. *Monogr. Surg. Sci. 3*: 1–34 (1968).

COMPLEX ANTIGENS

J. F. Ackroyd: Allergic purpura. *Am. J. Med. 14*: 605–32 (1953).

M. L. Rosenheim and R. Moulton (eds.): *Sensitivity Reactions to Drugs*. Blackwell, Oxford, 1958.

A. M. Kligman: Poison ivy (Rhus) dermatitis. *Arch. Derm. 77*: 149–80 (1958).

W. St. C. Symmers: The occurrence of angiitis and of other generalized diseases of connective tissue as a consequence of the administration of drugs (with a note on drug allergy as a cause of thrombotic purpura). *Proc. Roy. Soc. Med. 55*: 20–28 (1962).

B. B. Levine: Immunochemical mechanisms of drug allergy. *Ann. Rev. Med. 17*: 23–38 (1966).

B. B. Levine: Immunologic mechanisms of penicillin allergy. A haptenic model system for the study of allergic diseases of man. *New Engl. J. Med. 275*: 1115–25 (1966).

2. PHAGOCYTIC CELLS AND ANTIGEN UPTAKE

PHAGOCYTIC CELLS, MOBILIZATION, PROLIFERATION

A. H. E. Marshall: *An Outline of the Cytology and Pathology of the Reticular Tissue*. Thomas, Springfield, Ill., 1956.

G. J. Thorbecke and B. Benacerraf: The reticulo-endothelial system and immunologic phenomena. *Progr. Allergy 6*: 559–98 (1962).

Z. A. Cohn: The structure and function of monocytes and macrophages. *Adv. Immunol. 9*: 164–214 (1968).

J. S. Sutton: Ultrastructural aspects of in vitro development of monocytes into macrophages, epithelioid cells, and multinucleated giant cells. *Nat. Cancer. Inst. Monogr. 26*: 71–141 (1967).

A. Volkman and J. L. Gowans: The production of macrophages in the rat. The origin of macrophages from bone marrow in the rat. *Brit. J. Exp. Path. 46*: 50–61, 62–70 (1965).

D. M. Whitelaw: The intravascular life span of monocytes. *Blood 28*: 455–64 (1966).

B. Bennett: Isolation and cultivation in vitro of macrophages from various sources in the mouse. *Am. J. Path. 48*: 165–81 (1966).

M. Virolanien: Hematopoietic origin of macrophages as studied by chromosome markers in mice. *J. Exp. Med. 127*: 943–51 (1968).

G. Weissmann: Lysosomes. *New Engl. J. Med. 273*: 1084–90, 1143–49 (1965).

J. H. Jandl, N. M. Files, S. B. Barnett, and R. A. MacDonald: Proliferative response of the spleen and liver to hemolysis. *J. Exp. Med. 122*: 299–326 (1965).

BIBLIOGRAPHY

R. H. Drachman, R. K. Root, and W. B. Wood, Jr.: Studies on the effect of experimental nonketotic diabetes mellitus on antibacterial defense. *J. Exp. Med. 124*: 227–40 (1966).

W. G. Spector and D. A. Willoughby: The inflammatory response. *Bact. Rev. 27*: 117–54 (1963).

P. A. Ward: Chemotaxis of mononuclear cells. *J. Exp. Med. 128*: 1201–21 (1968).

PHAGOCYTOSIS

S. Mudd, M. McCutcheon, and B. Lucke: Phagocytosis. *Physiol. Rev. 14*: 210–75 (1934).

L. J. Berry and T. D. Spies: Phagocytosis. *Medicine 28*: 239–300 (1949).

E. Suter: Interaction between phagocytes and pathogenic microorganisms. *Bact. Rev. 20*: 94–132 (1956).

W. B. Wood, Jr.: Phagocytosis, with particular reference to encapsulated bacteria. *Bact. Rev. 24*: 41–49 (1960).

D. Rowley: Phagocytosis. *Adv. Immunol. 2*: 241–64 (1962).

M. L. Karnovsky, A. W. Shafer, R. H. Cagan, R. C. Graham, M. J. Karnovsky, E. A. Glass, and K. Saito: Membrane function and metabolism in phagocytic cells. *Trans. N.Y. Acad. Sci. 28*: 778–87 (1966).

M. Rabinovitch: The dissociation of the attachment and ingestion phases of phagocytosis by macrophages. *Exp. Cell Res. 46*: 19–28 (1967).

CLEARANCE

C. K. Drinker, M. E. Field, and H. K. Ward: The filtering capacity of lymph nodes. *J. Exp. Med. 59*: 393–405 (1934).

B. N. Halpern, B. Benacerraf, G. Biozzi, and S. A. Benos: Quantitative study of the granulopectic activity of the reticulo-endothelial system. *Brit. J. Exp. Path. 34*: 426–57 (1953); *35*: 97–106 (1954).

G. Biozzi, B. Benacerraf, and B. N. Halpern: The effect of *Salm. typhi* and its endotoxin on the phagocytic activity of the reticulo-endothelial system in mice. *Brit. J. Exp. Path. 36*: 206–35 (1955).

B. Benacerraf, E. Kivy-Rosenberg, M. M. Sebestyen, and B. W. Zweifach: The effect of high doses of X-irradiation on the phagocytic, proliferative and metabolic properties of the reticulo-endothelial system. *J. Exp. Med. 110*: 49–64 (1959).

F. J. Dixon, D. W. Talmage, P. H. Maurer, and M. Deichmiller: The half-life of homologous gamma globulin (antibody) in several species. *J. Exp. Med. 96*: 313–18 (1952).

W. O. Weigle and F. J. Dixon: The elimination of heterologous serum proteins and associated antibody responses in guinea pigs and rats. *J. Immunol. 79*: 24–33 (1957).

W. O. Weigle: Fate and biological action of antigen-antibody complexes. *Adv. Immunol. 1*: 283–317 (1961).

C. R. Jenkins and D. Rowley: The role of opsonins in the clearance of living and inert particles by cells of the reticulo-endothelial system. *J. Exp. Med. 114*: 363–74 (1961).

LOCALIZATION AND PERSISTENCE OF ANTIGEN

A. H. Coons: Labelled antigens and antibodies. *Ann. Rev. Microbiol. 8*: 333–52 (1954).

G. L. Ada, G. J. V. Nossal, et al.: Antigens in immunity. *Austral. J. Exp. Biol. Med. Sci. 42*: 267–82, 283–94, 295–310, 311–30, 331–46 (1964).

H. D. McDevitt, B. A. Askonas, J. H. Humphrey, I. Schechter, and M. Sela: The localization of antigen in relation to specific antibody producing cells. I. *Immunology 11*: 337–51 (1966).

G. J. V. Nossal, A. Abbot, and J. Mitchell: Antigens in immunity. XIV. Electron microscopic radioautographic studies of antigen capture in the lymph node medulla. *J. Exp. Med. 127*: 263–76 (1968).

G. J. V. Nossal, A. Abbot, J. Mitchell, and Z. Lummus: Antigens in immunity. XV. Ultrastructural features of antigen capture in primary and secondary lymphoid follicles. *J. Exp. Med. 127*: 277–90 (1968).

G. M. Williams: Antigen localization in lymphopenic states. *Immunology 11*: 467–74, 475–88 (1966).

G. J. V. Nossal and J. Mitchell: The thymus in relation to immunological tolerance. In CIBA Foundation Symposium: *The Thymus: Experimental and Clinical Studies.* Little, Brown, Boston, 1966, pp. 105–23.

Lord Florey: The uptake of particulate matter by endothelial cells. *Proc. Roy. Soc. B. 166*: 375–83 (1967).

PROCESSING OF ANTIGEN

M. B. Rittenberg and E. L. Nelson: Macrophages, nucleic acids, and the induction of antibody formation. *Am. Naturalist 94*: 321–42 (1960).

D. H. Campbell and J. S. Garvey: Nature of retained antigen and its role in immune mechanisms. *Adv. Immunol. 3*: 261–313 (1963).

M. Fishman and F. L. Adler: Antibody formation in vitro. *J. Exp. Med. 114*: 837–56 (1961); *117*: 595–602 (1963).

M. D. Schoenberg, V. R. Mumaw, R. D. Moore, and A. S. Weisberger: Cytoplasmic interactions between macrophages and lymphocytic cells in antibody synthesis. *Science 143*: 964–65 (1964).

B. A. Askonas and J. M. Rhodes: Immunogenicity of antigen-containing ribonucleic acid preparations from macrophages. *Nature 205*: 470–74 (1965).

A. A. Gottlieb, V. R. Glišin, and P. Doty: Studies on macrophage RNA involved in antibody production. *Proc. Nat. Acad. Sci. 57*: 1849–56 (1967).

E. R. Unanue and B. A. Askonas: Persistence of immunogenicity of antigen after uptake by macrophages. *J. Exp. Med. 127*: 915–26 (1968).

E. Kölsch and N. A. Mitchison: The subcellular distribution of antigen in macrophages. *J. Exp. Med. 128*: 1059–79 (1968).

D. W. Dresser: Adjuvanticity of vitamin A. *Nature 217*: 527–29 (1968).

H. O. McDevitt and A. Chinitz: Genetic control of the antibody response: Relationship between immune response and histocompatibility (H–2) type. *Science 163*: 1207–08 (1969).

D. E. Mosier: Cell interactions in the primary immune response in vitro: A requirement for specific cell clusters. *J. Exp. Med. 129*: 351–362 (1969).

3. Central Lymphoid Organs

general

T. Makinodan and J. F. Albright: Proliferative and differentiative manifestations of cellular immune potential. *Progr. Allergy 10*: 1–36 (1967).

K. B. Warren (ed.): *Differentiation and Immunology.* (Sympos. Intern. Soc. Cell Biology, vol. 7). Academic Press, New York and London, 1968.

D. McGregor: Bone marrow origin of immunologically competent lymphocytes in the rat. *J. Exp. Med. 127*: 953–66 (1968).

thymus

R. A. Good and A. E. Gabrielson (eds.): *The Thymus in Immunobiology.* Hoeber, New York, 1964.

Wistar Institute Symposium: *Thymus.* Wistar Inst. Press, Philadelphia, 1964.

I. R. MacKay and G. Goldstein: The thymus: Experimental physiology and pathology in man. *Australas. Ann. Med. 15*: 24–35 (1966).

CIBA Foundation Symposium: *The Thymus: Experimental and Clinical Studies.* Little, Brown, Boston, 1966.

H. A. Azar and J. Furth: The role of the thymus in lymphopoiesis and leukemogenesis. *Meth. Achievem. Exp. Path. 1*: 544–59 (1966).

D. Metcalf: *The Thymus.* Springer-Verlag, New York, 1966.

N. B. Everett and R. W. Tyler: Lymphopoiesis in the thymus and other tissues: Functional implications. *Int. Rev. Cytol. 22*: 205–37 (1967).

R. C. Ting and L. W. Law: Thymic function and carcinogenesis. *Progr. Exp. Tumor Res. 9*: 165–91 (1967).

E. A. Boyse, L. J. Old, and E. Stockert: The TL (thymus leukemia) antigen: A review. In *Fourth International Symposium on Immunopathology* (P. Grabar and P. A. Miescher, eds.). Grune and Stratton, New York, 1967, pp. 23–40.

J. F. A. P. Miller and D. Osoba: Current concepts of the immunological function of the thymus. *Physiol. Rev. 47*: 437–520 (1967).

M. D. Cooper, A. E. Gabrielson, and R. A. Good: Role of the thymus and other central lymphoid tissues in immunological disease. *Ann. Rev. Med. 18*: 113–38 (1967).

J. E. Kindred: A quantitative study of the lymphoid organs of the albino rat. *Am. J. Anat. 62*: 453–73 (1938); see also *67*: 99–149 (1940); *71*: 207–43 (1942).

U. von Haelst: Light and electron microscopic study of the normal and pathological thymus of the rat. I. The normal thymus. *Z. Zellforsch. 77*: 534–53 (1967).

C. E. Ford: Traffic of lymphoid cells in the body. In CIBA Foundation Symposium: *The Thymus: Experimental and Clinical Studies.* Little, Brown, Boston, 1966, pp. 131–52.

C. E. Ford, H. S. Micklem, E. P. Evans, J. G. Gray, and D. A. Ogden: The inflow of bone marrow cells to the thymus: Studies with part-body irradiated mice injected with chromosome-marked bone marrow and subjected to antigenic stimulation. *Ann. N.Y. Acad. Sci. 129*: Art. 1, 283–96 (1966).

M. A. S. Moore and J. J. T. Owen: Experimental studies on the development of the thymus. *J. Exp. Med. 126*: 715–25 (1967).

BURSA OF FABRICIUS; APPENDIX

N. L. Warner and A. Szenberg: The immunological function of the bursa of Fabricius. *Ann. Rev. Microbiol. 18*: 253–68 (1964).

N. L. Warner: The immunological role of the avian thymus and bursa of Fabricius. *Folia Biol. 13*: 1–17 (1967).

S. Konda and T. N. Harris: Effect of appendectomy and of thymectomy, with X-irradiation, on the production of antibodies to two protein antigens in young rabbits. *J. Immunol. 97*: 805–14 (1966).

G. N. Cooper and K. Turner: Immunological responses in rats following antigenic stimulation of Peyer's patches. I. Characteristics of the primary response. *Austral. J. Exp. Biol. Med. Sci. 45*: 363–78 (1967).

4. LYMPHOCYTES AND THEIR RECIRCULATION

PRECURSOR LYMPHOCYTES

J. M. Yoffey: The lymphocyte. *Ann. Rev. Med. 15*: 125–48 (1964).

M. W. Elves: *The Lymphocytes*. Lloyd-Luke, London, 1966.

P. H. Fitzgerald: The immunological role and long life-span of small lymphocytes. *J. Theoret. Biol. 6*: 13–25 (1964).

J. L. Gowans: The immunological activities of lymphocytes. *Progr. Allergy 9*: 1–78 (1965).

D. Zucker-Franklin: The ultrastructure of cells in human thoracic duct lymph. *J. Ultrastruct. Res. 9*: 325–39 (1963).

W. O. Reinhardt: Some factors influencing the thoracic duct output of lymphocytes. *Ann. N.Y. Acad. Sci. 113*: 844–66 (1964).

N. B. Everett, R. W. Caffrey, and W. O. Rieke: Recirculation of lymphocytes. *Ann. N.Y. Acad. Sci. 113*: 887–97 (1964).

J. L. Gowans and E. J. Knight: The route of recirculation of lymphocytes in the rat. *Proc. Roy. Soc. B. 159*: 257–82 (1964).

V. T. Marchesi and J. L. Gowans: The migration of lymphocytes through the endothelium of venules in lymph nodes: An electron microscopic study. *Proc. Roy. Soc. B. 159*: 283–90 (1964).

B. M. Gesner: Cell surface sugars as sites of cellular reactions: Possible role in physiological processes. *Ann. N.Y. Acad. Sci. 129*: 758–66 (1966).

J. J. Woodruff and B. M. Gesner: The effect of neuraminidase on the fate of transfused lymphocytes. *J. Exp. Med. 129*: 551–67 (1969).

D. F. Albright and T. Makinodan: Growth and senescence of antibody forming cells. *J. Cell Physiol. 67*, Suppl. *1*: 185–206 (1966).

J. D. Feldman and R. E. Nordquist: Immunologic competence of thoracic duct cells. *Lab. Invest. 16*: 564–79 (1967).

M. L. Tyan: Studies on the ontogeny of the mouse immune system. I. Cell-bound immunity. *J. Immunol. 100*: 535–42 (1968).

N. W. Nisbet, M. Simonsen, and M. Zaleski: The frequency of antigen-sensitive cells in tissue transplantation. A commentary on clonal selection. *J. Exp. Med. 129*: 459–67 (1969).

J. F. A. P. Miller, G. F. Mitchell, *et al*: Cell to cell interaction in the immune response. I–IV. *J. Exp. Med. 128*: 801–20, 821–37, 839–53, 853–76 (1968).

MEMORY CELLS

G. J. Thorbecke, R. M. Asofsky, G. M. Hochwald, and G. W. Siskind: Gamma globulin and antibody formation in vitro. III. Induction of secondary response at different intervals after the primary; the role of secondary nodules in the preparation for the secondary response. *J. Exp. Med. 116*: 295–310 (1962).

R. G. White: Functional recognition of immunologically competent cells by means of the fluorescent antibody technique. In CIBA Foundation Study Group No. 16: *The Immunologically Competent Cell*. Little, Brown, Boston, 1963, pp. 6–19.

J. L. Gowans and J. W. Uhr: The carriage of immunological memory by small lymphocytes in the rat. *J. Exp. Med. 124*: 1017–30 (1966).

F. Celada: Quantitative studies of the adoptive immunological memory in mice. I and II. *J. Exp. Med. 124*: 1–14 (1966); *125*: 199–211 (1967).

J. Radovich, H. Hemingsen, and D. W. Talmage: The immunologic memory of LAF$_1$ mice following a single injection of sheep red cells. *J. Immunol. 102*: 288–91 (1969).

ANTILYMPHOCYTE SERUM

G. E. W. Wolstenholme and M. O'Connor (eds.): CIBA Foundation Study Group No. 29: *Anti-Lymphocytic Serum.* Little, Brown, Boston, 1967.

K. James: Anti-lymphocyte antibody—A review. *Clin. Exp. Immunol. 2*: 615–31 (1967).

5. PERIPHERAL LYMPHOID ORGANS

Symposium: *Molecular and Cellular Basis of Antibody Formation*: Czechoslovak Acad. Sci. Prague, 1965.

H. Cottier, N. Odartchenko, R. Schindler, and C. C. Congdon (eds.): Symposium: *Germinal Centers in Immune Responses.* Springer Verlag, New York, 1967.

W. E. Ehrich and T. N. Harris: The formation of antibody in the popliteal lymph node in rabbits. *J. Exp. Med. 76*: 335–48 (1942).

A. H. E. Marshall and R. G. White: Reactions of the reticular tissues to antigens. *Brit. J. Exp. Path. 31*: 157–74 (1950).

N. Ringertz and C. A. Adamson: The lymph node response to various antigens. An experimental-morphological study. *Acta Path. Microbiol. Scand.* Suppl. 86: 1–69 (1950).

H. L. Langevoort: The histophysiology of the antibody response. *Lab. Invest. 12*: 106–18 (1963).

H. Z. Movat and N. V. P. Fernando: The fine structure of lymphoid tissue. *Exp. Mol. Path. 3*: 546–68 (1964). The fine structure of the lymphoid tissue during antibody formation. *Exp. Mol. Path. 4*: 155–88 (1965).

B. A. Askonas and J. H. Humphrey: Formation of specific antibodies and γ-globulin in vitro. A study of the synthetic ability of various tissues from rabbits immunized by different methods. *Biochem. J. 68*: 252–61 (1958).

G. J. Thorbecke: Gamma globulin and antibody formation in vitro. I. Gamma globulin formation in tissues from immature and normal adult rabbits. *J. Exp. Med. 112*: 279–92 (1960).

G. N. Cooper and K. Turner: Immunological responses in rats following antigenic stimulation of Peyer's patches. I. Characteristics of the primary response. *Austral. J. Exp. Biol. Med. Sci. 45*: 363–78 (1967).

C. L. Oakley, I. Batty, and G. H. Warrack: Local production of antibodies. *J. Path. Bact. 63*: 33–44 (1951).

L. Hulliger and E. Sorkin: Formation of specific antibody by circulating cells. *Immunology 9*: 391–401 (1965).

J. G. Hall, M. Morris, G. D. Moreno, and M. C. Bessis: The ultrastructure and function of the cells in the lymph following antigenic stimulation. *J. Exp. Med. 125*: 91–110 (1967).

6. CELLS MAKING THE IMMUNE RESPONSE

EFFECTOR CELLS

A. H. Coons et al.: Studies on antibody formation. *J. Exp. Med. 102*: 49–60, 61–72, 73–82 (1955); *117*: 1035–52, 1053–62, 1063–74, 1075–88 (1963).

J. J. Cebra, J. E. Colberg, and S. Dray: Rabbit lymphoid cells differentiated with respect to α, γ, and μ-heavy polypeptide chains and to allotypic markers Aa_1 and Aa_2. *J. Exp. Med. 123*: 547–58 (1966).

G. J. V. Nossal and O. Mäkelä: Autoradiographic studies on the immune response. *J. Exp. Med. 115*: 209–30, 231–44 (1961).

E. E. Capalbo, T. Makinodan, and W. D. Gude: Fate of H³-thymidine-labeled spleen cells in *in vivo* culture during secondary antibody response. *J. Immunol. 89*: 1–7 (1962).

G. Attardi, M. Cohn, K. Horibata, and E. S. Lennox: Antibody formation by rabbit lymph node cells. *J. Immunol. 92*: 335–45, 346–55, 356–71, 372–90 (1964).

N. K. Jerne, A. A. Nordin, and C. Henry: The agar plate technique for recognizing antibody-producing cells. In *Cell Bound Antibodies.* Wistar Inst. Press, Philadelphia, 1963, pp. 109–25.

J. A. Andre, R. S. Schwartz, W. J. Mitus, and W. Dameshek: The morphologic responses of the lymphoid system to homografts. *Blood 19*: 313–33, 334–47 (1962).

T.-W. Tao and J. W. Uhr: Primary-type antibody response *in vitro. Science 151*: 1096–98 (1966).

R. W. Dutton: In vitro studies of immunological responses of lymphoid cells. *Adv. Immunol. 6*: 253–336 (1967).

ANTIBODY FORMATION AS PROTEIN SYNTHESIS

E. Helmreich, M. Kern, and H. N. Eisen: Observations on the mechanism of secretion of γ-globulins by isolated lymph node cells. *J. Biol. Chem. 237*: 1925–31 (1962).

B. Mach and P. Vassalli: Template activity of RNA from antibody-producing tissues. *Science 150*: 622–26 (1965).

BIBLIOGRAPHY

V. Lazda and J. L. Starr: The stability of messenger ribonucleic acid in antibody synthesis. *J. Immunol. 95*: 254–61 (1965).

B. A. Askonas and A. R. Williamson: Biosynthesis of immunoglobulins. Free light chain as an intermediate in the assembly of γ-G molecules. *Nature 211*: 369–72 (1966).

S. Tawde, M. D. Scharff, and J. W. Uhr: Mechanisms of γ-globulin synthesis. *J. Immunol. 96*: 1–7 (1966).

Oak Ridge Symposium: *Differentiation and Growth of Hemoglobin- and Immunoglobin-Synthesizing Cells.* Wistar Inst. Press, Philadelphia, 1966.

P. M. Knopf, R. M. E. Parkhouse, and E. S. Lennox: Biosynthetic units of an immunoglobulin heavy chain. *Proc. Nat. Acad. Sci. 58*: 2288–95 (1967).

TOLERANCE

M. W. Cohen and G. J. Thorbecke: Specificity of reaction to antigenic stimulation in lymph nodes of immature rabbits. II. Suppression of local morphologic reactions to alum precipitated bovine serum albumin by intraperitoneal injections of soluble bovine serum albumin in neonatal rabbits. *J. Immunol. 93*: 629–36 (1964).

F. M. Dietrich and W. O. Weigle: Immunologic unresponsiveness to heterologous serum proteins induced in adult mice and transfer of the unresponsive state. *J. Immunol. 92*: 167–72 (1964).

H. Friedman: Adoptive tolerance to Shigella antigen in irradiated mice receiving spleen cell transplants from unresponsive donors. *J. Immunol. 94*: 352–57 (1965).

D. D. McGregor, P. J. McCullagh, and J. L. Gowans: The role of lymphocytes in antibody formation. I. Restoration of the haemolysin response in X-irradiated rats with lymphocytes from normal and immunologically tolerant donors. *Proc. Roy. Soc. B. 168*: 229–93 (1967).

D. W. Scott and B. H. Waksman: Mechanism of immunologic tolerance. I. Induction of tolerance to bovine γ-globulin by injection of antigen into intact organs in vitro. *J. Immunol. 102*: 347–54 (1969).

E. Diener and W. D. Armstrong: Immunological tolerance in vitro. Kinetic studies at the cellular level. *J. Exp. Med. 129*: 591–603 (1969).

S. Britton: Regulation of antibody synthesis against *Escherichia coli* endotoxin. IV. Induction of paralysis in vitro by treating normal lymphoid cells with antigen. *J. Exp. Med. 129*: 469–82 (1969).

A. Morris and G. Möller: Regulation of cellular antibody synthesis. Effect of adoptively transferred antibody-producing spleen cells on cellular antibody synthesis. *J. Immunol. 101*: 439–45 (1968).

AGENTS AFFECTING IMMUNE RESPONSE

C. A. Leone (ed.): *Effect of Ionizing Radiations on Immune Processes.* Gordon and Breach, New York, 1962.

W. H. Taliaferro, L. G. Taliaferro, and B. N. Jaroslow: *Radiation and Immune Mechanisms.* Academic Press, New York, 1964.

G. H. Hitchings and G. B. Elion: Chemical suppression of the immune response. *Pharm. Rev. 15*: 365–405 (1963).

C. T. Ambrose: Biochemical agents affecting the inductive phase of the secondary antibody response initiated in vitro. *Bact. Rev. 30*: 408–17 (1966).

R. Schwartz (ed.): Symposium on immunosuppressive drugs. *Fed. Proc. 26*: 877–960 (1967).

A. E. Gabrielson and R. A. Good: Chemical suppression of adaptive immunity. *Adv. Immunol. 6*: 91–229 (1967).

J. Munoz: Effect of bacteria and bacterial products on antibody response. *Adv. Immunol. 4*: 397–440 (1964).

7. PHYLOGENY AND ONTOGENY OF LYMPHOID ORGANS

PHYLOGENY

C. G. Huff: Immunity in invertebrates. *Physiol. Rev. 20*: 68–87 (1940).

A. M. Heimpel and J. C. Harshbarger: Immunity in insects. *Bact. Rev. 29*: 397–405 (1965).

Symposium on Defense Reactions in Invertebrates. *Fed. Proc. 26*: 1664–1715 (1967).

W. H. Hildemann: Immunogenesis of homograft reactions in fishes and Amphibia. *Fed. Proc. 22*: 1145–51 (1963).

R. A. Good and B. W. Papermaster: Ontogeny and phylogeny of adaptive immunity. *Adv. Immunol. 4*: 1–115 (1964).

R. T. Smith, P. A. Miescher, and R. A. Good (eds.): *Phylogeny of Immunity.* Univ. of Florida Press, Gainesville, 1966.

J. Šterzl and A. M. Silverstein: Developmental aspects of immunity. *Adv. Immunol. 6*: 337–459 (1967).

E. Diener and G. J. V. Nossal: Phylogenetic studies on the immune response. I. Localization of antigens and immune response in the toad, *Bufo marinus. Immunology 10*: 535–42 (1966).

E. Diener, R. Wistar, and E. H. M. Ealey: Phylogenetic studies on the immune response. II. The immune response of the Australian echidna, *Tachyglossus aculeatus. Immunology 13*: 329–37 (1967).

B. N. Jaroslow and D. E. Smith: Effects of hibernation on the latent period in normal and X-irradiated ground squirrels. *J. Immunol. 93*: 649–55 (1964).

ONTOGENY

F. W. R. Brambell: The passive immunity of the young mammal. *Biol. Rev. 33*: 488–531 (1958).

A. M. Silverstein: Ontogeny of the immune response. *Science 144*: 1423–28 (1964).

W. A. Altemeier and R. T. Smith: Immunologic aspects of resistance in early life. *Ped. Clin. N. Am. 12*: 663–86 (1965).

C. A. Janeway: The immunological system of the child. *Arch. Dis. Child. 41*: 358–74 (1966).

R. T. Smith, R. A. Good, and P. A. Miescher (eds.): *Ontogeny of Immunity.* Univ. of Florida Press, Gainesville, 1967.

J. Sri Ram: Aging and immunological phenomena—A review. *J. Gerontol. 22*: 92–107 (1967).

T. D. Luckey: *Germfree Life and Gnotobiology.* Academic Press, New York, 1963.

G. J. V. Nossal: Studies on the transfer of antibody-producing capacity. *Immunology 2*: 137–47 (1959); *3*: 109–16 (1960).

S. E. Kalmutz: Antibody production in the opossum embryo. *Nature 193*: 851–53 (1962).

D. Mitchie and J. G. Howard: Transplantation tolerance and immunological immaturity. *Ann. N.Y. Acad. Sci. 99*: 670–78 (1962).

A. M. Silverstein, C. J. Parshall, Jr., and J. W. Uhr: Immunologic maturation in utero: Kinetics of the primary antibody response in the fetal lamb. *Science 154*: 1675–77 (1966).

J. W. Uhr, J. Dancis, E. C. Franklin, M. S. Finkelstein, and E. W. Lewis: The antibody response to bacteriophage ϕX174 in newborn premature infants. *J. Clin. Invest. 41*: 1509–13 (1962).

R. T. Smith and D. V. Eitzman: The development of the immune response. Characterization of the response of the human infant and adult to immunization with Salmonella vaccines. *Pediatrics 33*: 163–83 (1964).

D. Gitlin: Protein metabolism, cell formation, and immunity. *Pediatrics 34*: 198–210 (1964).

8. DEFICIENCY STATES AND NEOPLASMS OF LYMPHOID ORGANS

DEFICIENCY STATES

D. Gitlin, P. A. M. Gross, and C. A. Janeway: The gamma globulins and their clinical significance. *New Engl. J. Med. 260*: 21–27, 72–76, 121–25 (1959).

Das Antikörpermangelsyndrom. *Helv. Med. Acta 26*: 109–539 (1959).

R. A. Good, W. D. Kelly, J. Rötstein, and P. L. Varco: Immunological deficiency diseases. Agammaglobulinemia, hypoglobulinemia, Hodgkin's disease and sarcoidosis. *Progr. Allergy 6:* 187–319 (1962).

R. D. A. Peterson, M. D. Cooper, and R. A. Good: The pathogenesis of immunologic deficiency diseases. *Am. J. Med. 38*: 579–604 (1965).

F. S. Rosen, D. Gitlin, and C. A. Janeway: Alymphocytosis, agammaglobulinemia, homografts and delayed hypersensitivity. Study of a case. *Lancet 2*: 380–81 (1962).

P. Fireman, M. Boesman, and D. Gitlin: Ataxia telangiectasia. A dysgammaglobulinemia with deficient γ_{1A} (β_{2A})-globulin. *Lancet 1*: 1193–95 (1964).

W. F. Barth et al.: An antibody-deficiency syndrome. Selective immunoglobulin deficiency with reduced synthesis of γ and α immunoglobulin polypeptide chains. *Am. J. Med. 39*: 319–34 (1965).

G. Karpati, A. H. Eisen, F. Audermann, H. L. Bacal, and P. Rabb: Ataxia-telangiectasia. Further observations and report of eight cases. *Am. J. Dis. Child. 110*: 51–63 (1965).

O. Hansson, S. G. O. Johansson, and B. Vahlquist: Vaccinia gangrenosa with normal humoral antibodies. *Acta Paed. 55*: 264–72 (1966).

NEOPLASMS AND RETICULOSES

J. F. Heremans, M.-Th. Heremans, A. H. F. Laurell, C.-B. Laurell, L. Mårtensson, J. Sjöquist, and J. Waldenström: Studies on "abnormal" serum globulins (M-components) in myeloma, macroglobulinemia and related diseases. *Acta Med. Scand.* Suppl. 367: 1–126 (1961).

L. Korngold: Abnormal plasma components and their significance in disease. *Ann. N.Y. Acad. Sci. 94*, Art. 1: 110–30 (1961).

E. C. Franklin, J. Lowenstein, B. Bigelow, and M. Meltzer: Heavy chain disease—a new disorder of serum γ-globulins. *Am. J. Med. 37*: 332–50 (1964). (See also pp. 351–73.)

D. D. Porter, F. J. Dixon, and A. E. Larsen: The development of a myeloma-like condition in mink with Aleutian disease. *Blood 25*: 736–42 (1965). Metabolism and function of gamma globulin in Aleutian disease of mink. *J. Exp. Med. 121*: 889–900 (1965).

L. Cone and J. W. Uhr: Immunological deficiency disorders associated with chronic lymphocytic leukemia and multiple myeloma. *J. Clin. Invest. 43*: 2241–48 (1964).

H. H. Fudenberg: Immunologic deficiency, autoimmune disease, and lymphoma: Observations, implications, and speculations. *Arthr. and Rheum. 9*: 464–72 (1966).

Conference on Murine Leukemias. *Nat. Cancer. Inst. Monogr. 22*: 1–712 (1966).

P. B. Dent, R. D. A. Peterson, and R. A. Good: A defect in cellular immunity during the incubation period of passage A leukemia in C3H mice. *Proc. Soc. Exp. Biol. Med. 119*: 869–71 (1965).

Symposium: Obstacles to the Control of Hodgkin's Disease. *Cancer Res. 26*: 1043–1311 (1966). See articles by M. W. Chase, L. W. Law, R. A. McBride, A. C. Aisenberg, and M. D. Cooper.

A. C. Aisenberg: Immunologic status of Hodgkin's disease. *Cancer 19*: 385–94 (1966).

R. S. Schwartz and L. Beldotti: Malignant lymphomas following allogenic disease: Transition from an immunological to a neoplastic disorder. *Science 149*: 1511–14 (1965).

R. C. Mellors: Autoimmune and immunoproliferative diseases of NZB/B1 mice and hybrids. *Int. Rev. Exp. Path. 5*: 217–52 (1967).

J. B. Howie and B. J. Helyer: The immunology and pathology of NZB mice. *Adv. Immunol. 9*: 215–66 (1968).

P. J. Staples and N. Talal: Relative inability to induce tolerance in adult NZB and NZB/NZW F_1 mice. *J. Exp. Med. 129:*123–39 (1969).

9. Neutralization by Antibody

CIBA Foundation Colloquia on Endocrinology: *Immunoassay of Hormones*, vol. 14. Little, Brown, Boston, 1962.

C. G. Pope: The immunology of insulin. *Adv. Immunol. 5*: 209–44 (1966).

J. B. Field: Insulin resistance in diabetes. *Ann. Rev. Med. 13*: 249–60 (1962).

L. Lowenstein, B. A. Cooper, L. Brinton, and S. Gartha: An immunologic basis for acquired resistance to oral administration of hog intrinsic factor and vitamin B_{12} in pernicious anemia. *J. Clin. Invest. 40*: 1656–62 (1961).

J. M. Fisher and K. B. Taylor: A comparison of autoimmune phenomena in pernicious anemia and chronic atrophic gastritis. *New Engl. J. Med. 272*: 499–503 (1965).

A. Prader, H. Wagner, J. Széky, R. Illig, J. L. Touber, and D. Maingay: Acquired resistance to human growth hormone caused by specific antibodies. *Lancet 2*: 378–82 (1964).

R. Levi-Montalcini and B. Booker: Destruction of the sympathetic ganglia in mammals by an antiserum to a nerve growth protein. *Proc. Nat. Acad. Sci. 46*: 384–91 (1960).

S. Lieberman, B. F. Erlanger, S. M. Beiser, and F. J. Agate, Jr.: Steroid-protein conjugates: Their chemical, immuno-chemical, and endocrinological properties. *Recent Progr. Hormone Res. 15*: 165–96 (1959).

L. Sánchez Medal and R. Lisker: Circulating anticoagulants in disseminated lupus erythematosus. *Brit. J. Haematol. 5*: 284–93 (1959).

A. Svejgård: Circulating anticoagulant in a hemophiliac (evidence for antibody nature). *Scand. J. Haematol. 3*: 227–35 (1966).

10. Single Cell Lesions

SINGLE CELL LESIONS

G. Möller and E. Möller: Phenotypic expression of mouse isoantigens. *J. Cell Comp. Physiol. 60*, Suppl. 1: 107–28 (1962).

E. J. Ambrose (ed.): *Cell Electrophoresis*. Little, Brown, Boston, 1965.

CIBA Foundation Symposium: *Complement*. Little, Brown, Boston, 1965.

H. J. Müller-Eberhard: Chemistry and reaction mechanisms of complement. *Adv. Immunol. 8*: 1–80 (1968).

R. I. Weed and C. F. Reed: Membrane alterations leading to red cell destruction. *Am. J. Med. 41*: 681–98 (1966).

H. Green and B. Goldberg: The action of antibody and complement on mammalian cells. *Ann. N.Y. Acad. Sci. 87*: 352–61 (1960).

W. F. Rosse, R. Dourmashkin, and J. H. Humphrey: Immune lysis of normal human and paroxysmal nocturnal hemo-globulinuria (PNH) red blood cells. III. The membrane defects caused by complement lysis. *J. Exp. Med. 123*: 969–84 (1966).

J. H. Jandl, A. Richardson Jones, and W. B. Castle: The destruction of red cells by antibodies in man. I. Observations on the sequestration and lysis of red cells altered by immune mechanisms. *J. Clin. Invest. 36*: 1428–59 (1957).

P. L. Mollison: Destruction of incompatible red cells in vivo in relation to antibody characteristics. In *Mechanism of Cell and Tissue Damage Produced by Immune Reactions* (P. Grabar and P. Miescher, eds.), B. Schwabe, Basel/Stuttgart, 1962, pp. 267–82.

J. Dausset and L. Contu: Drug-induced hemolysis. *Ann. Rev. Med. 18*: 55–70 (1967).

J. S. Scott: Immunological diseases and pregnancy. *Brit. Med. J. 1*: 1559–67 (1966).

D. S. Nelson: Immune adherence. *Adv. Immunol. 3*: 131–80 (1963).

R. R. A. Coombs and D. Franks: Immunological reactions involving two cell types. *Progr. Allergy. 13*: 174–272 (1969).

FEVER

E. Atkins: Pathogenesis of fever. *Physiol. Rev. 40*: 580–646 (1960).

I. V. Allen: The cerebral effects of endogenous serum and granulocytic pyrogen. *Brit. J. Exp. Path. 46*: 25–34 (1965).

P. D. Mott and S. M. Wolff: The association of fever and antibody response in rabbits immunized with human serum albumin. *J. Clin. Invest. 45*: 373–79 (1966).

C. P. Engelfriet and J. J. van Loghem: Studies on leucocyte iso- and auto-antibodies. *Brit. J. Haematol. 7*: 223–38 (1961).

J. H. Jandl and A. S. Tomlinson: The destruction of red cells by antibodies in man. II. Pyrogenic, leukocytic and dermal responses to immune hemolysis. *J. Clin. Invest. 37*: 1202–28 (1958).

J. W. Uhr and M. W. Brandriss: Delayed hypersensitivity. IV. Systemic reactivity of guinea pigs sensitized to protein antigens. *J. Exp. Med. 108*: 905–24 (1958).

I. V. Allen: The effect of irradiation on the fever of delayed hypersensitivity. *Immunology 8*: 475–83 (1965).

11. Anaphylaxis and Related Phenomena

ANAPHYLAXIS

C. A. Dragstedt: Anaphylaxis. *Physiol. Rev. 21*: 563–87 (1941).

Z. Ovary: Immediate reactions in the skin of experimental animals provoked by antibody-antigen interaction. *Progr. Allergy 5*: 459–508 (1958).

K. Ishizaka: Gamma globulin and molecular mechanisms in hypersensitivity reactions. *Progr. Allergy 7*: 32–106 (1963).

J. L. Mongar and H. O. Schild: Cellular mechanisms in anaphylaxis. *Physiol. Rev. 42*: 226–70 (1962).

K. F. Austen and J. H. Humphrey: *In vitro* studies of the mechanism of anaphylaxis. *Adv. Immunol. 3*: 3–96 (1963).

R. Keller: *Tissue Mast Cells in Immune Reactions.* Monographs in Allergy, Elsevier, N.Y., 1966.

N. M. Vaz and A. Prouvost-Danon: Behaviour of mouse mast cells during anaphylaxis in vitro. *Progr. Allergy 13*: 111–73 (1969).

CIBA Foundation Symposium *Histamine.* Little, Brown, Boston, 1956.

K. F. Austen and E. L. Becker (eds.): *Biochemistry of the Acute Allergic Reactions.* F. A. Davis, Philadelphia, 1968.

R. P. Orange, M. D. Valentine, and K. F. Austen: Antigen-induced release of slow reacting substance of anaphylaxis (SRS-A^{rat}) in rats prepared with homologous antibody. *J. Exp. Med. 127*: 767–82 (1968).

A. G. Osler et al.: Some relationships between complement, passive cutaneous anaphylaxis, and anaphylatoxin. In Henry Ford Hospital Symposium: *Mechanisms of Hypersensitivity.* Little, Brown, Boston, 1959, pp. 281–304.

W. Dias da Silva, J. W. Eisele, and I. H. Lepow: Complement as a mediator of inflammation. *J. Exp. Med. 125*: 921–46 (1967); *126*: 1027–48 (1967).

R. P. Siraganian, A. G. Secchi, and A. G. Osler: The allergic response of rabbit platelets. *J. Immunol. 101*: 1130–39, 1140–47 (1968).

ATOPY

D. R. Stanworth: Reaginic antibodies. *Adv. Immunol. 3*: 181–260 (1963).

K. J. Bloch: The anaphylactic antibodies of mammals including man. *Progr. Allergy 10*: 84–150 (1967).

A. G. Osler, L. M. Lichtenstein, and D. A. Levy: In vitro studies of human reaginic allergy. *Adv. Immunol. 8*: 183–231 (1968).

R. Patterson: Laboratory models of reaginic allergy. *Progr. Allergy. 13*: 332–407 (1969).

L. L. Layton, E. Yamanoka, and C. W. Denko: Demonstration of human reagins to foods, cat dander, an insect, and ragweed and grass pollens. *J. Allergy 33*: 271–75 (1962).

R. Patterson, J. N. Fink, E. T. Nishimura, and J. J. Pruzansky: The passive transfer of immediate type hypersensitivity from man to other primates. *J. Clin. Invest. 44*, 140–48 (1965).

B. Z. Rappaport: Antigen-antibody reactions in allergic human tissues. II. Studies by fluorescence technique of the localization of reagins in human skin and their relation to globulins. *J. Exp. Med. 112*: 725–34 (1960).

M. E. Fitzpatrick, R. C. Connolly, D. J. Lea, S. A. O'Sullivan, R. Augustin, and M. B. MacCaulay: In vitro detection of human reagins by double layer leucocyte agglutination: Method and controlled blind study. *Immunology 12*: 1–12 (1967).

K. Ishizaka and T. Ishizaka: Identification of γE-antibodies as a carrier of reaginic activity. *J. Immunol. 99*: 1187–98 (1967).

K. Ishizaka, T. Ishizaka, and M. M. Hornbrook: Allergen-binding activity of γE, γG, and γA antibodies in sera from atopic patients. *In vitro* measurements of reaginic antibody. *J. Immunol. 98*: 490–501 (1967).

S. G. O. Johansson, H. Bennich, and L. Wide: A new class of immunoglobulin in human serum. *Immunology 14*: 265–72 (1968).

E. A. Caspary and J. S. Comaish: Release of serotonin from human platelets in hypersensitivity states. *Nature 214*: 286–87 (1967).

C. E. Reed: Pertussis sensitization as an animal model for the abnormal bronchial sensitivity of asthma. *Yale J. Biol. Med. 40*: 507–15 (1968).

OTHER LESIONS

V. H. Donaldson and F. S. Rosen: Hereditary angioneurotic edema: A clinical survey. *Pediatrics 37*: 1017–27 (1966).

K. F. Austen and A. L. Sheffer: Detection of hereditary angioneurotic edema by demonstration of a reduction in the second component of human complement. *New Engl. J. Med. 272*: 649–56 (1965).

J. Pepys: Hypersensitivity diseases of the lungs due to fungi and organic dusts. *Monogr. Allergy 4*: 1–147 (1969).

J. Rankin, W. H. Jaeschke, Q. C. Callies, and H. A. Dickie: Farmer's lung. Physiopathologic features of the acute interstitial granulomatous pneumonitis of agricultural workers. *Ann. Intern. Med. 57*: 606–26 (1962).

J. E. Salvaggio, H. A. Buechner, J. H. Seabury, and P. Arquembourg: Bagassosis. I. Precipitins against extracts of crude bagasse in the serum of patients. *Ann. Intern. Med. 64*: 748–58 (1966).

12. LOCAL PHENOMENA OF ARTHUS TYPE

C. G. Cochrane: Mediators of the Arthus and related reactions. *Progr. Allergy 11*: 1–35 (1967).

C. G. Cochrane: Immunologic tissue injury mediated by neutrophilic leukocytes. *Adv. Immunol. 9*: 97–162 (1968).

J. H. Humphrey: The mechanism of Arthus reactions. *Brit. J. Exp. Path. 36*: 268–82, 283–89 (1955).

W. T. Daems and J. Oort: Electron microscopic and histochemical observations on polymorphonuclear leucocytes in the reversed Arthus reaction. *Exp. Cell Res. 28*: 11–20 (1962).

H. S. Movat and N. V. P. Fernando: Allergic inflammation. I. The earliest fine structural changes at the blood-tissue barrier during antigen-antibody interaction. *Am. J. Path. 42*: 41–59 (1963).

I. van den Berg, J. Oort, and T. G. van Rijssel: Fluorescent protein tracer studies in allergic reactions. III. Distinguishing characteristics of direct and reversed passive Arthus reactions: The influence of size of antigen and of animal species. *Immunology 10*: 1–8 (1966).

P. A. Ward, C. G. Cochrane, and H. J. Müller-Eberhard: The role of serum complement in chemotaxis of leukocytes in vitro. *J. Exp. Med. 122*: 327–46 (1965).

C. G. Cochrane and B. S. Aikin: Polymorphonuclear leukocytes in immunologic reactions. The destruction of vascular basement membrane *in vivo* and *in vitro*. *J. Exp. Med. 124*: 733–52 (1966).

A. Janoff and B. W. Zweifach: Production of inflammatory changes in the microcirculation by cationic proteins extracted from lysosomes. *J. Exp. Med. 120*: 747–64 (1964).

13. SYSTEMIC PHENOMENA OF ARTHUS TYPE (IMMUNE COMPLEX DISEASE)

C. F. von Pirquet and B. Schick: *Serum Sickness* (B. Schick, trans.). Williams and Wilkins, Baltimore, 1951.

F. J. Dixon, J. J. Vazquez, W. O. Weigle, and C. G. Cochrane: Pathogenesis of serum sickness. *Arch. Path. 65*: 18–28 (1958).

C. E. Arbesman, N. R. Rose, E. Witebsky, et al.: Serum sickness. I, II, and III. *J. Allergy 31*: 257–72 (1960); *32*: 531–43 (1961); *33*: 250–58 (1962).

B. Benacerraf, R. T. McCluskey, and D. Patras: Localization of colloidal substances in vascular endothelium. A mechanism of tissue damage. I. Factors causing the pathologic deposition of colloidal carbon. II. Experimental serum sickness with acute glomerulonephritis induced passively in mice by antigen-antibody complexes in antigen excess. *Am. J. Path. 35*: 75–91, 275–95 (1959).

J. H. Vaughan, E. V. Barnett, and J. P. Leddy: Immunologic and pathogenetic concepts in lupus erythematosus, rheumatoid arthritis and hemolytic anemia. *New Engl. J. Med. 275*: 1426–32, 1486–94 (1966).

E. R. Unanue and F. J. Dixon: Experimental glomerulonephritis: Immunological events and pathogenetic mechanisms. *Adv. Immunol. 6*: 1–90 (1967).

W. S. Rodman, R. C. Williams, Jr., B. J. Bilke, and H. J. Müller-Eberhard: Immunofluorescent localization of the third and the fourth component of complement in synovial tissue from patients with rheumatoid arthritis. *J. Lab. Clin. Med. 69*: 141–50 (1967).

D. Koffler, P. H. Schur, and H. G. Kunkel: Immunological studies concerning the nephritis of systemic lupus erythematosus. *J. Exp. Med. 126*: 607–24 (1967).

P. H. Lambert and F. J. Dixon: Pathogenesis of the glomerulonephritis of NZB/W mice. *J. Exp. Med. 127*: 507–22 (1968).

14. Lesions Produced By Antibody against Extracellular Tissue Antigens: Nephrotoxic Nephritis

W. E. Ehrich, R. E. Wolf, and G. M. Bartol: Acute experimental glomerular nephritis in rabbits: A correlation of morphological and functional changes. *J. Exp. Med. 67*: 769–90 (1938).

L. G. Ortega and R. C. Mellors: Analytical Pathology. IV. The role of localized antibodies in the pathogenesis of nephrotoxic nephritis in the rat. *J. Exp. Med. 104*: 151–70 (1956).

P. Vassalli and R. T. McCluskey: The pathogenetic role of the coagulation process in rabbit Masugi nephritis. *Am. J. Path. 45*: 653–77 (1964).

J. D. Feldman, D. Hammer, and F. J. Dixon: Experimental glomerulonephritis. III. Pathogenesis of glomerular ultrastructural lesions in nephrotoxic serum nephritis. *Lab. Invest. 12*: 748–63 (1963).

R. A. Lerner, R. J. Glassock, and F. J. Dixon: The role of antiglomerular basement membrane antibody in the pathogenesis of human glomerulonephritis. *J. Exp. Med. 126*: 989–1004 (1967).

S. Liebowitz *et al.*: Cerebral vascular damage in guinea pigs induced by various heterophile antisera injected by the Forssman intracarotid technique. *Brit. J. Exp. Path. 42*: 455–63 (1961).

C. A. Krakower and S. Greenspon: Skin reactions with heterologous antitissue serums and the probable sites of the principal antigens. *Am. J. Path. 43*: 55–71 (1963).

R. L. Brent: The production of congenital malformations using tissue antisera. IV. Evaluation of the mechanism of teratogenesis by varying the route and time of administration of anti-rat-kidney antiserum. *Am. J. Anat. 119*: 555–62 (1966).

15. Endotoxin and the Local and General Shwartzman Reactions

endotoxin

L. Thomas: The physiologic disturbances produced by endotoxins. *Ann. Rev. Physiol. 16*: 467–90 (1954).

Symposium on Molecular Biology of Gram-Negative Bacterial Lipopolysaccharides. *Ann. N.Y. Acad. Sci., 133*: 277–786 (1966).

A. Nowotny: Molecular aspects of endotoxic reactions. *Bact. Rev. 33*: 72–98 (1969).

C. A. Stetson: Studies on the mechanism of Shwartzman phenomenon. Similarities between reactions to endotoxins and certain reactions of bacterial allergy. *J. Exp. Med. 101*: 421–36 (1955).

W. W. Spink: Endotoxin shock. *Ann. Intern. Med. 57*: 538–52 (1962).

E. Suter: Hyperreactivity to endotoxin in infection. *Trans. N.Y. Acad. Sci., Ser. 2, 24*: 281–90 (1962).

D. H. Heilman: In vitro studies on changes in the reticuloendothelial system of rabbits after an injection of endotoxin. *J. Reticuloendothelial Soc. 2*: 89–104 (1965).

Y. B. Kim and D. W. Watson: Role of antibodies in reactions to Gram-negative bacterial endotoxins. *Ann. N.Y. Acad. Sci. 133*: 727–45 (1966).

H. Gewurz, H. S. Shin, and S. E. Mergenhagen: Interactions of the complement system with endotoxic lipopolysaccharide: Consumption of each of the six terminal complement components. *J. Exp. Med. 128*: 1049–57 (1968).

SHWARTZMAN REACTIONS

P. F. Hort and S. I. Rapaport: The Shwartzman reaction: Pathogenic mechanisms and clinical manifestations. *Ann. Rev. Med. 16*: 135–68 (1965).

D. G. McKay: Diseases of hypersensitivity. Disseminated intravascular coagulation. *Arch. Internal Med. 116*: 83–94 (1965).

J. D. Wells, E. G. Margolin, and E. A. Gall: Renal cortical necrosis. Clinical pathological features in twenty-one cases. *Am. J. Med. 29*: 257–67 (1960).

C. A. Stetson: Similarities in the mechanisms determining the Arthus and Shwartzman phenomena. *J. Exp. Med. 94*: 347–58 (1951).

L. Thomas, R. A. Good, et al: Studies on the generalized Shwartzman phenomenon. *J. Exp. Med. 96*: 605–41 (1952); *97*: 751–66, 871–88 (1953); *102*: 249–78 (1955).

J. J. Vazquez and F. J. Dixon: Immunopathology of hypersensitivity. *Ann. N.Y. Acad. Sci. 86*: Art. 4, 1025–32 (1960).

W. Margaretten and D. G. McKay: The role of the platelet in the generalized Shwartzman reaction. *J. Exp. Med. 129*: 585–90 (1969).

16. LOCAL REACTIONS DUE TO DELAYED OR CELLULAR HYPERSENSITIVITY

BACTERIAL ALLERGY

B. H. Waksman: Delayed hypersensitive reactions: A growing class of immunologic phenomena. *J. Allergy 31*: 468–75 (1960).

P. G. H. Gell: Cellular hypersensitivity. *Int. Arch. Allergy 18*: 39–54 (1961).

B. Amos and H. Koprowski (eds.): *Cell Bound Antibodies*. Wistar Inst. Press, Philadelphia, 1963.

J. H. Uhr: Delayed hypersensitivity. *Physiol. Rev. 46*: 359–419 (1966).

J. L. Turk (ed.): Delayed hypersensitivity: Specific cell-mediated immunity. *Brit. Med. Bull. 23*: 1–104 (1967).

J. L. Turk: *Delayed Hypersensitivity*. North Holland, Amsterdam, 1967.

CONTACT ALLERGY

K. Landsteiner: Hypersensitivity to substances of simple composition. In *The Specificity of Serological Reactions*. Harvard Univ. Press, Cambridge, 1947, pp. 197–210.

M. W. Chase: Models for hypersensitivity studies. In *Cellular and Humoral Aspects of the Hypersensitive States* (H. S. Lawrence, ed.). Hoeber, New York, 1959, pp. 251–78.

H. N. Eisen: Hypersensitivity to simple chemicals. In *Cellular and Humoral Aspects of the Hypersensitive States* (H. S. Lawrence, ed.). Hoeber, New York, 1959, pp. 89–122.

PASSIVE TRANSFER

B. R. Bloom and M. W. Chase: Transfer of delayed-type hypersensitivity. *Progr. Allergy 10*: 151–255 (1967).

H. S. Lawrence: The transfer in humans of delayed skin sensitivity to streptococcal M substance and to tuberculin with disrupted leucocytes. *J. Clin. Invest. 34*: 219–30 (1955).

P. Baram, L. Yuan, and M. M. Mosko: Studies on the transfer of human delayed-type hypersensitivity. I. Partial purification and characterization of two active components. *J. Immunol. 97*: 407–20 (1966).

MORPHOLOGIC AND LABELING STUDIES

B. H. Waksman: A comparative histopathologic study of delayed hypersensitive reactions. CIBA Foundation Symposium: *Cellular Aspects of Immunity*. Churchill, London, 1960, pp. 280–322.

T. U. Kosunen, B. H. Waksman, M. H. Flax, and W. S. Tihen: Radioautographic study of cellular mechanisms in delayed hypersensitivity. I. Delayed reactions to tuberculin and purified proteins in the rat and guinea pig. *Immunology 6*: 276–90 (1963).

M. H. Flax and J. B. Caulfield: Cellular and vascular components of allergic contact dermatitis. Light and electron microscopic observations. *Am. J. Path. 43*: 1031–53 (1963).

R. T. McCluskey, B. Benacerraf, and J. W. McCluskey: Studies on the specificity of the cellular infiltrate in delayed hypersensitivity reactions. *J. Immunol. 90*: 466–77 (1963).

D. M. Lubaroff and B. H. Waksman: Bone marrow as source of cells in reactions of cellular hypersensitivity. I and II. *J. Exp. Med. 128*: 1425–35, 1437–49 (1968).

17. DISSEMINATED LESIONS DUE TO CELLULAR HYPERSENSITIVITY

BACTERIAL LESIONS

G. E. Murphy and H. F. Swift: The induction of rheumatic-like cardiac lesions in rabbits by repeated focal infections with group A streptococci. Comparison with the cardiac lesions of serum disease. *J. Exp. Med. 91*: 485–98 (1950).

C. M. Pearson, B. H. Waksman, and J. T. Sharp: Studies of arthritis and other lesions induced in rats by injection of mycobacterial adjuvant. V. Changes affecting the skin and mucous membranes. Comparison of the experimental process with human disease. *J. Exp. Med. 113*: 485–510 (1961).

C. M. Pearson: Experimental joint disease. Observations on adjuvant-induced arthritis. *J. Chron. Dis. 16*: 863–74 (1963).

J. H. Schwab, W. J. Cromartie, S. H. Ohanian, and J. G. Craddock: Association of experimental chronic arthritis with the persistence of group A streptococcal cell walls in the articular tissue. *J. Bact. 94*: 1728–35 (1967).

D. M. Angevine and S. Rothbard: The significance of the synovial villus and the ciliary process as factors in the localization of bacteria in the joints and eyes of rabbits. *J. Exp. Med. 71*: 129–36 (1940).

ALLERGIC GRANULOMATOSIS

G. H. Curtis: Cutaneous hypersensitivity due to beryllium. *Arch. Derm. Syph. 64*: 470–82 (1951).

W. B. Shelley and H. J. Hurley: The allergic origin of Zirconium deodorant granulomas. *Brit. J. Derm. 70*: 75–101 (1958).

M. W. Chase: Disseminated granulomata in the guinea pig. In Henry Ford Hospital Symposium: *Mechanisms of Hypersensitivity*. Little, Brown, Boston, 1959, pp. 673–78.

W. L. Epstein: Granulomatous hypersensitivity. *Progr. Allergy 11*: 36–88 (1967).

18. REACTIONS OF "SENSITIZED CELLS" IN VITRO

GENERAL

Symposium: In Vitro Correlates of Delayed Hypersensitivity. *Fed. Proc. 27*: 3–48 (1968).

ANTIGEN UPTAKE BY "SENSITIZED CELLS"

J. L. Turk: Some quantitative aspects of the uptake of antigens in vitro by the lymphocytes of hypersensitive guinea pigs. *Int. Arch. Allergy 17*: 338–51 (1960).

C. Steffen and M. Rosak: In vitro demonstration of anti-ovalbumin specificity of lymph node cells in delayed type hypersensitivity. *J. Immunol. 90*: 337–46 (1963).

H. C. Rauch and S. Raffel: Antigen uptake by specifically reactive cells in experimental allergic encephalomyelitis. *Ann. N.Y. Acad. Sci., 122*: 297–307 (1965).

BLAST TRANSFORMATION

J. H. Robbins: Tissue culture studies of the human lymphocyte. Science *146*: 1648–54 (1964).

R. W. Dutton: Significance of the reaction of lymphoid cells to homologous tissue. *Bact. Rev. 30*: 397–407 (1966).

G. Pearmain, R. R. Lycette, and P. H. Fitzgerald: Tuberculin-induced mitosis in peripheral blood leucocytes. *Lancet 1*: 637–38 (1963).

B. Bain, M. R. Vas, and L. Lowenstein: The development of large immature mononuclear cells in mixed leukocyte cultures. *Blood 23*: 108–16 (1964).

J. J. Oppenheim, J. W. Long, and E. Frei, III: The effect of skin homograft rejection on recipient and donor mixed leukocyte cultures. *J. Exp. Med. 122*: 651–54 (1965).

D. B. Wilson, W. K. Silvers, and P. C. Nowell: Quantitative studies on the mixed lymphocyte interaction in rats. *J. Exp. Med. 126*: 625–54, 655–65 (1967).

D. C. Cowling, D. Quaglino, and P. K. M. Barrett: Effect of Kveim antigen and old tuberculin on lymphocytes in culture from sarcoid patients. *Brit. Med. J. 1*: 1481–82 (1964).

E. M. Hersh and J. J. Oppenheim: Impaired in vitro lymphocyte transformation in Hodgkin's disease. *New Engl. J. Med. 273*: 1006–12 (1965).

BIBLIOGRAPHY

INHIBITION OF MACROPHAGE MIGRATION

A. R. Rich and M. R. Lewis: The nature of allergy in tuberculosis as revealed by tissue culture studies. *Johns Hopkins Hosp. Bull. 50*: 115–31 (1932).

C. B. Favour: In vitro effect of tuberculin on cells. *Adv. Tuberc. Res. 4*: 219–35 (1951).

F. A. Kapral and W. R. Stinebring: The effect of glucose on the tuberculin reaction in tissue culture. *Am. Rev. Tuberc. 78*: 712–24 (1958).

B. H. Waksman and M. Matoltsy: The effect of tuberculin on peritoneal exudate cells of sensitized guinea pigs in surviving cell culture. *J. Immunol. 81*: 220–34 (1958).

R. C. Carpenter and M. W. Brandriss: *In vitro* studies of cellular hypersensitivity. I and II. *J. Immunol. 91*: 807–18 (1963); *J. Exp. Med. 120*: 1231–43 (1964).

J. R. David, S. Al-Askari, H. S. Lawrence, and L. Thomas: Delayed hypersensitivity in vitro. I, II, and III. *J. Immunol. 93*: 264–73, 274–78, 279–82 (1964).

J. R. David and P. Y. Paterson: In vitro demonstration of cellular sensitivity in allergic encephalomyelitis. *J. Exp. Med. 122*: 1161–71 (1965).

J. R. David: Suppression of delayed hypersensitivity in vitro by inhibition of protein synthesis. *J. Exp. Med. 122*: 1125–34 (1965).

B. R. Bloom and B. Bennett: Mechanism of a reaction in vitro associated with delayed type hypersensitivity. *Science 153*: 80–82 (1966).

B. Bennett and B. R. Bloom: Reactions in vivo and in vitro produced by a soluble substance associated with delayed-type hypersensitivity. *Proc. Nat. Acad. Sci. 59*: 756–62 (1968).

D. E. Thor and S. Dray: The cell-migration-inhibition correlate of delayed hypersensitivity. Conversion of human nonsensitive lymph node cells to sensitive cells with an RNA extract. *J. Immunol. 101*: 469–80 (1968).

N. H. Ruddle and B. H. Waksman: Cytotoxicity mediated by soluble antigen and lymphocytes in delayed hypersensitivity. I, II, and III. *J. Exp. Med. 128*: 1237–54, 1255–65, 1267–79 (1968).

P. A. Ward, H. G. Remold, and J. R. David: Leukotactic factor produced by sensitized lymphocytes. *Science 163*: 1079–81 (1969).

CYTOTOXIC EFFECTS ON TARGET CELLS

D. B. Wilson and R. E. Billingham: Lymphocytes and transplantation immunity. *Adv. Immunol. 7*: 189–273 (1967).

J. M. Weaver, G. H. Algire, and R. T. Prehn: The growth of cells *in vivo* in diffusion chambers. II. The role of cells in the destruction of homografts in mice. *J. Nat. Cancer Inst. 15*: 1737–67 (1955).

G. D. Snell, H. J. Wihn, and A. A. Kandutsch: A quantitative study of cellular immunity. *J. Immunol. 87*: 1–17 (1961).

W. Rosenau and H. D. Moon; Lysis of homologous cells by sensitized lymphocytes in tissue culture. *J. Nat. Cancer Inst. 27*: 471–83 (1961).

O. Berg and B. Källén: White blood cells from animals with experimental allergic encephalomyelitis tested on glia cells in tissue cultures. *Acta Path. Microbiol. Scand. 58*: 33–42 (1963).

P. Perlmann and O. Broberger: In vitro studies of ulcerative colitis. II. Cytotoxic action of white blood cells from patients on human fetal colon cells. *J. Exp. Med. 117*: 717–33 (1963).

H. Bondevik and J. A. Mannick: RNA-mediated transfer of lymphocyte vs. target cell activity. *Proc. Soc. Exp. Biol. Med. 129*: 264–68 (1968).

L. F. Speel, J. E. Osborn, and D. L. Walker: An immunocytopathogenic interaction between sensitized leukocytes and epithelial cells carrying a persistent noncytocidal myxovirus infection. *J. Immunol. 101*: 409–17 (1968).

G. A. Granger and R. S. Weiser: Homograft target cells: Contact destruction in vitro by immune macrophages. *Science 151*: 97–99 (1965).

A. Berken and B. Benacerraf: Properties of antibodies cytophilic for macrophages. *J. Exp. Med. 123*: 119–44 (1966).

B. Bennett: Specific suppression of tumor growth by isolated peritoneal macrophages from immunized mice. *J. Immunol. 95*: 656–64 (1965).

ALLOGENEIC INHIBITION

K. E. Hellström and I. Hellström: Allogeneic inhibition of transplanted tumor cells. *Progr. Exp. Tumor Res. 9*: 41–76 (1967).

K. E. Hellström, I. Hellström, and C. Bergheden: Allogeneic inhibition of tumor cells by in vitro contact with cells containing foreign H-2 antigens. *Nature 208*: 458–60 (1965).

G. Möller and E. Möller: Plaque formation by non-immune and x-irradiated lymphoid cells on monolayers of mouse embryo cells. *Nature 208*: 260–63 (1965).

"CELLULAR IMMUNITY"

S. E. Elberg: Cellular immunity. *Bact. Rev. 24*: 67–95 (1960).

C. R. Jenkin and D. Rowley: Basis for immunity to typhoid in mice and the question of "cellular immunity." *Bact. Rev. 27*: 391–404 (1963).

E. Suter and H. Ramseier: Cellular reactions in infection. *Adv. Immunol. 4*: 117–73 (1964).

G. B. Mackaness and R. V. Blanden: Cellular immunity. *Progr. Allergy 11*: 89–140 (1967).

E. Suter: Multiplication of tubercle bacilli within mononuclear phagocytes in tissue cultures derived from normal animals and animals vaccinated with BCG. *J. Exp. Med. 97*: 235–45 (1953).

E. Suter: Passive transfer of acquired resistance to infection with Mycobacterium tuberculosis by means of cells. *Am. Rev. Resp. Dis. 83*: 535–43 (1961).

H. Ramseier and E. Suter: An antimycobacterial principle of peritoneal mononuclear cells. I and II. *J. Immunol. 93* 511–17, 518–23 (1964).

K. Saito and S. Mitsuhashi: Experimental salmonellosis. VI. *In vitro* transfer of cellular immunity of mouse mononuclear phagocytes. *J. Bact. 90*: 629–34 (1965).

G. B. Mackaness: The influence of immunologically committed lymphoid cells on macrophage activity in vivo. *J. Exp. Med. 129*: 973–92 (1969).

I. Gresser and J. F. Enders: Alteration of cellular resistance to Sindbis virus in mixed cultures of human cells attributable to interferon. *Virology 16*: 428–35 (1962).

L. A. Glasgow: Leukocytes and interferon in the host response to viral infections. II. Enhanced interferon response of leukocytes from immune animals. *J. Bact. 91*: 2185–91 (1966).

19. HOMOGRAFT REJECTION

REJECTION OF NORMAL TISSUES

G. D. Snell: The homograft reaction. *Ann. Rev. Microbiol. 11*: 439–58 (1957).

P. B. Medawar: The immunology of transplantation. *Harvey Lect. 52*: 144–76 (1958).

F. Albert and P. B. Medawar (eds.): *Biological Problems of Grafting.* Blackwell, Oxford, 1959.

R. E. Billingham and W. K. Silvers (eds.): *Transplantation of Tissue and Cells.* Wistar Inst. Press, Philadelphia, 1961.

CIBA Foundation Symposium : *Transplantation.* Little, Brown, Boston, 1962.

Transplantation of tissues and organs. *Brit. Med. Bull. 21*: 97–182 (1965).

Wistar Institute Symposium: *Isoantigens and Cell Interactions.* Wistar Inst. Press, Philadelphia, 1965.

H. S. Micklem and J. F. Loutit: *Tissue Grafting and Radiation.* Academic Press, New York, 1966.

Seventh International Transplantation Conference. *Ann. N.Y. Acad. Sci., 129*: 1–884 (1966).

J. P. Merrill: Human tissue transplantation. *Adv. Immunol. 7*: 275–327 (1967).

D. M. Hume: Renal homotransplantation in man. *Ann. Rev. Med. 18*: 229–68 (1967).

F. T. Rapaport and J. Dausset (eds.): *Human Transplantation.* Grune and Stratton, New York and London, 1968.

B. H. Waksman: The pattern of rejection in rat skin homografts and its relation to the vascular network. *Lab. Invest. 12*: 46–57 (1963).

I. Wiener, D. Spiro, and P. S. Russell: An electron microscopic study of the homograft reaction. *Am. J. Path. 44*: 319–47 (1964).

TUMOR IMMUNITY

Conference on Tumor Immunity. *Ann. N.Y. Acad. Sci. 101*: Art. 1, 1–326 (1962).

K. E. Hellström and G. Möller: Immunological and immunogenetic aspects of tumor transplantation. *Progr. Allergy 9*: 158–245 (1965).

J. G. Kidd and H. W. Toolan: The association of lymphocytes with cancer cells undergoing distinctive necrobiosis in resistant and immune hosts. *Am. J. Path. 26*: 672–73 (1950).

20. GRAFT-VERSUS-HOST REACTIONS

M. Simonsen: Graft versus host reactions. Their natural history, and applicability as tools in research. *Progr. Allergy 6*: 349–467 (1962).

BIBLIOGRAPHY

L. Brent, J. Brown, and P. B. Medawar: Skin transplantation immunity in relation to hypersensitivity *Lancet. 2*: 561–64 (1958).

H. F. Dvorak, T. U. Kosunen, and B. H. Waksman: The "transfer reaction" in the rabbit. I and II. *Lab. Invest. 12*: 58–68, 628–37 (1963).

F. M. Burnet and G. S. Boyer: The chorio-allantoic lesion in the Simonsen phenomena. *J. Path. Bact. 81*: 141–50 (1961).

H. Ramseier and J. W. Streilein: Homograft sensitivity reactions in irradiated hamsters. *Lancet 1*: 622–24 (1965).

W. L. Elkins: The interaction of donor and host lymphoid cells in the pathogenesis of renal cortical destruction induced by a local graft versus host reaction. *J. Exp. Med. 123*: 103–18 (1966).

21. EXPERIMENTAL AUTOALLERGIES

EXPERIMENTAL LESIONS

F. J. Dixon: Autoimmunity in disease. *Ann. Rev. Med. 9*: 257–86 (1958).

M. W. Kies and E. C. Alvord, Jr. (eds.): "*Allergic*" *Encephalomyelitis*. Thomas, Springfield, 1959.

B. H. Waksman: Experimental allergic encephalomyelitis and the autoallergic diseases. *Int. Arch. Allergy 14*, Suppl.: 1–87 (1959).

B. H. Waksman: Auto-immunization and the lesions of auto-immunity. *Medicine 41*: 93–141 (1962).

M. H. Flax: Experimental allergic thyroiditis. *Meth. Achievem. Exp. Path. 1*: 493–513 (1966).

P. Y. Paterson: Experimental allergic encephalomyelitis and autoimmune disease. *Adv. Immunol. 5*: 131–208 (1966).

T. U. Kosunen, B. H. Waksman, and I. K. Samuelsson: Radioautographic study of cellular mechanisms in delayed hypersensitivity. II. Experimental allergic encephalomyelitis in the rat. *J. Neuropath. 22*: 367–80 (1963).

P. Lampert and S. Carpenter: Electron microscopic studies on the vascular permeability and the mechanism of demyelination in experimental allergic encephalomyelitis. *J. Neuropath. 24*: 11–24 (1965).

AUTOIMMUNIZATION

P. G. H. Gell and A. S. Kelus: Anti-antibodies. *Adv. Immunol. 6*: 461–78 (1967).

P. J. Lachmann: Conglutinin and immunoconglutinins. *Adv. Immunol. 6*: 479–527 (1967).

J. E. M. St. Rose and B. Cinader: The effect of tolerance on the specificity of the antibody response and on immunogenicity. Antibody response to conformationally and chemically altered antigens. *J. Exp. Med. 125*: 1031–55 (1967).

W. O. Weigle: The induction of autoimmunity in rabbits following injection of heterologous or altered homologous thyroglobulin. *J. Exp. Med. 121*: 289–308 (1965).

J. Lindenmann and P. A. Klein: *Immunological Aspects of Viral Oncolysis*. Springer, New York, 1967.

P. Isacson: Myxoviruses and autoimmunity. *Progr. Allergy 10*: 256–92 (1967).

W. Erwin, R. W. Weber, and R. T. Manning: Complications of infectious mononucleosis. *Am. J. Med. Sci. 238*: 699–712 (1959).

R. C. Mellors and C. Y. Huang: Immunopathology of NZB/B1 mice. V. Virus-like (filtrable) agent separable from lymphoma cells and identifiable by electron microscopy. *J. Exp. Med. 124*: 1031–38 (1966).

22. AUTOANTIBODIES IN HUMAN DISEASE

Conference on Immuno-Reproduction. Population Council, New York, 1962.

I. R. MacKay and F. M. Burnet: *Autoimmune Diseases. Pathogenesis, Chemistry and Therapy*. Thomas, Springfield, Ill., 1963.

L. E. Glynn and E. J. Holborow: *Autoimmunity and Disease*. Davis, Philadelphia, 1965.

Symposium on Autoimmunity-Experimental and Clinical Aspects. *Ann. N. Y. Acad. Sci. 124*: 1–890 (1965).

J. R. Anderson, W. W. Buchanan, and R. B. Goudie: *Autoimmunity*. Thomas, Springfield, Ill., 1967.

H. G. Kunkel and E. M. Tan: Autoantibodies and disease. *Adv. Immunol. 4*: 351–95 (1964).

L. A. Sternberger: Electron microscopic immunocytochemistry: A review. *J. Histochem. 15*: 139–59 (1967).

POSTSCRIPT: IMMUNITY AND HOST-PARASITE RELATIONSHIPS

HOST–ORGANISM INTERACTION

Mechanisms of Microbial Pathogenicity. Cambridge Univ. Press, Cambridge, 1965.

Symposium on Relationship of Structure of Microorganisms to Their Immunological Properties. *Bact. Rev. 27*: 325–90 (1963).

Symposium: *Host-Parasite Relationships in Living Cells*. Thomas, Springfield, Ill., 1957.

Symposium on Non-Specific Resistance to Infection. *Bact. Rev. 24*: 1–200 (1960).

D. E. Rogers: Host mechanisms which act to remove bacteria from the blood stream. *Bact. Rev. 24*: 50–65 (1960).

F. M. Burnet: *The Integrity of the Body*. Harvard Univ. Press, Cambridge, Mass., 1962.

Symposium on Some Biochemical and Immunological Aspects of Host-Parasite Relationships. *Ann. N.Y. Acad. Sci. 113*: 1–510 (1963).

C. A. Mims: Aspects of the pathogenesis of virus diseases. *Bact. Rev. 28*: 30–71 (1964).

WHO Expert Committee: *Immunology and Parasitic Diseases. Wld Hlth Org. Techn. Rep. Ser.* (1965).

E. H. Kass, G. M. Green, and E. Goldstein: Mechanisms of antibacterial action in the respiratory system. *Bact. Rev. 30*: 488–97 (1966).

"NON-SPECIFIC" HUMORAL AGENTS IN IMMUNITY

R. J. Dubos: *Biochemical Determinants of Microbial Diseases*. Harvard Univ. Press, Cambridge, Mass., 1954.

R. C. Skarnes and D. W. Watson: Antimicrobial factors of normal tissues and fluids. *Bact. Rev. 21*: 273–94 (1957).

J. G. Hirsch: Antimicrobial factors in tissues and phagocytic cells. *Bact. Rev. 24*: 133–39 (1960).

L. H. Muschel: The antibody complement system and properdin. *Vox Sang. 6*: 385–97 (1961).

SPECIFIC IMMUNOLOGIC MEDIATORS IN IMMUNITY

L. Dienes: The specific immunity response and healing of infectious diseases. Significance of active immunity and the connections between the immunity response and the anatomic lesions. *Arch. Path. 21*: 357–86 (1936).

A. A. Miles: Some aspects of antibacterial immunity. *Lect. Sci. Basis Med. 1*: 192–213 (1951–52).

R. M. Friedman et al.: The role of antibody, delayed hypersensitivity and interferon production in recovery of guinea pigs from primary infection with vaccinia virus. *J. Exp. Med. 116*: 347–56 (1962).

K. F. Austen and Z. A. Cohn: Contribution of serum and cellular factors in host defense reactions. *New Engl. J. Med. 268*: 933–38, 994–1000, 1056–64 (1963).

C. R. Jenkin: Heterophile antigens and their significance in the host–parasite relationship. *Adv. Immunol. 3*: 351–76 (1963).

J. B. Zabriskie: Mimetic relationships between group A streptococci and mammalian tissues. *Adv. Immunol. 7*: 147–88 (1967).

Index